Clinical Audiology

An Introduction

A Singular Audiology Text
Jeffrey L. Danhauer, Ph.D.
Audiology Editor

Clinical Audiology

An Introduction

Brad A. Stach, Ph.D.

President and Chief Executive Officer
Nova Scotia Hearing and Speech Clinic
Halifax, Nova Scotia

Professor
School of Human Communication Disorders
Dalhousie University
Halifax, Nova Scotia

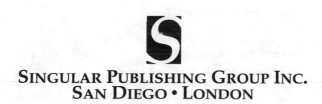

SINGULAR PUBLISHING GROUP INC.
SAN DIEGO • LONDON

Cover artwork by Bob Lanig of Lanig Associates reproduced with kind permission of ReSound Corporation, Palo Alto, California.

Singular Publishing Group, Inc.
401 West A Street, Suite 325
San Diego, California 92101-7904

Singular Publishing Ltd.
19 Compton Terrace
London N1 2UN, UK

Singular Publishing Group, Inc., publishes textbooks, clinical manuals, clinical reference books, journals, videos, and multimedia materials on speech-language pathology, audiology, otorhinolaryngology, special education, early childhood, aging, occupational therapy, physical therapy, rehabilitation, counseling, mental health, and voice. For your convenience, our entire catalog can be accessed on our website at http://www.singpub.com. Our mission to provide you with materials to meet the daily challenges of the ever-changing health care/educational environment will remain on course if we are in touch with you. In that spirit, we welcome your feedback on our products. Please telephone **(1-800-521-8545),** fax **(1-800-774-8398),** or e-mail(singpub@mail.cerfnet.com) your comments and requests to us.

Second Printing May 1998
Typeset in 11/14 Palatino by Thompson Type
Printed in the United States of America by McNaughton and Gunn

Library of Congress Cataloging-in-Publication Data

Stach, Brad A.
    Clinical audiology : an introduction / Brad A. Stach.
      p. cm.
    Includes index.
    ISBN 1-56593-346-X (softcover : alk. paper)
    1. Audiology. 2. Hearing disorders—Treatment. I. Title.
RF290.S755   1998
  617.8—dc21   97-51972
                                          CIP

Contents

Preface

This introductory textbook provides an overview of the broad field of audiology, a clinical profession devoted to the evaluation and rehabilitation of communication disorders that result from hearing impairment. The aim of the book is to provide general familiarization with the many different evaluative and rehabilitative technologies and to demonstrate how these technologies are integrated into answering the many challenging clinical questions facing an audiologist.

It is the intention of this book to introduce audiology as a clinical profession, to introduce the clinical questions and challenges that an audiologist faces, and to provide an overview of the various technologies that the audiologist can bring to bear on these questions and challenges. It is hoped that this type of approach will be of benefit to all students who might take an introductory course. For those students who will not pursue a career in audiology, the book will provide an understanding of the nature of hearing impairment, the challenges in its assessment and rehabilitation, and an appreciation of the existing and emerging technologies related to hearing. For those who will be pursuing the profession, the book will also provide a basis for more advanced classes in each of the various areas, with the added advantage of a clinical perspective on why and how such information fits into the overall scheme of their professional challenge.

Rather than writing another introductory textbook focused on rudimentary details, I have attempted in this book to provide a "big picture" of the field of audiology. My assumptions were: (1) that the basics of hearing and speech sciences are covered in other textbooks and in other classes; (2) that teaching a basic skill in one of the audiometries is not as useful as a broader perspective; (3) that each of the topic areas in the book will be covered in significant depth in advanced classes; and (4) that by introducing young students to the broad scope of the field, they will be better prepared to understand the relevance of what they learn later. For the nonaudiology major, this will promote an understanding of the clinical usefulness of audiology, without undue attention to the details of implementation.

I have tried to provide equivalent depth across topics, although some lend themselves better to specific clinical examples and others to a more didactic approach. This was particularly challenging in some areas. For example, I am rather fond of immittance audiometry as a clinical tool and do not find a cursory overview, even at the introductory level, to be satisfactory. Yet the intricacies of reflex and tympanogram patterns can easily overwhelm the novice. In cases such as this, I tried to use a number of clinical examples in the hope that repetition would bring some level of understanding.

In each of the clinical areas, I have included Clinical Notes, which are descriptions of particular techniques that the student might consider using. Knowing that there are as many ways to establish a speech threshold as there are people teaching the technique, for example, I was reluctant to burden the beginning student with arguments about the merits of the various methods. Rather, I used the Clinical Notes to express an opinion about clinical strategies that I have used successfully. I would expect that the contrary opinions of a professor would serve as an excellent teaching opportunity.

This publication is intended primarily for beginning-level students in the fields of audiology and speech-language pathology. This book is intended for the first major course in audiology, whether it be at the undergraduate or graduate level. Both intentions challenged the depth and scope of the content, and I can only hope that I reached an appropriate balance.

Acknowledgments

For the most part, I wrote this book off the top of my head. But I had to learn all of this somewhere. Much came from clinical colleagues, and much came from my professors and supervisors. When necessary, I filled in with the details that I had long since forgotten or never knew. The sources I used to obtain those details are included in the Recommended Reading section of each chapter.

Dr. James Jerger has been the biggest single influence on my career. Much of what is written here is based on what I have learned from him as his student and colleague. He has the best clinical mind that I have ever known. We have written several book chapters and articles together, and much of that work is reflected here. The historical perspective in Chapter 1 is his, and his influence permeates the remainder of the book. I am better than he is at racquetball and, arguably, sheepshead, but that's all.

I have worked with a number of remarkably talented clinicians in my career. Each has contributed to my knowledge in some way, and that knowledge is reflected in this book. Louise Loiselle directed the clinical audiology program at The Methodist Hospital while I was there and taught me a great deal. Other clinicians at The Methodist Hospital and Baylor College of Medicine in Houston included Michele Barr, Rose Chmiel, Leighanne Davis, Gloria Delgado-Vilches, Kathy Fleming-Hoskins, Mary Hudson, Karen

Johnson, Marcy McCoy, Sandy Mintz, Jeff Nye, Terrey Oliver Penn, Jeanine Pruitt, Kerry Roesch, Kathy Saucedo, Sheri Smith, Maureen Spretnjak, Renae Stoner, and Amy Wilson. The staff at Georgetown University Medical Center, under the apt leadership of Susan Morgan, included Regina Gilbert, Jody Livermore-Hughes, Lisa Smeallie, and Sheryl Wolf. The clinical staff at the California Ear Institute at Stanford included Lara Alessandrelli, Stefani Cozine, Dana Latham, Geri Miller, Lori Ratto, Jennifer Sauer, Valerie Saul, Jeni Sauter, Mont Stong, Lisa Tonokawa, and Cindi Warner-Urquhart. All of these clinicians have taught me something about audiology, and I am grateful to each of them. The audiology staff at the Nova Scotia Hearing and Speech Clinic is currently seeing to it that my clinical education continues.

I am also grateful to a number of teachers, clinical supervisors, and colleagues who over the years have contributed to the knowledge base necessary to write a textbook of this breadth, including Chris Bauch, Fred Bess, Gene Bratt, Bertha Clarke, Roberta DiDonato, Barry Freeman, Judy Farmer, Steve Farmer, Edgar Garrett, Makoto Igarashi, Jim Jerger, Susan Jerger, Sabina Kurdziel, Wayne Olson, Rodney Perkins, Joe Roberson, Darrell Rose, Jay Sanders, Ann Sitton, Glenn Thompson, and Brian Westerberg.

Dr. H. Gustav Mueller contributed substantially to this project by helping me with Chapters 10 through 13. He provided suggestions for the organization of the chapters and provided wit, criticism, and constructive suggestions after reviewing their content. I appreciate his insight and friendship.

Dr. Jeffrey Danhauer talked me into this project. His enthusiasm assisted greatly in its completion. His constructive review helped this book considerably.

Dr. Judith Scheinberg from San Diego State University reviewed the first draft of the completed text. Her suggestions improved the final version significantly.

A number of friends in industry were called upon to find me pictures of equipment and hearing instruments. They did, and I appreciate their efforts. Audiologist Chris Santilli helped with the OAE graphics and Steven Pugsley with the hearing aid graphics.

Chapter 9 contains a report-writing glossary, consisting of a number of descriptors of audiometric outcomes that can be used for computer-generated reports. These descriptors were first developed around 1980 by Dr. Jerger and his colleagues at the Baylor College of Medicine and The Methodist Hospital in Houston. The audiology staff at the Methodist and I fine-tuned them over the years. In addition, the audiology staffs at Georgetown University Medical Center and the California Ear Institute at Stanford contributed by adding descriptors of their own.

A number of professors reviewed the initial outline of the textbook as a first step in the project. They included Jane Baran, Carmen Brewer, Rochelle Cherry, Carl Crandell, Stephanie Davidson, Robert DeJonge, Kris English, John Ferraro, Mary Florentine, Vic Gladstone, Teri Hamill, William Hodgson, Ben Kelly, Douglas Laws, Toni Maxon, Marvin Mazor, James McCartney, June McCullough, Robert Muzzarelli, Michael Nerbonne, Gerald Popelka, Lloyd Price, Beth Prieve, Robert Redden, William Rintelmann, Lynn Root, Judith Scheinberg, Carol Silverman, Tom Simpson, Carol Sommer, Richard Sweetman, Janice Trent, Lida Wall, and Mike Wynne. I appreciate their efforts and the feedback that they provided.

Marie Linvill at Singular Publishing Group was responsible for the overall orchestration of this project. Her guidance and patience were remarkable. Candice Janco saw the project to its completion. Sandy Doyle made the text come alive with her copyediting and production. Their assistance was invaluable.

The photograph on the cover is of a creation by my very talented friend Bob Lanig and his staff at Lanig Associates in Palo Alto, California. The original artwork was commissioned by ReSound Corporation. I am grateful to both Bob and ReSound for their permission to use this stunning piece.

Casey Stach contributed to this project in a number of ways. She generated the margin notes, reviewed the manuscript in progress and upon completion, and made innumerable suggestions that improved this textbook. She also provided the support necessary for completion of the project and understood its value, despite the considerable toll it took on early mornings, late evenings, and weekends. Thanks Casey.

To Mike Crum, who guided my career
To Edgar Garrett, who taught me the rules of thought
To Jay Sanders, who taught me how to teach
To James Jerger, my mentor and friend

I wondered, I guessed, and I tried
They just knew

The Profession of Audiology in the United States

In this context, **amelioration** means to make better or improve.

A **hearing disorder** is a disturbance of the function of hearing.

A **communication disorder** is an impairment resulting from a speech, language, or hearing disorder.

Hearing aid amplification refers to any electronic prosthetic device used to provide amplified sound to the ear.

Rehabilitation is a program or therapy designed to help a person with hearing impairment redevelop abilities or skills he or she *once* had.

Habilitation is a program or therapy designed to help a person with hearing impairment develop abilities or skills he or she *never* had.

Electroacoustic means conversion of an acoustical signal to an electrical signal.

Electrophysiologic refers to measuring the electrical activity of the brain and body.

The portion of the ear from the tympanic membrane (or eardrum) to the oval window is called the **middle ear**.

The **inner ear** contains the sensory organs of hearing.

The portion of the hearing mechanism from the auditory nerve to the auditory cortex is called the **central auditory nervous system**.

Audiology is the health-care profession devoted to hearing. It is a clinical profession that has as its unique mission the evaluation of hearing ability and the **amelioration** of impairment that results from **hearing disorders**. Most practitioners in the field of audiology practice their profession in health-care settings or in private practice. Others practice in educational settings, rehabilitation settings, and industry. Regardless of setting, the mission of the audiologist is the prevention of hearing loss, identification of hearing loss, and amelioration of **communication disorder** that may result from hearing loss. Specifically, audiologists play a crucial role in early identification of hearing impairment in infants, evaluation of hearing ability in people of all ages, and assessment of communication disorders that may result from hearing impairment. In addition, audiologists evaluate the need for **hearing aid amplification** and assess, fit, and dispense hearing aids and other assistive listening devices. Audiologists are also involved in postfitting **rehabilitation** and in educational programming and facilitation.

In the grand scheme of things, audiology is a relatively new profession. Its roots took hold following World War II, when clinics were developed to test the hearing of soldiers returning from the front lines who developed hearing loss as a result of exposure to excessively loud sounds. In those days, audiologic services consisted of measuring how much hearing impairment was present and instruction in lipreading and auditory rehabilitation. Hearing aid technology was only beginning to emerge. If we fast-forward to today, the profession's challenges remain the same, but our ability to meet them has changed dramatically.

Today, using **electroacoustic** and **electrophysiologic** techniques, we screen the hearing of infants on their first day of life. We accurately quantify the hearing ability of even the most rambunctious 2-year-old during a single visit to the clinic. Today we routinely assess **middle-ear** function, **inner-ear** function, and **central auditory nervous system** function with ever-evolving precision. Our questions about hearing aid amplification now go well beyond that of yes or no. We can measure, with great precision, the amount of amplification that we deliver to an eardrum. And we can alter that amplification in a number of ways to tailor it to the degree and nature of an individual's hearing loss.

But the main questions remain the same:

■ Does a hearing loss exist?
■ What is the extent of the hearing loss?

- Is the loss causing impairment in communication ability?
- Can the impairment be overcome to some extent with hearing aid amplification?
- What kind of amplification and how much?
- How can success with this amplification be verified?
- How much additional rehabilitation is necessary?

These questions form the basis for the profession of audiology. They encompass the issues that represent the unique purview of the profession.

WHAT IS AN AUDIOLOGIST?

An audiologist is a professional who, by virtue of academic and clinical training, and appropriate **certification** and/or **licensure**, is uniquely qualified to provide a comprehensive array of professional services related to the prevention, evaluation, and rehabilitation of hearing impairment and its associated communication disorder. The audiologist may play a number of different roles:

- clinician,
- therapist,
- teacher,
- research investigator,
- administrator, and
- consultant.

The audiologist provides clinical and academic training in all aspects of hearing impairment and its rehabilitation to students of audiology and personnel in medicine, nursing, and other related professions.

Certification is typically awarded by the governing body of a profession to individuals who have met certain academic and clinical requirements.

Licensure is a permit to practice a profession, typically awarded by a state or province to individuals who have met certain criteria.

WHAT IS AN AUDIOLOGIST'S ROLE?

The audiologist assesses hearing, evaluates and fits hearing aids, and assists in the implementation of rehabilitation.

Evaluation

The audiologist serves as the primary expert in the assessment and nonmedical diagnosis of auditory impairment. Assessment includes, but is not limited to, the administration and interpretation of **behavioral**, electroacoustic, and electrophysiologic mea-

Behavioral measures pertain to the observation of the activity of a person in response to some stimuli.

Nerve endings in the inner ear and the VIIIth nerve constitute the **peripheral auditory nervous system**.

Hearing sensitivity is the ability of the ear to detect faint sound.

A **cochlear implant** is a device that is implanted in the inner ear to provide hearing for individuals with profound deafness.

The portion of the inner ear that consists of a fluid-filled shell-like structure is called the **cochlea**.

A **neural system** is a system containing nerve cells, in this case the VIIIth cranial nerve or auditory nerve.

A hearing loss of 90 dB HL or greater, typically considered deaf, is called a **profound hearing loss**.

Auditory training is a rehabilitation method designed to train people to use their remaining hearing.

sures of the status of the **peripheral** and central **auditory nervous systems**. Evaluation typically involves assessment of both the type of hearing loss and the extent or degree of hearing loss. The evaluation process reveals whether or not a hearing loss is of a type that can be medically treated with surgery or drugs or of a more permanent type that can be treated only by the use of hearing aid amplification. Once the nature of the loss is determined, the extent of the impairment is evaluated in terms of both **hearing sensitivity** and the ability to use hearing for the perception of speech. Results of this evaluation are then placed into the context of the patient's life-style and communication demands to determine the extent to which a loss of hearing becomes an impairment and impacts communication function.

Rehabilitation

Academic preparation and clinical experience qualify the audiologist to provide a full range of auditory rehabilitative services to patients of all ages. Rehabilitative services include those related to hearing aids, **cochlear implants**, and aural rehabilitation.

The audiologist is the primary individual responsible for the evaluation and fitting of all types of amplification devices, including hearing aids and assistive listening devices. The audiologist determines whether the patient is a suitable candidate for an amplification system, evaluates the benefit that the patient may expect to derive from such systems, and recommends an appropriate system to the patient. In conjunction with these recommendations, the audiologist may take ear impressions, fit the hearing aid devices, provide counseling regarding its use, and ultimately dispense the device.

The audiologist is also the primary individual responsible for the nonmedical evaluation of candidates for cochlear implants. Cochlear implants provide direct electrical stimulation of the inner ear of hearing, or the **cochlea**, and to the **neural system** of hearing. They are used for individuals with **profound hearing loss**. Prior to implant surgery, the audiologist carries out audiologic testing to determine candidacy for the device and provides counseling to the candidate about appropriateness of implantation and viability of other amplification options. After implant surgery, the audiologist is responsible for programming implant devices, providing **auditory training** and other rehabilitation services, trouble-shooting and maintaining implant hardware, and counseling both implant users and their families.

The audiologist also provides rehabilitative services and education to individuals with hearing impairment, family members, and the public. The audiologist provides information concerning hearing and hearing loss, the use of **prosthetic devices**, and strategies for improving speech recognition by exploiting auditory, visual, and tactile avenues for information processing. The audiologist also counsels patients regarding the effects of auditory disorder on communicative and psychosocial status in the personal, social, and vocational arenas.

A device that assists or replaces a missing or dysfunctional system is called a **prosthetic device**.

Education

Audiologists involved in educational settings administer screening and evaluative programs in schools to identify hearing impairment and ensure that all students receive appropriate follow-up and **referral** services. The audiologist also trains and supervises nonaudiologists who perform hearing screening in educational settings. The audiologist serves as the resource for school personnel in matters pertaining to classroom acoustics, assistive listening systems, and communicative strategies. The audiologist maintains both classroom assistive systems and personal hearing devices. The audiologist serves on the team that makes decisions concerning an individual child's educational setting and special requirements. The audiologist also participates actively in the management of all children with hearing disorders of all varieties in the educational setting.

Referral means to direct someone for additional services.

Prevention

The audiologist designs, implements, and coordinates industrial and military hearing conservation programs in an effort to prevent hearing loss that may occur from exposure to excessively loud noises. These programs include identification and amelioration of hazardous noise conditions, identification of hearing loss, employee education, and training and supervision of nonaudiologists performing hearing screening in the industrial setting.

Related Activities

Some audiologists, by virtue of employment setting, education, experience, and personal choice, may engage in health-care activities in areas related to, but outside of, the profession. For ex-

Vestibulometry is the measurement of balance function and dizziness.

Multimodality sensory evoked potentials is a collective term used to describe the measurement of electrical activity of the ears, eyes, and other systems of the body.

ample, some audiologists in medical settings carry out **vestibulometry**, the measurement of balance function and dizziness. Other audiologists elect to practice in hospital intensive care units and operating rooms, where **multimodality sensory evoked potentials** are used to monitor the function of sensory systems during surgery.

Scope of Practice

It is incumbent on all professions to define their boundaries. They must delineate the professional activities that lie within their territory and, by exclusion, the activities outside their territory. This is not always easy to do. In a dynamic profession like audiology, boundaries that once were clear become blurred by advances in technology and the consequent expansion of activities that audiologists are called on to handle.

To function independently, means you are **autonomous**.

It is important to understand scope of practice issues. Audiology is an **autonomous** profession. As long as audiologists are practicing within their boundaries, they are acting as experts in their field. Decisions about evaluative approaches and about hearing aids and other rehabilitative strategies are theirs to make. A patient with a hearing loss can choose to enter the health-care door through the audiologist, without referral from a physician or other health-care provider. This is a very important status to have and to preserve. As long as audiologists are providing services that fall within their true mission, they are the most qualified practitioners to provide these services and are afforded the autonomy to do so.

Approximately 85% of all audiologists today in the U.S. **dispense hearing aids**.

Defining the scope of practice for any profession remains a fairly dynamic process. Not so very long ago, in the 1970s, official scope of practice guidelines for the profession of audiology did not delineate the **dispensing of hearing aids** as being within the scope of the profession. Because the dispensing of hearing aids was such a natural extension of the central theme of the profession, audiologists began expanding their practices into this area as a routine matter of course. Soon, it became a common part of professional practice, and today dispensing hearing aids is considered an integral part of an audiologist's responsibilities.

Professional practices have also expanded in other ways, some of which have been short-lived, some of which will be, and others of which will probably become a routine part of the profession of audiology. Several examples may illustrate the dynamic nature of professional practice.

One example of an expanding activity is in the area of ear canal inspection and **cerumen** management. In order to evaluate hearing, make **ear impressions**, and fit hearing protection devices and hearing aids, the ear canals of patients need to be relatively free of debris and excessive cerumen. In the past, assessment and management of cerumen was relegated to physicians or nursing staff. Recently, **otoscopic** examination and external ear canal management for cerumen removal has become a more routine part of audiologists' practices.

Another example of expanding roles is in the area of auditory electrophysiology. Since the late 1970s, audiologists have used what are termed electrophysiologic procedures to estimate hearing ability in infants and other patients who could not cooperate with behavioral testing strategies. The main electrophysiologic procedure is termed the **auditory brain stem response**, or ABR. This technique measures electrical activity of the brain in response to sound and provides an objective assessment of hearing ability. Audiologists have embraced this technology as an excellent means of helping them to assess hearing ability. But the ABR is useful for something else as well. It provides an exquisite means for evaluating the integrity of the neural elements of the **VIIIth cranial nerve** and the auditory brain stem. Thus, it is a technique that is very useful to the medical professions that diagnose and treat brain disease, such as **neurology, neurosurgery**, and **otolaryngology**. Because audiologists were already using these techniques to evaluate hearing, they were called on to extend their use to assist in the diagnosis of neurologic disorders. Throughout the 1980s, audiologists obligingly engaged in assisting the medical professions in this way, and the scope of practice expanded to include such activities. Then an interesting phenomenon occurred. Imaging and **radiographic techniques** kept improving until they reached a point where they became more sensitive to neurologic disorders than the ABR. When that happened, the use of ABR for neurologic diagnostic purposes diminished rapidly. Today, the ABR technique still enjoys widespread use in hearing assessment, but is used to ever diminishing degrees in medical diagnosis.

There is a moral to the ABR story that is worth noting. The moral is that, if a particular practice you are currently engaged in lies outside of the central theme of your profession, it is likely to be relatively short-lived within the scope of your profession. Audi-

Cerumen is earwax, the waxy secretion in the external ear canal. When it accumulates, it can become impacted and block the external ear canal.

An **ear impression** is a cast made of the ear and ear canal for creating a customized earplug or hearing aid.

Otoscopic pertains to an otoscope. An **otoscope** is an instrument used to visually examine the ear canal and eardrum.

An **auditory brain stem response** is an electrophysiologic response to sound, consisting of five to seven identifiable peaks that represent neural function of auditory pathways.

The **VIIIth cranial nerve** refers to the auditory and vestibular nerves.

Neurology is the medical specialty that deals with the nervous system.

Neurosurgery is the medical specialty that deals with operating on disorders of the nervous system.

Otolaryngology is the medical specialty that deals with the ear, nose, and throat.

Techniques used to view the structures of the body through X rays are called **radiographic techniques**.

ologists engaged in diagnostic ABR because they were familiar with the equipment and willingly agreed to assist in the medical diagnostic tasks. Once the technology was replaced, so too was the audiologist's role in providing this assistance. Perhaps the second part of the moral to the story is that, if what you are doing is only being done because a particular technology is at your disposal, then what you are doing may be destined to obsolescence.

We see other parallels today. Audiologists became involved in balance and dizziness testing because of physicians' interests in documenting this type of function in their patients. Audiologists actually became involved because they happened to be present in physician's offices and were technically competent to carry out such procedures. The most common type of testing is called **electronystagmography**, or ENG, and you will often find it in scope of practice documents for audiologists. But two trends are occurring. First, the technique is becoming increasingly less sensitive as other diagnostic strategies have developed. Thus, in many parts of the country, its use is diminishing in value. Second, audiologists are beginning to see it as a drain on their resources, which are committed to helping those with communication disorders, and are beginning to delegate the testing to more technical staff.

Electronystagmography measures eye movements to assess vestibular (balance) function.

Another direction that audiologists have taken is in the area of **multisensory modality** monitoring in the operating room. From what you have read about the definition of an audiologist, you might be wondering what an audiologist is doing in the operating room. This practice was an extension of the use of ABR for assisting in the diagnosis of neurologic impairment. Remember that the ABR is useful for evaluating function of the VIIIth cranial nerve and the auditory brain stem. Surgeons found that, if they monitored function of the VIIIth nerve and other nerves during surgery for removal of a tumor on that nerve, they could often preserve the nerve's function. Because audiologists knew how to use the equipment and because of their technical expertise, often they were asked to participate in the surgical monitoring of patients undergoing tumor removal. Because they were there, these audiologists were also asked to monitor other nervous system responses as well. As a result of this activity, intraoperative monitoring is often mentioned as being within the scope of practice of audiologists.

Multisensory modality means incorporating the auditory, visual, and tactile senses.

It is important to keep in mind that this issue of scope of practice goes beyond what a particular profession says that it does or wants to do. There is a tendency to want to define a profession by what people do on a daily basis rather than on the central theme of the profession. Thus, if audiologists are carrying out dizziness testing or monitoring spinal-cord function during surgery, those procedures may be included within the scope of practice simply because audiologists are doing them. There are two problems with this approach. One is that, although a group of professionals can claim a territory because some of them happen to be doing it, that territory probably has another owner if it is not within the central theme of the profession. For example, diagnosis of dizziness problems is a medical question, not a communication-disorders question. As a result, although audiologists may be carrying out dizziness testing, they are truly in the territory of physicians and are acting as their assistants when they are doing this type of testing. Similarly, when audiologists are monitoring nervous-system function in the operating room, they are providing assistance to the surgeons, anesthesiologists, and neurophysiologists. Their autonomy in each of these cases lasts only as long as the primary territory-keeper wishes it to.

This is not to say that providing services in other professions' arenas is not useful or important. Indeed, audiologists have been helping otolaryngologists in their surgical practices for many years. But it is important to understand that, if the practice in which audiologists are engaging falls outside of the true theme of their profession, then those involved are acting in someone else's behalf and necessarily lose their autonomy. Stated another way, when audiologists are in the operating room, they are in the territory of the surgeon and they do what they are told to do. When audiologists are fitting hearing aids, they are in their own unique territory, and they do what they are professionally trained to do.

The scope of practice of any profession may expand or contract, but the key to success lies in understanding whether or not what you are doing is within the central theme of your profession. If it is, then what you are doing is your decision. If it is not, then you are assisting another profession and must necessarily follow that profession's rules. Sometimes you will be using the same audiologic procedures in both cases. For example, you may be testing a patient's hearing sensitivity to determine the degree of hearing loss so that you can estimate hearing impairment for the purposes of fitting a hearing aid. You might also be testing hearing sensitivity to see if an otolaryngologist's surgery on the ear was successful in restoring that sensitivity. Even though you are carrying out exactly the same procedure, you are practicing in two very distinct territories. In the former, you have been consulted by the patient to practice the autonomous profession of audiology. The decisions as to how to best evaluate and treat this patient are yours to make. In the latter, you have been consulted by the physician to assist in his or her surgical practice. The decisions as to how to best evaluate this patient are left up to mutual agreement between the audiologist and the physician.

What, then, is the scope of practice of audiology? Audiologists are uniquely qualified to evaluate hearing and hearing impairment and to ameliorate communication disorders that result from that impairment. To do this, audiologists may be involved in:

Screening the hearing of an infant during the first 4 weeks of life is called neonatal hearing screening.

- hearing loss prevention programs,
- **neonatal hearing screening,**
- ear canal inspection and cleaning,
- pediatric and adult assessment of hearing,
- determination of hearing handicap,
- fitting of hearing aids,
- aural rehabilitation, and
- educational programming.

In addition, some audiologists, by virtue of education, experience, and personal choice, may ethically engage in activities outside of the central theme or boundaries of the profession. Thus, some audiologists may elect to practice in environments such as the hospital intensive care unit and the operating arena, where the use of multimodality sensory evoked potentials augments patient care. Others may elect to provide evaluative and rehabilitative services related to balance function.

WHERE DO AUDIOLOGISTS PRACTICE?

Audiologists practice their profession in a number of different settings. The largest growth area over the past two decades has been in the area of private practice and other nonresidential health-care facilities. Because audiology is primarily a health-care profession, most audiologists practice in health-care settings. An estimate of the distribution of settings is shown in Figure 1–1. Nearly half of all audiologists work in some type of nonresidential health-care facility, such as a private clinic, a community speech and hearing center, or a physician's practice. About 20% of audiologists work in a hospital or medical center facility, and about 10% of audiologists work in a school setting. The remain-

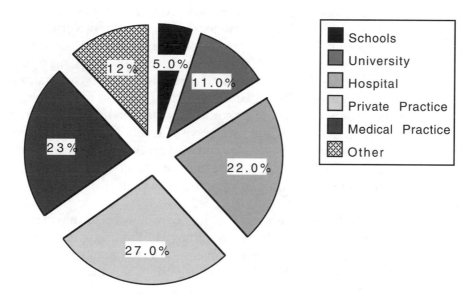

Figure 1-1. The distribution of primary settings in which audiologists practice.

ing 20% of audiologists work in university settings, residential health-care facilities, industry, and other related agencies.

With regard to primary employment function, most audiologists, nearly 80%, are **clinical service providers**, regardless of employment setting. Nearly 10% are involved primarily in administration, and about 5% are college or university professors. The remaining audiologists serve as researchers, consultants, and in other related capacities. Thus, a typical audiologist would provide clinical services in a private practice, hospital, or other health-care facility.

Eighty percent of audiologists are **clinical service providers**.

Private Practice

Nearly 40% of all audiologists have some type of **private practice arrangement**. Of those, nearly 60% are in private practice on a full-time basis. The remaining 40% have a part-time practice, typically as a supplement to their primary employment.

Forty percent of audiologists have some type of **private practice arrangement**.

Private-practice arrangements take on a number of forms. Some audiologists have their own stand-alone offices. The offices are often located in commercial office space that is oriented to outpatient health care. In other instances, the offices are located in retail shopping space to provide convenient access for patients. Some private practices are located adjacent to or within practices of related health-care professionals. For example, some audiologists have practices in conjunction with speech-language pathologists. More often, though, audiologists have practices in conjunction with otolaryngologists. This type of arrangement is of practical value in that some patients who have hearing impairment for which they would visit an audiologist also have ear disease for which they would visit an otolaryngologist, and vice versa. Thus, offices that are in close proximity allow for easy and convenient referrals and continuity of care.

A **gerontologist** is a physician specializing in the health of the aging.

A **pediatrician** is a physician specializing in the health of children.

Audiologists in private practices typically provide a wide range of services, from evaluative audiology to the fitting and dispensing of hearing aids. If there is an emphasis for private practitioners, it is usually on the rehabilitative rather than the diagnostic side, although that may vary depending on the location of the practice. Private practices may serve as the entry point for a patient into the health-care system, or they may serve as consultative services after the patient has entered the system through a primary-care physician or a specialist. Audiologists in private practice, then, work closely with **gerontologists, pediatricians**, family-medicine physicians, and otolaryngologists to assure good referral relationships and good lines of communication. Audiologists in private practice also provide contract services to hospitals, clinics, school systems, and physicians' offices. Services that are contracted range from specialty testing, such as infant hearing screening in a hospital neonatal intensive care unit, to hearing screening of children in school or preschool settings. Some private practitioners also contract with industry to provide screening and testing of individuals who are exposed to potentially damaging noise.

The challenges and risks associated with private practice are often high, but so are the rewards. Private practices are small businesses that carry all of the responsibilities and challenges associated with small-business ownership. Sound business practices related to cash management, personnel management, accounting, marketing, advertising, and so on are all essential to the success of a private practice. Successful private practices are usually more financially rewarding than other types of practices. For example, data suggest that median earnings of private practitioners are 33 to 100% higher than salaries of other audiologists. But if you talk with audiologists in private practice, you will learn that perhaps the greatest rewards are related to being an autonomous practitioner, without the institutional and other constraints related to working for hospitals or physicians' practices.

Physician's Practices

Many audiologists are employed by physicians to provide audiologic services. Most often, they are employed by otolaryngologists. Audiologists working in physicians' offices can be private practitioners, but more often are employees of the corporation. Physicians' offices range in size considerably, and audiology practices can vary from single audiologist arrangements to audiology-clinic arrangements.

Audiologic services provided within a physician's practice are usually strongly oriented to the evaluative side of the profession. This relates to the nature of medical practices as the entry point for all types of disorders, including both ear disease and communication complaints. In many cases, however, hearing aid services are included as a means of attaining continuity of care for patients.

Audiologists providing services in physicians' practices are usually compensated on a salaried basis. Some practices also provide incentives based on performance of the overall practice or performance of the audiologic aspects of the practice.

Hospitals and Medical Centers

Approximately one fifth of all audiologists work in a hospital or medical center facility. Of those who do, most (70%) work in general medical hospitals; the remainder work in rehabilitation hospitals or other specialized facilities. Within a hospital or medical center structure, audiology services can stand alone as their own administrative entities or can fall under the auspices of a more general medical department, typically otolaryngology, surgery, or physical medicine. Audiologists may be employees of the hospital or, in the case of a medical center, may be faculty members of a medical school department and part of a professional practice plan.

Audiologic activities in a hospital facility can be nearly as broad as the field. Because of the nature of the setting, emphasis in hospitals is on the evaluative or diagnostic side of the profession. Audiologists evaluate the hearing of patients who have complaints such as hearing impairment, ear disease, ear pain, and dizziness. They also evaluate patients who are undergoing **chemotherapy** that is potentially toxic to the auditory system. Most hospital settings also provide in-depth electroacoustic, electro-

Chemotherapy refers to treating a disease, such as cancer, with chemicals or drugs.

The hospital unit designed to take care of newborns needing special care is the **neonatal intensive care unit.**

The hospital unit designed to take care of normal newborns is called the **well-baby nursery**.

The **facial nerve** is the VIIth cranial nerve.

The **vestibular nerve** is part of the VIIIth cranial nerve.

A **for-profit practice** is a privately owned commercial business.

physiologic, and behavioral assessment of infants and children. In many hospitals, audiologists are also responsible for carrying out or directing the hearing screening of newborns in **neonatal intensive care units** or **well-baby nurseries**.

Audiologists also provide a number of services related to assisting physicians in the diagnosis of ear disease and neurologic disorder. In addition, some audiologists are called on to help monitor auditory or other sensory function during surgery. An example of this is the electrophysiologic monitoring of auditory nerve and **facial nerve** function during surgical removal of a tumor that impinges on the auditory and **vestibular nerves**.

Although the major emphasis is diagnostic, many hospital settings provide hearing-device services as well. It is not uncommon for audiologists to dispense hearing aids either through the hospital or through a **for-profit practice** within a hospital setting. Many hospital and medical center facilities serve as the centers for cochlear-implant evaluation, surgery, and device programming. For patients of all ages, audiologists have the primary role in determining implant candidacy and in programming the implant device as a first step in the rehabilitative process.

Audiologists in medical-center practices typically do not provide extensive rehabilitative services. This usually relates to sizable caseloads and reduced facility access. As a result, audiologists in these settings are involved in the development and implementation of outreach programs so that patients who receive evaluative and hearing aid services can be referred appropriately for any necessary rehabilitative services. Most outreach networks include local educational audiologists, schools for the deaf, vocational rehabilitation counselors, and self-help groups.

Hearing and Speech Clinics

In the 1950s and 1960s, a number of prestigious speech and hearing centers were developed and built that provided a wide range of communication services to their communities. These centers were often associated with universities, and many were partially supported with funding from organizations such as Easter Seals or the United Way. Clinics such as these remain today, and audiologic practices are usually broadly based, including a full range of diagnostic and rehabilitative activities. If there is an emphasis, it is usually on the rehabilitative side. One common strength of such a setting is a commitment to the team approach to evaluation and treatment. This is particularly important for children who have both hearing and speech-language disorders. Approximately 6% of audiologists work in a speech and hearing clinic.

Schools

One of every 10 audiologists works in an educational setting. In most cases, educational audiologists work in public schools at the primary-grade level. Some also work at the preschool level. Responsibilities of the educational audiologist are not unlike those of audiologists in general, except that they are oriented more toward a consultative role in assuring optimal access to education by students with hearing impairment.

Educational audiologists' roles in the schools range from the actual provision to the overall coordination of services. For example, in some settings the educational audiologist may be responsible for evaluative audiology services, whereas in others the audiologist is responsible for ensuring that those services are adequately provided through resources within the community.

The role of educational audiologists usually begins with oversight of hearing screening programs, which are commonplace in school settings. The role extends to the provision of diagnostic audiologic services to children who have failed the screening or, on an annual basis, to those who have been identified with hearing impairment. Educational audiologists are also responsible for ensuring that students have proper amplification devices and that those devices are functioning appropriately in the classroom. One major role of an educational audiologist is the education of school personnel about:

■ the nature of hearing impairment,
■ the effects of hearing impairment on classroom ability,
■ the way that amplification devices work, and
■ the fundamentals of hearing device trouble-shooting.

Audiologists who work in educational settings serve as advocates for students with hearing impairment and are involved in decisions about appropriate classroom placement and the necessity for itinerant assistance.

Universities

Eight to 10% of audiologists are employed in university settings, either as professors of audiology or clinical supervisors. Many audiology faculty members have teaching and research as their main responsibilities. Their primary roles are:

■ the graduate-level education of audiology students,
■ the procurement and maintenance of grant funds, and
■ the provision of audiologic research.

Other faculty members have as their primary role the supervision of students in the university clinical setting. It is usually these individuals who provide students with their first exposure to the clinical activities that constitute their future profession.

Hearing Instrument Manufacturers

Some audiologists work for manufacturers of hearing devices or audiometric equipment. They tend to work in one of two areas, research and development or professional education and sales. Those who work in research and development are responsible for assisting engineers and designers in the development of products for use in hearing assessment or rehabilitation. They bring to the development process the expertise in clinical matters that is so critical to the design of instrumentation and hearing devices. Those who work in professional education and sales typically represent a single manufacturer and are responsible for educating clinical audiologists in the types of devices available, new technologies that have been developed, and new devices that have been brought to market.

The role of audiologists in this area has been expanding over the past few decades. Audiologists bring to the design and manufacturing process an understanding of the needs of both clinical audiologists and patients with hearing impairment. This has greatly enhanced the applicability of instruments and devices to the clinical setting. In addition, the complexity and sophistication of hearing instruments have grown dramatically over the years, and the need for professional education has grown accordingly. As a result, manufacturers' representatives provide important continuing education to audiology practitioners.

Industrial hearing conservation is the area of audiology devoted to protecting the ears from hearing loss due to exposure to noise in the workplace.

Industry

Audiologists often play an important role in what is known as **industrial hearing conservation**. Exposure to noise in job settings is pervasive. For example, estimates suggest that as many as nine million workers in the United States are exposed to hazardous levels of noise. As a result, occupational safety and health standards have been developed to protect workers from noise exposure, and audiologists are often involved in assisting industry in meeting those standards. Audiologists' roles in hearing conservation include:

- assessment of noise exposure,
- provision or supervision of baseline and annual audiometric assessment,
- provision of appropriate follow-up services,
- recommendations about appropriate noise protection devices, and
- employee education about noise exposure and hearing loss prevention.

Audiologists also work with industry personnel to devise methods for engineering or administrative controls over noise exposure.

The majority of audiologists who work in industry do so on a **consultative** basis. Some audiologists contract to provide a full range of services to a particular company. Others contract only to provide hearing-test review or follow-up audiologic services. Regardless, hearing conservation is a very important aspect of comprehensive hearing health care, and audiologists often play a major role in the provision of these services.

An individual hired on an hourly or contract basis for expertise in a profession is called a **consultant**.

RELATION TO OTHER PROFESSIONS

As broadly based health care professionals assessing and treating hearing impairment, audiologists come into contact with many other professionals on a daily basis. Much of their work in assessment involves referrals from and to physicians in various specialties and other health-care professions. Much of the work in rehabilitation involves referrals from and to social services, educational personnel, and other professionals involved in outreach programs. The following is an overview of the professions that are most closely related to audiology.

Otolaryngology

Otolaryngology, or otorhinolaryngology, is the medical specialty devoted to the diagnosis and treatment of diseases of the ear, nose, and throat. The focus of the profession has evolved over the years, and now it is routinely referred to as *otolaryngology— head and neck surgery,* which is a title that accurately reflects the current emphasis of the specialty. Physicians who are otolaryngologists have completed medical school and at least a four- or five-year residency in the specialty. The residency program usually includes a year or two in general surgery, followed by an emphasis on surgery of the head and neck. One component of the otolaryngology specialty is otology.

Otology is the subspecialty devoted to the diagnosis and treatment of ear disease. In contrast, audiology is the profession devoted to the nonmedical diagnosis and treatment of communication disorders that results from hearing loss. Although the roles are clearly defined, the overlap between the professions in daily practice can be substantial. As a result, the two professions are closely aligned.

An **otologist** is a physician specializing in the ear.

The relationship between audiology and otology is perhaps best defined by considering the route that patients might take if they have hearing problems. If a patient has a complaint of hearing impairment, that patient is likely to seek guidance from a general medical practitioner, who is likely to refer the patient to either an audiologist or an **otologist**. If the general practitioner does not detect any ear disease, the patient is likely to be referred to the audiologist, who will evaluate the hearing of the patient in an effort to determine the need for rehabilitation. The audiologist's first question is whether or not the hearing loss is treatable medically. If any suspicion of ear disease is detected, the audiologist will recommend to the general practitioner that the patient receive an otologic consultation to rule out a treatable condition. If the general practitioner detects the presence of ear disease at the initial consult, the patient is likely to be referred first to the otologist, who will diagnose the problem and implement treatment as necessary. As part of the otologic assessment, the otologist may consult the audiologist to determine if the medical condition is resulting in a hearing loss and if that hearing loss is of a medically treatable nature. If ear disease is present, the otologist will treat it with appropriate drugs or surgery. The audiologist may be involved in quantifying hearing ability before and after treatment. If ear disease is not present, the otologist will consult with the audiologist to determine the extent of hearing impairment and the prognosis for successful hearing aid use.

From these examples, it is easy to see how the professions of audiology and otology are closely related. *Many patients with ear disease have hearing impairment,* at least until the ear disease is treated. Thus, otologists will diagnose and treat the ear disease. They will consult with audiologists to evaluate the extent to which that ear disease affects hearing and the extent to which their treatment has eliminated any hearing problem. Conversely, *many patients with hearing impairment have ear disease.* Estimates suggest that as many as 5–10% of individuals with hearing impairment have **treatable medical conditions**. Thus, the medical discipline of otology and the communication-disorder discipline of audiology are often called on to evaluate the same patients.

Understanding the unique contributions of the two disciplines is important in defining territories and roles in the assessment and treatment of patients with hearing impairment. Overlap of roles can occur in some patients with hearing loss complaints. For example, audiologists call on otologists to rule out or treat active ear disease in patients with hearing impairment. Once completed, the audiologists can continue their assessment and amelioration of any residual communication disorder that may be present. Similarly, otologists call on audiologists to provide pre- and post-treatment assessment of hearing sensitivity in patients with ear disease. Thus, the two disciplines work together to help patients who have complaints related to ears or hearing.

Other Medical Specialties

Audiologists also work closely with other medical specialties that treat patients who are at risk for hearing impairment. These specialties include:

- pediatrics,
- neonatology,
- neurology,
- neurosurgery,
- oncology,
- infectious diseases,
- community and family medicine, and
- gerontology.

Many infants in the neonatal intensive care units are at risk for significant hearing impairment. As a result, audiologists work closely with **neonatologists** to provide or oversee hearing screening and follow-up hearing assessment of neonates who might be at risk. In recent years, screening efforts have been extended to well-babies, and audiologists are working closely with all medical

Approximately 5–10% of individuals with hearing impairment have **treatable medical conditions**.

A **neonatologist** is a physician specializing in the care of newborns.

personnel who have the nursery as part of their professional territory. As children get older, their pediatricians are among the first professionals consulted by parents if a hearing problem is suspected. As a result, audiologists often have close referral relationships with pediatricians.

A **tumor** is an abnormal growth of tissue, which can occur on or around the auditory nerve.

A **cerebrovascular accident** (CVA) is an interruption of the blood supply to the brain resulting in a loss of function, a stroke for example.

Patients with neurologic disorders sometimes have hearing impairment as a result. **Tumors, cerebrovascular accidents**, or trauma to the central nervous system can affect the central auditory system in ways that result in hearing problems. Audiologists may be called on by neurologists or neurosurgeons to assist in diagnosis, monitor cranial nerve function during surgery, or manage residual communication disorders.

An **oncologist** is a physician specializing in the treatment of cancer.

When a substance is poisonous to the ear, it is **ototoxic**.

Audiologists also work closely with **oncologists** and specialists in infectious diseases to monitor hearing function in patients undergoing certain types of drug therapies. Some chemotherapy drugs and antibiotics are toxic to the auditory system, or **ototoxic**. Ingestion of high doses of these drugs may result in permanent damage to the hearing mechanism. Sometimes this is an inevitable consequence of saving someone's life. Drugs used to treat cancer or serious infections may need to be administered in doses that will harm the hearing mechanism. But in many cases, the dosage can be adjusted to remain effective in its purpose without causing ototoxicity. Patients undergoing such treatment will often be referred to the audiologist for monitoring of hearing function throughout the treatment.

Half of all individuals over the age of 65 years have at least **some degree of hearing impairment**.

Audiologists also work closely with family-medicine specialists and those specializing in aging, the gerontologists. One pervasive consequence of the aging process is a loss in hearing sensitivity. Estimates of prevalence suggest that as many as half of all individuals over the age of 65 years have at least **some degree of hearing impairment**, and the prevalence increases with increasing age. Family-medicine physicians are often the first professionals consulted by patients who have hearing impairment. As a result, audiologists often develop close referral relations with physicians who work with aging individuals.

Speech-Language Pathology

Audiology and speech-language pathology were considered by many to be one profession in the early years. This evolved from the educational model in which one individual would be responsible for hearing, speech, and language assessment and treatment in school-age children. Some professionals are actually certified and licensed in both audiology and speech-language pathology. Today, although some overlap remains, the two areas have evolved into separate and independent professions. Nevertheless, because of historical ties and because of a common theme of communication disorders, the two professions remain inextricably linked.

The unique role of speech-language pathology is the nonmedical diagnosis and treatment of communication disorders that result from speech and/or language impairment. **Speech-language pathologists** are responsible for evaluation of disorders in:

A **speech-language pathologist** is a professional who diagnoses and treats speech and language disorders.

- oral-motor function,
- articulation,
- voice,
- fluency,
- and language

in patients of all ages. Following assessment, speech-language pathologists design and implement treatment programs for individuals with impairments in any of these various areas.

There are at least three groups of patients with whom audiologists and speech-language pathologists work closely together. First, because good speech and oral-language development requires good hearing, auditory disorders in children often result in speech and/or language developmental delays. Thus, children with hearing impairment are usually referred to speech-language pathologists for speech and language assessment and treatment following hearing aid fitting. Second, some children have auditory perceptual problems as a consequence of impaired central auditory nervous systems. These problems result, most importantly, in difficulty discerning speech in a background of noise. The problem is usually referred to as **central auditory processing disorder** (CAPD). Many children with CAPD have concomitant **receptive language processing** problems, learning disabilities, and attention deficits. As a result, adequate diagnosis of CAPD usually requires a multidisciplinary assessment. Third, many older individuals who have language disorders due to **stroke** or other neurologic insult also have some degree of hearing sensitivity loss or central auditory problem. The audiologist and speech-language pathologist work together in such instances in an effort to determine the extent to which hearing impairment is impacting on receptive language ability.

A disorder of the central auditory structures, which can result in difficulty understanding speech in the presence of noise, is called a **central auditory processing disorder** (CAPD).

Receptive language processing is the ability to understand spoken language.

A **stroke** is a cerebrovascular accident that can result in problems with processing language.

With these exceptions, the majority of individuals who have hearing impairment do not have speech and language disorders. Similarly, the majority of individuals who have speech and language disorders do not have hearing impairment. Nevertheless, professionals in both disciplines understand the interdependence of hearing, speech, and language. Thus, during audiologic evaluations, particularly in children, it is important to include an informal screening of speech and language. During speech-language evaluations, it is important to include a screening of hearing sensitivity.

Nonaudiologist Hearing Aid Dispensers

The American Speech-Language-Hearing Association (ASHA) was founded in 1925. The original name of the Association (used from 1927 –1929) was the American Academy of Speech Correction. The 25 charter members were primarily university faculty members in Iowa and Wisconsin. The primary professional focus of the Association was on stuttering.

Prior to 1977, it was against the Code of Ethics of **the American Speech-Language-Hearing Association (ASHA)** for audiologists to dispense hearing aids. Although some audiologists dropped their memberships in ASHA so that they could provide these services, hearing aids were dispensed mostly by hearing aid dispensers. Nonaudiologist hearing aid dispensers are individuals who dispense hearing aids as their main focus. They usually have no formal education in the field. Most states have developed licensure regulation of hearing aid dispensers, and requirements vary significantly across states.

In the 1970s, audiologists began assuming a greater role in hearing aid dispensing. By the 1990s, audiologists who were licensed to dispense hearing aids outnumbered hearing aid dispensers in many states. Most individuals wishing to dispense hearing aids as a career now pursue the profession of audiology as the entry point. Nevertheless, there remain many individuals who began dispensing hearing aids before these trends were pervasive.

Although the number of traditional hearing aid dispensers is diminishing in proportion to the number of dispensing audiologists, there is considerable overlap in territory. As a result, dispensing audiologists and hearing aid dispensers may take opposing stands on regulations aimed at controls over hearing aid dispensing. In many settings, however, audiologists and hearing aid dispensers work together in an effort to provide comprehensive hearing rehabilitation services.

Other Professionals

Audiologists work with many other professionals to ensure that patients with hearing impairment are well served. For children, audiologists often work with educational diagnosticians, neuro-psychologists, and teachers to assure complete assessment for educational placement. Audiologists also refer parents of children with hearing impairment to **geneticists** for counseling regarding possible familial causes of hearing loss. Family counselors, whether social workers, psychologists, or other professionals, are often called on to assist families of children with hearing impairment. For adults with hearing impairment, referrals are often made to professionals for counseling about vocational or coping skills related to the hearing loss.

A **geneticist** is a physician specializing in the identification of hereditary diseases.

PROFESSIONAL REQUIREMENTS AND ISSUES

A typical audiologist in the late 1990s:

- holds a Bachelor's degree in communication disorders or other health-related areas,
- has completed a Master's degree in audiology,
- has completed 1 year of supervised employment,
- has passed a national examination in audiology,
- holds national certification,
- has a state license to practice audiology, and
- has a state license to dispense hearing aids.

The nature and extent of academic preparation and clinical training is driven by the certification process, which in turn provides a standard for state licensure.

Certification and Licensure

Most health-care professions are governed on the state level by state boards of examiners. Qualifications are promulgated from national organizations or boards for consideration by the states. Audiology is slightly different in this regard. To be an audiologist currently requires national certification first, followed by licensure at the state level. Audiology and speech-language pathology are among only a few professions that have this type of arrangement.

In general, in order to practice audiology, an individual must hold the Certificate of Clinical Competence in Audiology (CCC-A) from the American Speech-Language-Hearing Association. In most states, individuals must also be licensed by the state in which they work. This licensure, however, is contingent on the

CCC-A. Thus, the CCC-A is usually the first step toward state licensure. This system may seem somewhat confusing, and much of this is understandable only in historical terms. If trends continue as they have in the 1990s, all states will eventually have licensure for audiology, and the CCC-A will no longer be a necessary precursor. Meanwhile, the certification process is an important first step to practice audiology.

To obtain the CCC-A, an individual must be granted a master's or doctoral degree from an academic institution that meets requirements set forth by the ASHA. The candidate must then complete a Clinical Fellowship Year (CFY). A CFY is a specified period of time during which the candidate must be employed and supervised in a specified way by someone who holds the CCC-A. The candidate must also pass a national examination in audiology. On completion of the CFY and after passing the national examination, the candidate becomes eligible for certification. Once certified, the audiologist is usually automatically eligible for state licensure. Licensure is usually renewed on an annual basis and usually requires evidence of active involvement in continuing education. Some audiologists are exempt from state licensure because of the nature of their employment setting. As a general rule, audiologists who work in public school settings or who work for government agencies are exempt from state licensure.

Requirements necessary to dispense hearing aids vary across states. In some states, licensure in audiology also automatically grants licensure to dispense hearing aids. Although there is a growing trend for this type of arrangement, most states still require a separate license to dispense hearing aids. Most dispensing-licensure requirements are less stringent than requirements to practice audiology. Thus, most individuals who meet requirements for audiology licensure have the necessary requirements for a dispensing license. A separate examination, usually written and practical, is required by most state dispensing boards.

Academic and Clinical Requirements

Academic and clinical requirements for audiology are determined by individual academic institutions, based on guidelines offered by the ASHA. In order for students to be considered for the CCC-A, they must graduate from an institution that is accredited by the ASHA. These requirements are intended to ensure educational quality and provide uniformity across programs.

Academic requirements include minimum number of classroom hours of exposure to different aspects of audiology and related bodies of knowledge. In general, audiology students are required or encouraged to take classes in general science areas such as acoustics, anatomy and physiology, electronics, and computer technology. Classes are required in normal processes of hearing, speech, and language development as well as in pathologies of the auditory system. Audiologic evaluation is usually covered in a number of classes, including those on basic testing, electroacoustic and electrophysiologic measurement, and pediatric assessment. Audiologic rehabilitation is usually covered in classes on aural rehabilitation, amplification, counseling, and so on.

Clinical requirements include a minimum number of hours of hands-on testing and rehabilitation in a variety of settings. Some minimum requirements of speech and language evaluation and remediation serve as a precursor to the audiologic experience. In audiology, clinical hours are necessary in basic and advanced assessment of children and adults and in hearing aid assessment and fitting.

Following graduation, the aspiring audiologist must embark on the clinical fellowship year. This "year" is actually a 9-month experience during which the audiology candidate serves in a clinical capacity under the supervision of a certified audiologist. The goal of the CFY is to enhance and polish the clinical abilities of the audiology candidate. Some clinical settings hire CFY-level audiologists into full-time positions, so that the candidate continues in the position following completion of the CFY. Other clinics have rotating CFY positions, where a new CFY-level audiologist is employed annually to fill the position.

Academic Models

Historically, academic training in audiology has been based on an educational model. There are many reasons why this model became predominant, but the most important contributor is audiology's close association with speech pathology. As the clinical profession of audiology has evolved, however, it has strained the boundaries of the educational model, and fundamental changes in the nature of academic training are occurring.

The Educational Model

Academic training in audiology has mirrored that in speech-language pathology since the two professions developed from a single profession in the middle 1900s. Governance of the professions has been the auspices of the ASHA since those early days. Most of the members of ASHA are speech-language pathologists (83%), and most speech-language pathologists work in educational settings. Therefore, the logical model for academic training was the educational model, as most of the graduates of training programs would eventually work in school settings. In the early days of the profession, a speech-language pathologist or audiologist needed only a bachelor's degree to be eligible for certification and practice credentials. When it became apparent that the body of knowledge necessary to practice exceeded that which could be adequately addressed at the undergraduate level, master's degree programs developed to provide advanced academic training. Because most training programs were in Colleges of Education or Colleges of Arts and Sciences, the master's degree was the next logical choice for an advanced degree.

The model for audiologic education today remains this educational model, and its influence is pervasive. Undergraduate education tends to be general, with a focus on communication sciences and disorders. Graduate education is at the master's level. Most graduate education has an academic focus. Clinical training comes under the purview of centers that are a part of university programs and clinical and hospital programs that are loosely affiliated with university programs. This evolved from the "student-teaching" concept of educational training. Even the CFY is influenced by the educational model, with its 9-month duration.

Additional training in audiology can be gained at the doctoral level. Most audiologists who hold advanced degrees beyond the master's, hold doctorates. Traditionally, the Ph.D. degree has been a research degree, preparing an individual for the academic rigors of scholarship in teaching and research. In the early days of the profession, those who pursued Ph.D.s usually went on to lives in academic teaching and research institutions. More recently, however, the need has emerged for more advanced education in clinical matters. Because the Ph.D. has been the only advanced degree available, both students who desire advanced training in clinical audiology and students who wish to pursue careers in university teaching and research pursue the Ph.D. in audiology.

In recent years, the educational model for the training of audiologists has come under scrutiny for several reasons. First, most audiologists provide clinical services in health-care settings. Only one in 10 audiologists is involved directly in a school setting. Second, the realization has emerged that audiology is a clinical profession, not an academic discipline. The educational model may not provide adequately the rigorous clinical training necessary to prepare students to practice their profession autonomously. As a result, training programs are beginning to assess other models of academic training for the profession of audiology.

The Professional Doctorate Model

Attention has turned to other professional educational models as potential substitutes for the educational model. In the medical model, a physician attends medical school for 3 or 4 years following completion of the bachelor's degree. Medical school involves intensive academic training during the early years, followed by clinical rotations during the later years. After graduation, physicians usually seek residencies for specialty training. Residency involves intensive clinical training, with additional academic training in the specialty area. This model of education, while promoting academic rigor, also provides extensive clinical training so that physicians are prepared to practice independently on completion of their training.

Other clinical professions have based their educational training on this medical model. Examples of this are the nonphysician health-care professions of dentistry and optometry. In both cases, 3- or 4-year programs begin following completion of the bachelor's degree. The early years are devoted to rigorous academic training, and the later years are devoted to rigorous clinical training. On completion, students are granted professional doctorate degrees and are prepared to practice independently.

This model of the professional doctorate, based on the medical model rather than the educational model, has gained popularity in audiology in recent years. A comparison of the two models is depicted in Figure 1–2. Under the educational model, students gain their academic training during the master's degree program. Clinical practica are scattered throughout. Because the programs are usually of a short, 2-year duration, most students are not prepared to practice independently. The CFY is then used to round out their education. Under the professional doctorate model, students enroll in a 3- or 4-year program. As in optometry

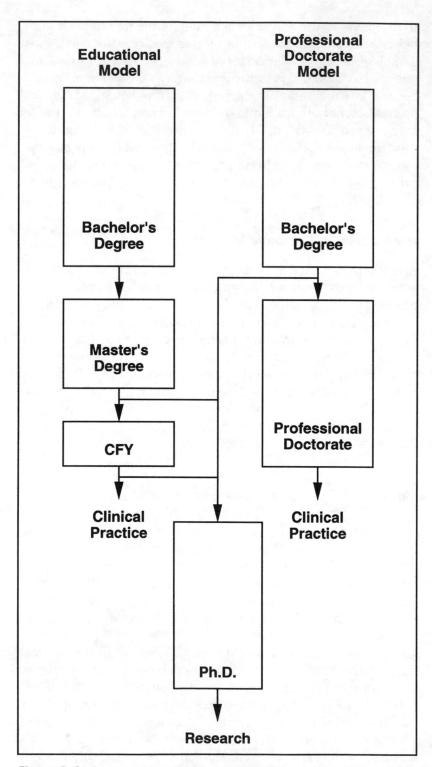

Figure 1-2. A comparison of the educational model and the professional doctorate model.

or dentistry, the early years are devoted mostly to academic training and the later years to clinical training. Upon completion of the program, students are awarded a professional doctorate degree, the **Au.D.**, and are prepared to practice independently.

Au.D. designates the professional doctorate in the field of audiology.

By the middle of the 1990s, Au.D. programs began to appear, the first being at the Baylor College of Medicine in Houston, Texas. Traditional master's level programs also began to adapt their programs in response to the need for more extensive clinical training. Several audiology professional organizations challenged academic institutions to develop professional-doctorate programs so that in future years, students who graduate from audiology programs will be granted Au.D. degrees.

A PERSPECTIVE ON THE PAST AND THE FUTURE

At the beginning of this chapter, audiology was defined as the health-care profession devoted to hearing. This definition has its roots in clinical activities that go back as far as the 1920s and 1930s. The term audiology can be traced back to the 1940s when it was used to describe clinical practices related to serving hearing care needs of soldiers returning from World War II. Following the war, graduate training programs were developed to teach the academic discipline of audiology. Definitions of audiology during the 1950s and 1960s reflected this academic perspective, in which audiology was often defined as the study of hearing and hearing disorders. Tremendous strides were made in the 1970s in the technologies available for evaluating hearing. Similarly, tremendous strides were made in the 1980s in hearing aid amplification technologies. As the decades progressed, the number of practitioners of the profession of audiology grew substantially. Audiology had evolved from an academic discipline to a clinical profession.

Audiology's Beginnings (Before 1950)

Credit for the genesis of audiology should be given to a number of individuals, but a few stand out as true leaders in the early years of the profession. Perhaps the first individual to whom credit should go is **C. C. Bunch**. Bunch, first at the University of Iowa and later at Washington University in St. Louis, used the newly developed Western Electric 1-A audiometer to assess the

C. C. Bunch developed the **pure-tone audiogram**.

hearing of patients with otologic problems. He did so in the 1920s and 1930s. Working with an otologist, Dr. L. W. Dean, he showed how the electric audiometer could be used as an enhancement to tuning forks to quantify hearing loss. In doing so, he developed what we now know as the pure-tone audiogram and was the first to describe audiometric patterns of many different types of auditory disorders.

The profession of audiology can be traced back to the 1940s. Near the end of World War II, the Army established three aural rehabilitation centers to provide medical and rehabilitative services to returning soldiers who had developed hearing impairment during the war. The three centers were the Borden General Hospital at Chickasha, Oklahoma; Hoff General Hospital at Santa Barbara, California; and Deshon General Hospital at Butler, Pennsylvania. The Navy also established a center at the Naval Hospital in Philadelphia. Perhaps the most notable of the centers was Deshon hospital, where a young captain in the Army Medical Corps, Raymond Carhart, developed a protocol for the fitting and evaluation of hearing aids that became a model for clinical practice for many years. Carhart had been a student of C. C. Bunch at Northwestern University, where Bunch was a visiting professor late in his career.

Following World War II, Carhart returned to Northwestern University, where he developed a graduate training program that was to produce many of the leaders of the audiology profession for the remainder of the century. Other leaders emerged from the aural rehabilitation centers as well. Grant Fairbanks, from the Borden Hospital, went to the University of Illinois and established a model program for the training of hearing scientists. William G. Hardy, from the Naval Hospital, went to Johns Hopkins Medical School and pioneered pediatric hearing testing. Also during the post-war era, three pioneers joined together at the Central Institute for the Deaf in St. Louis. Hallowell Davis, a physiologist from Harvard, S. Richard Silverman, an educator of the deaf, and Ira Hirsh, from the psychology department at Harvard, created a powerful program of basic and applied research that provided the basis for many clinical concepts in use today.

Audiology as an Academic Discipline (1950s and 1960s)

In the early 1950s, fewer than 500 individuals considered themselves audiologists. Most worked in otologists' offices, Veteran's

Administration hospitals, universities, and speech and hearing centers. The graduate programs at Northwestern University and then at other midwestern universities dominated the academic scene. In 1958, the first textbook on audiology was written by Hayes Newby of Stanford University. In parallel developments in Washington D.C., Kenneth O. Johnson, the Executive Secretary of the ASHA, was working to establish the profession of speech and hearing in the political realm. During the 1960s, the quality of academic programs was measured by the number and productivity of Ph.D. students.

Practitioners were beginning to expand services, although hearing aid dispensing was considered to be unethical. In the 1960s, James Jerger, a student of Carhart's at Northwestern, traveled south to Houston, where his clinical efforts ushered in the concept of diagnostic audiology. In those days, radiographic techniques were still relatively crude and not very sensitive to neurologic disorders. Jerger led the way in showing how behavioral measures of auditory function could be used to assist in the diagnosis of these disorders. His highly innovative work, beginning in the middle 1950s, continued throughout the century. In the 1960s, he ushered in new concepts in speech audiometry and other diagnostic techniques. In the 1970s, he brought clinical relevance to **impedance audiometry**. In the 1980s, he started the **American Academy of Audiology**. In the 1990s, he established the first Au.D. program. His tireless work over these years will undoubtedly be remembered for its influence on the clinical practice of audiology.

> By the late 1990s approximately 12,000 **audiologists** were practicing in the U.S.

> **Speech audiometry** pertains to measurement of the hearing of speech signals.
> **Impedance audiometry** is now referred to as **immittance audiometry.**
> The **American Academy of Audiology** was established in 1988, as an organization of, by, and for audiologists.

Audiology as a Clinical Profession (1970s and Beyond)

By the 1970s, clinical audiology began to flourish. Major technological advances helped to enhance both diagnostic and rehabilitative efforts. Impedance audiometry, later to become known as **immittance audiometry**, enhanced the testing of middle-ear function substantially. Discovery of the auditory brain stem response led to major breakthroughs in diagnostic measures and in pediatric audiology.

Another milestone also occurred in the 1970s. Hearing devices, once relegated to the retail market, were declared to be medical devices by the United States Food and Drug Administration. This had a substantial impact on the nature of devices and delivery systems. In the latter part of the 1970s, ethical restrictions to audiologists dispensing hearing aids fell to the concept of comprehensive patient care, and audiologists began dispensing hearing devices routinely.

If the 1970s was the decade of diagnostic breakthroughs, the 1980s was the decade of rehabilitative breakthroughs. Hearing-device amplification improved dramatically. In-the-ear devices that were both reliable and of good sound quality were introduced early in the decade and were embraced by hearing aid users. Computer-based hearing devices that permitted programmability of features were introduced later in the decade and began to set new standards for amplification. By the end of the decade, cochlear implants were becoming routine care for adults with profound hearing loss and were beginning to be used successfully by young children.

The 1990s brought other challenges and other successes. The use of audiologic techniques to assist in the medical diagnosis of neurologic disease, which began to decline in the 1980s, diminished further in the 1990s. The sensitivity of imaging and radiographic techniques outpaced the capabilities of electrophysiologic techniques in identifying tumors and other disorders. Yet the evaluative side of clinical audiology was boosted by two trends. First, the introduction of clinically feasible measures of **otoacoustic emissions** led to the notion of hearing screening of all infants born in the United States. By the mid-1990s, efforts to achieve this goal were well under way. Also on the evaluative side, a great deal more attention was being focused on disorders of central auditory processing abilities. As diagnostic strategies were enhanced, the practicality of measuring these abilities became apparent.

Otoacoustic emissions (OAEs) are measurable sounds emitted by the normal cochlea, which are related to the function of the outer hair cells.

On the rehabilitative side, the 1990s brought renewed enthusiasm for hearing device dispensing as user satisfaction grew dramatically with enhancements in sound processing technology. The 1990s also brought a healthy emphasis on consumerism, which led to renewed calls by the Food and Drug Administration and the Federal Trade Commission for enhanced delivery systems to consumers and a crackdown on misleading advertising by some manufacturers. Programmable and digital hearing devices began to impact the market in a significant way. Cochlear implants became increasingly common in young children.

As the century draws to a close, the profession of audiology can look forward with great expectations. Efforts to screen the hearing of all infants at birth should lead to substantial improvement in early identification. Enhancements in diagnostic strategies allow an understanding of patients' hearing impairment from the peripheral system to the central nervous system. Hearing devices, once passive amplifiers, are of a sophistication that is beginning to have a substantial impact on the quality with which patients can be served.

SUMMARY

- Audiology is the health-care profession devoted to hearing. It is a clinical profession that has as its unique mission the evaluation of hearing ability and the amelioration of impairment that results from hearing disorders.
- An audiologist is a professional who, by virtue of academic and clinical training, and appropriate certification and/or licensure, is uniquely qualified to provide a comprehensive array of professional services related to the prevention, evaluation, and rehabilitation of hearing impairment and its associated communication disorder.
- The audiologist assesses hearing, evaluates and fits hearing aids, and assists in the implementation of rehabilitation.
- Audiology is an autonomous profession. A patient with a hearing loss can choose to enter the health-care door through the audiologist, without referral from a physician or other health-care provider. Audiologists are the most qualified practitioners to assess hearing and provide hearing rehabilitative services and are afforded the autonomy to do so.
- Audiologists are employed in a number of different settings, including private practices, physicians' practices, hospitals and medical centers, hearing and speech clinics, schools, universities, hearing instrument manufacturers, and industry.
- As broadly based health-care professionals assessing and treating hearing impairment, audiologists come into contact with many other professionals on a daily basis, including otolaryngologists, other physicians, speech-language pathologists, nonaudiologist hearing aid dispensers, and other health-care and education professionals.
- A typical audiologist holds a bachelor's degree in communication disorders or other health-related areas, has

completed a master's degree in audiology, has completed 1 year of supervised employment, has passed a national examination in audiology, holds national certification, has a state license to practice audiology, and has a state license to dispense hearing aids.

■ In the grand scheme of things, audiology is a relatively new profession. The term audiology can be traced back to the 1940s when it was used to describe clinical practices related to serving hearing care needs of soldiers returning from World War II. Tremendous strides were made in the 1970s in the technologies available for evaluating hearing and in the 1980s in hearing aid amplification technologies. As the decades progressed, the number of practitioners of the profession of audiology grew substantially, and audiology evolved from an academic discipline to a clinical profession.

INFORMATION SOURCES

Organizations

American Academy of Audiology
8201 Greenboro Drive, Suite 300
McLean, Virginia 22102
703/610-9022 (phone)
800/222-2336 (toll free)
703/610-9005 (fax)
http://www.audiology.org (website)

American Speech-Language-Hearing Association
10801 Rockville Pike
Rockville, MD 20852-3279
301/897-5700 (phone)
http://www.asha.org (website)

Canadian Association of Speech-Language Pathologists
and Audiologists
2006-130 Albert Street
Ottawa, Ontario K1P 5G4
613/567-9968 (phone)
800/259-8519 (toll free)
613/567-2859 (fax)
caslpa@caslpa.ca (email)

Books

Minifie, F. D. (Ed.). (1994). *Introduction to communication sciences and disorders.* San Diego: Singular Publishing Group.

Stach, B. A. (1997). *Comprehensive dictionary of audiology.* Baltimore: Williams & Wilkins.

2

The Nature of Hearing

Hydraulic energy is related to the movement and force of liquid.

Sensory cells are hair cells in the cochlea.

The term **cortex** is commonly used to describe the cerebral cortex or outer layer of the brain.

The hearing mechanism is an amazingly intricate system. Sound is generated by a source that sends out air pressure waves. These pressure waves reach the eardrum, or tympanic membrane, which vibrates at a rate and magnitude proportional to the nature of the waves. The tympanic membrane transforms this vibration into mechanical energy in the middle ear, which in turn converts it to **hydraulic energy** in the fluid of the inner ear. The hydraulic energy stimulates the **sensory cells** of the inner ear, which send electrical impulses to the auditory nerve, brain stem, and **cortex**. But the passive reception of auditory information is only the beginning. The listener brings to bear upon these acoustic waves attention to the sound, differentiation of the sound from background noise, and experience with similar sounds. The listener then puts all of these aspects of audition into the context of the moment to identify the nature of a sound.

That simple sounds can be identified is testimony to the exquisite sensitivity of the auditory system. Now imagine the intricacy of identifying numerous sounds that have been molded together to create speech. These sounds of speech are made up of pressure waves that by themselves carry no meaning. When they are put together in a certain order and processed by a normally functioning auditory system, they take on the characteristics of speech, which is then processed further to reveal the meaning of what has been said.

When you think about the auditory system, it is easy to become amazed that it serves both as an obligatory sense and as a very specialized means of communication. That is, the auditory system simultaneously monitors the environment for events that might alert the listener to danger, opportunity, or change, while focusing on the processing of acoustic events as complicated as speech. The importance of continual environmental monitoring, the intricacy of turning pressure waves into meaningful constructs, and the complexity of doing all of this at once speaks to the extraordinary capability of the auditory system.

This chapter provides an overview of the nature of sound and its characteristics, the structure and function of the auditory system, and the way in which sound is processed by the auditory system to allow us to hear.

THE NATURE OF SOUND

You have undoubtedly heard the question about whether or not a tree that falls in a forest makes a sound if no one is around to hear it. The question is of interest because it serves to illustrate the difference between the physical properties that we know as **sound** and the psychological properties that we know as **hearing**.

> **Sound** is vibratory energy transmitted by pressure waves in the air or other media.
> **Hearing** is the perception of sound.

What is Sound?

Sound is a common type of energy that occurs as a result of *pressure waves* that emanate from some force being applied to a sound source. For example, a hammer being applied to a nail results in vibrations that propagate through the air, the hammer, the nail, and the wood. Sound results from the compression of molecules in the medium through which it is traveling. In this example, the sound that emanates through the air results from a disturbance of air molecules. Groups of molecules are compressed, which, in turn, compress adjacent groups of molecules. This results in waves of pressure that emanate from the source.

There are several requirements for sound to exist. Initially there must be a source of vibratory energy. This energy must then be delivered to and cause a disturbance in a medium. Any medium will do, actually, as long as it has mass and is compressible, or elastic, which most are. The disturbance is then propagated in the medium in the form of sound waves that carry energy away from the source. These waves occur from a *compression* of the medium, or **condensation**, followed by an *expansion* of the medium, or **rarefaction**. This compression and expansion of particles results in pressure changes propagated through the medium. The waves are considered longitudinal in that the motion of the medium's particles is in the same direction as the disturbance.

> During **condensation**, the density of air molecules is increased.
> During **rarefaction**, the density of air molecules is decreased.

Thus, sound results from a force acting on an elastic mass that is then propagated through a medium in the form of longitudinal condensation and rarefaction waves that create pressure changes and create sound. Got it? I didn't think so. Let's see if we can clarify.

Suppose for a moment that you are an air molecule. You are surrounded on all sides by other air molecules. Your position in space is fixed (the analogy is not perfect, but bear with me). You are free to move in any direction, but because of your elasticity, you always move back to your original position after you have been displaced. That is, your movement will always be opposed by a restoring force that will bring you back to where you were. This movement of yours is illustrated in Figure 2–1.

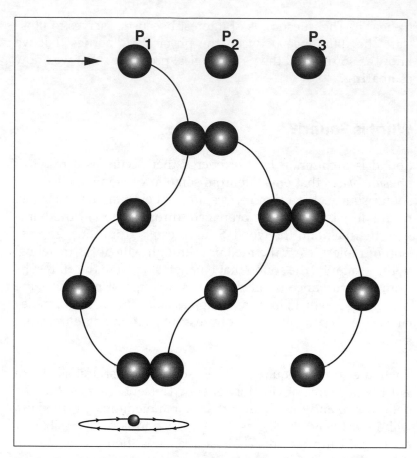

Figure 2-1. Schematic representation of the motion of particles in a medium. Here, a sound wave, designated by an arrow, moves particle P1 into its neighbor, P2. Due to elasticity, P1 moves back to its original position after displacement, and P2 continues the energy transfer by moving into P3. The small inset shows the displacement of a single particle. The lines connecting particles trace the movement over time.

Okay, now an earphone diaphragm moves outward from behind you. You and your neighbors to your left and right get pushed from behind by those neighbors behind you. This causes you to bump into your neighbors in front of you, who in turn push those in front of them. Your elasticity keeps you from moving too far, and so basically, you get squished or compressed in the crowd. You haven't really moved much, but the energy from the loudspeaker has been passed by the action of you bumping into those in front of you, who bump into those in front of them, and so on. Thus the pressure caused by the loudspeaker movement is passed on in a wave of compression. But wait, now the diaphragm moves back and you are pulled backwards by a low pres-

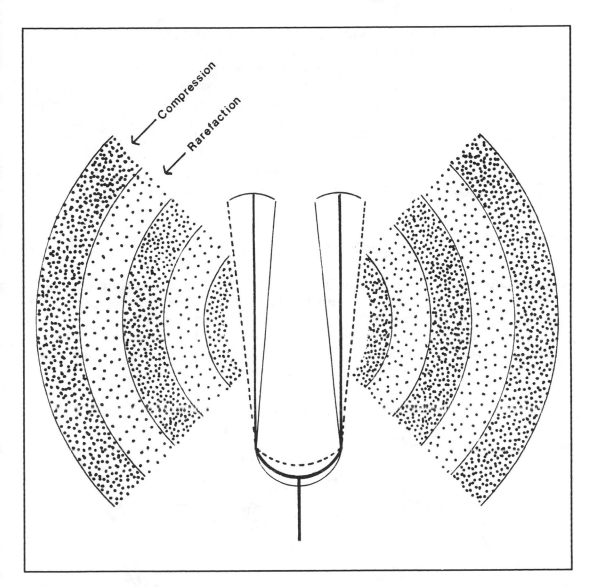

Figure 2–2. Alternate regions of compression and rarefaction waves move away from a vibratory source, in this case a tuning fork. (From *Introduction to Sound*, 2nd ed., by C. Speaks, 1997, p. 13, San Diego: Singular Publishing Group. Reprinted with permission.)

sure area, resulting in an expansion (rarefaction) of space between you and the neighbors behind and in front of you. Then, just as the elbow room is feeling good, the diaphragm moves back the other way and squishes you back together, and so on. This series of compression and expansion waves is depicted in Figure 2–2.

Of course, it doesn't work exactly like this. Air molecules are constantly moving in a random manner, but you get the gist. You do not move along because your net displacement, or movement from your original place, is zero (i.e., you are going nowhere) due to the elasticity restoring your original position; rather the energy in the wave of disturbance gets passed along as a chain reaction. That is, it is your motion that is passed on to your neighboring molecule rather than you being displaced. You pass on the wave of disturbance rather than move with it.

You have **mass**, you are **elastic**, and you pass **energy** along in the form of pressure waves. What could be simpler.

Properties of Sound

Your back and forth movement is referred to as **simple harmonic motion**, or **sinusoidal motion**. Now suppose that we wanted to graph your movement. We give you a pencil and ask you to hold it as we plot your movement over time. The result is shown in Figure 2–3. This graphic representation is called a waveform, and

Mass is the quantity of matter in a body.

The restoring force of a material that causes it to return to its original shape after displacement is called **elasticity**.

Energy is the ability to do work.

The continuous, periodic back and forth movement of an object is called **simple harmonic motion**. **Sinusoidal motion** is harmonic motion plotted as a function of time.

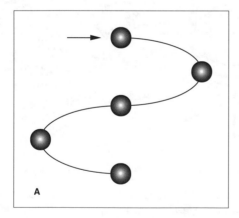

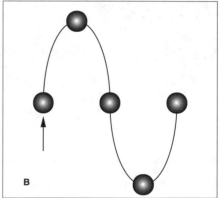

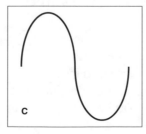

Figure 2–3. The back and forth movement of an air molecule over time can be represented as harmonic or sinusoidal motion. In A, the particle is set into motion by sound vibration, and its course is traced over time. The graph is replotted in B to show time along the x-axis. The line in C is a sinusoid that describes the movement.

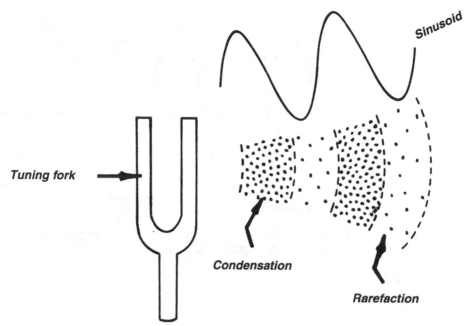

Figure 2–4. The relation between condensation and rarefaction waves and the sinusoidal function. (From *The Speech Sciences*, by R. Kent, 1997, p. 30, San Diego: Singular Publishing Group. Reprinted with permission.)

your simple harmonic motion produces a sinusoidal **waveform**, or sine wave. Because your displacement as an air molecule is propagated, or passed on, through the pressure wave, your simple harmonic motion also describes the condensation and rarefaction of the sound wave. Thus, a sine wave is a graphic way of representing the pressure waves of sound. This is illustrated in Figure 2–4.

> A **waveform** is a form or shape of a wave, represented graphically as magnitude versus time.

This sinusoidal waveform is used as a means of describing the various properties of sound, as shown in Figure 2–5. The magnitude or amplitude of displacement dictates the intensity of the sound. How often a complete **cycle** of displacement occurs dictates the frequency of a sound. The point along the displacement path describes the **phase** element of a waveform.

> A **cycle** is one complete period of compression and rarefaction of a sound wave.

> A **phase** is any stage of a cycle.

Intensity

The magnitude of a sound is described as its **intensity**. Intensity is related to the perception of loudness. As described above, an air molecule that is displaced will be moved a certain distance, return past its original location to an equal displacement in the opposite

> **Intensity** is the quantity or magnitude of sound.

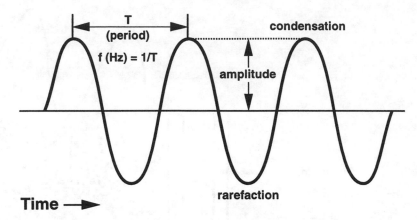

Figure 2–5. A sinusoidal waveform, describing the various properties of sound, including amplitude and frequency (f).

direction, and then return to its original location. The total displacement can be thought of as one cycle in the movement of the molecule. The magnitude of the cycle, or the distance that the molecule moves, is called its intensity. The higher the force or magnitude of the compression wave, the higher the intensity of the signal. Figure 2–6 illustrates two waveforms that are identical in frequency and phase but vary in amplitude or intensity.

The range of intensity of sound is quite large. For example, the pressure level of a sound that is just barely audible is approximately 20 μPa (or microPascals, a unit of measure of pressure). The pressure level of a sound that is so intense that it is painful is 200,000,000 μPa. This relationship is shown in Figure 2–7. As a result of this large range, the description of sound pressure level in absolute units would be rather intractable. Instead, intensity has come to be described in units called **decibels** (dB).

The decibel was the eventual result of the necessity to describe the magnitude of sound in the early days of telephone. The convention used was to describe intensity as the **logarithm** of the ratio of a measured power to a reference power. Power was used rather than pressure because of the nature of measuring the output of telephone lines. But the concept held, and the unit of measure used was referred to as a **Bel**, named after **Alexander Graham Bell**. Because of using logarithms, the large intensity range was made to vary between 1 and 14 Bels. This proved to be too small a resolution, and the notion of a decibel was created so

A **decibel** (dB) is one tenth of a Bel.

The exponent expressing the power to which a fixed number, the base, must be raised to produce a given number is the **logarithm**.

A **Bel** is a unit of sound intensity relative to a reference intensity.

Alexander Graham Bell, who invented the telephone, also championed aural education of the deaf. The A.G. Bell museum is located in Baddeck, Nova Scotia.

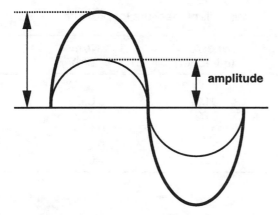

Figure 2-6. Two waveforms that are identical in frequency and phase but vary in magnitude.

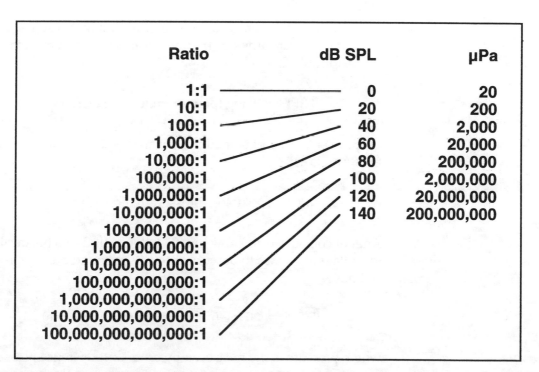

Figure 2-7. The relationship of the ratio of sound magnitude to the range of sound intensity expressed in sound pressure level. Sound ranges from barely audible at 20 μPa to painful at 200,000,000 μPa.

Table 2-1. Various units of measure for pressure.

dB SPL	dynes/cm² (microbar)	Nt/m² (Pa)	μNt/m² (μPa)
0	0.0002	0.00002	20
20	0.002	0.0002	200
40	0.02	0.002	2,000
60	0.2	0.02	20,000
80	2.0	0.2	200,000
100	20.0	2.0	2,000,000

that 1 Bel would equal 10 decibels, 2 Bels would equal 20 decibels, and so on.

Sound pressure level (SPL) = magnitude of sound energy relative to a reference pressure .0002 dyne/cm² or 20 μPa

Today, we most often express intensity in decibels **sound pressure level**, or SPL. Here's how we got there. First, intensity level (IL), or the magnitude of sound expressed as power, is described by the following formula:

$$dB\ IL = 10 \log (\text{power/reference power})$$

But we don't want to measure power, we want to measure sound pressure. Well, it turns out that power equals pressure squared, so the formula that applies is:

$$dB\ SPL = 10 \log (\text{pressure/reference pressure})^2$$

Of course, the log of something squared is 2, so we can restate the formula as:

$$dB\ SPL = 2 \times 10 \log (\text{pressure/reference pressure})$$

And, of course, we all know that 2×10 equals 20, so the decibel formula that we use to describe intensity is sound pressure level is, finally:

$$dB\ SPL = 20 \log (\text{pressure/reference pressure})$$

where pressure is the measured pressure and reference pressure is a chosen standard against which to compare the measured pressure. This reference pressure is expressed in various units of measure as described in Table 2–1.

This is probably not as difficult as it seems. There are at least two important points to remember that should make this easier and more useful to comprehend.

> *Important Point #1.* The logarithm idea is a way of reducing the range of pressure levels to a tractable one. By using this approach, pressures that vary from 1:1 to a hundred-million:1 can be expressed as varying from 0 to 140 dB.

> *Important Point #2.* Decibels are expressed as a ratio of a measured pressure to a reference pressure. This means that *0 dB does not mean no sound.* It simply means that the measured pressure is equal to the reference pressure, as follows:

dB SPL = 20 log (20 μPa/20 μPa)
dB SPL = 20 log (1)
dB SPL = 20 × 0
dB SPL = 0

So, if the measured pressure is 20 μPa, and 20 μPa is the standard reference pressure, then 20/20 equals 1, and we all remember that the log of 1 is 0 and that 20 times 0 equals 0. Therefore, as you can see, 0 dB SPL does not mean no sound. It also means that having a sound with an intensity of −10 dB is possible.

As you will learn later in this section when we get to the **audiogram**, we are not content to stop with SPL as a way of expressing decibels. In fact, one of the most common referents for decibels in audiometry is known as **hearing level (HL)**, which represents decibels according to *average normal hearing.* Thus, 0 dB HL would refer to the intensity of a signal that could just barely be heard by the human ear. Human hearing ranges from the threshold of audibility, around 0 dB HL, to the threshold of pain, around 140 dB HL. Normal conversational speech occurs at around 40 to 50 dB HL, and the point of discomfort is approximately 90 dB HL.

An **audiogram** is a graph of thresholds of hearing sensitivity as a function of frequency.

Hearing level (HL) refers to the dB level of a sound referenced to audiometric zero.

Frequency

The second major way that sound is characterized is by its frequency. **Frequency** is the speed of vibration and is related to the perception of **pitch**. Recall that, as an air molecule, you were pushed in one direction, pulled in the other, and then returned

Frequency is the number of cycles occurring in 1 second, expressed in Hertz (Hz).

Pitch is the perception of frequency.

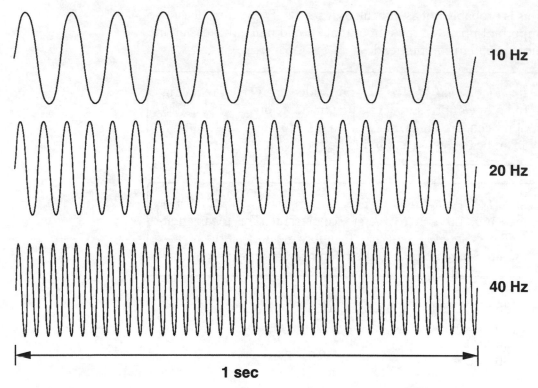

Figure 2-8. Three waveforms that are identical in amplitude and phase but vary in frequency.

The length of time for a sine wave to complete one cycle is called the **period**.

to your original position. This constitutes one cycle of displacement. Frequency is the speed with which you moved. One way to describe this speed is by the time elapsed for one complete cycle to occur. This is called the **period**. Another way is by the number of cycles that a molecule moves in a specified period of time, which can be calculated as 1/period. Figure 2–8 illustrates three waveforms that are identical in amplitude and phase but vary in frequency.

Hertz (Hz) is unit of measure of frequency, named after physicist Heinrich Hertz.

The frequency interval between one tone and a tone of twice the frequency is called an **octave**.

Frequency is usually expressed in cycles-per-second or **Hertz** (Hz). Human hearing in young adults ranges from 20 Hz to 20,000 Hz. Middle C on the piano has a frequency of 500 Hz. For audiometric purposes, frequency is not expressed in a linear form (i.e., with equal intervals), rather it is partitioned into **octave** intervals. An octave is simply twice the frequency of a given frequency. For audiometry, convention sets the lowest frequency at 125 Hz. Octave intervals then are 250, 500, 1000, 2000, 4000, and 8000 Hz.

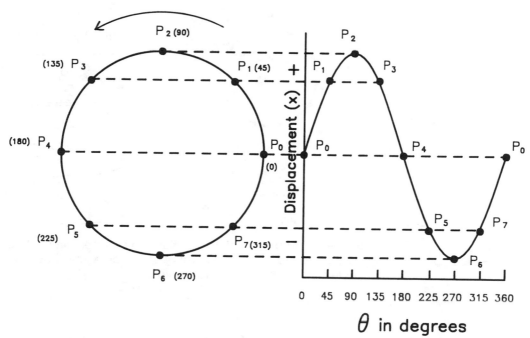

Figure 2-9. Schematic representation of a turning wheel undergoing simple harmonic motion. Points on the wheel are projected on a sinusoidal function, showing the magnitude of displacement corresponding to the angle of rotation and expressed in degrees of a circle. (From *Introduction to Sound*, 2nd ed., by C. Speaks, 1997, p. 52, San Diego: Singular Publishing Group. Reprinted with permission.)

Phase

Phase is the description of your location at any point in time in your displacement as an air molecule during simple harmonic motion. Phase is expressed in degrees of a circle, as shown in Figure 2–9. That back and forth vibratory motion can be equated to circular motion may not be altogether intuitive. Figure 2–10 shows what would happen to you as an air molecule if you were being moved by the motion of a wheel. As the wheel approached 90°, you would be maximally displaced away from the vibrating source; as the wheel approached 270°, you would be maximally displaced toward the vibrating source, and so on.

One important aspect of phase is in its description of the starting point of a waveform. Figure 2–11 illustrates two waveforms that are identical in amplitude and frequency but vary in starting phase.

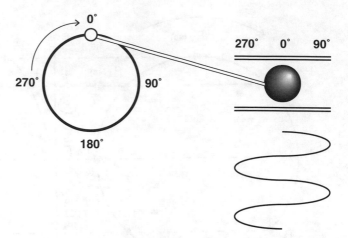

Figure 2-10. Schematic of the relationship between circular motion and the back and forth movement of an air molecule. Movement of the molecule results in sinusoidal motion.

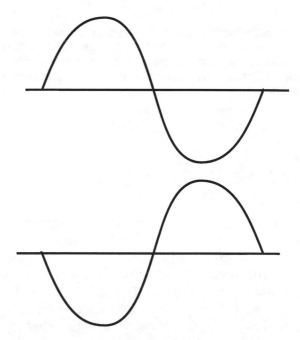

Figure 2-11. Two waveforms that are identical in amplitude and frequency but vary in starting phase.

Spectrum

A **pure tone** is a sound wave having only one frequency of vibration.

Thus far, sound has been described in it simplest form, that of a sinusoid or **pure tone** of one frequency. Simplifying to this level is helpful in describing the basic aspects of sound. Although pure tones are not commonly found in nature, they are used extensively in audiometry as a method of assessing hearing sensitivity. A sinusoid is a *periodic* wave in that it repeats itself at regular intervals over time.

Waves that are not sinusoidal are considered *complex,* as they are composed of more than one sinusoid that differ in amplitude, frequency, and/or phase. Complex waves can be periodic, in which some component repeats at regular intervals, or they can be *aperiodic,* in which the components occur randomly.

Sounds in nature are usually complex, and they are rarely sufficiently described on the basis of the intensity of a single frequency. For these more complex sounds, the interaction of intensity and frequency is referred to as the sound's **spectrum**. The spectral content of a complex sound can be expressed as the intensity of the various frequencies that are represented at a given moment in time. An example is shown in Figure 2–12.

The distribution of the magnitude of frequencies in a sound is called the **spectrum**.

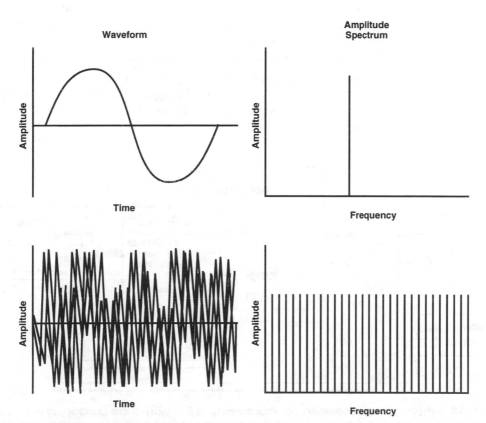

Figure 2-12. The spectral content of a single-frequency tone *(top)* and of a complex sound *(bottom)* are expressed as amplitude spectra, or amplitude of the individual frequency components.

THE AUDITORY SYSTEM

Hearing is an obligatory function; it cannot be turned off. Hearing is also a distance sense that functions mostly to monitor the external environment. In most animals, hearing serves a protective function, locating potential predators and other danger. In most animals, it also serves a communication function, with varying levels of sophistication.

The auditory system is an amazingly intricate system, which has high sensitivity, sharp frequency tuning, and wide dynamic range. It is sensitive enough to perceive **acoustic** signals with pressure wave amplitudes of minuscule magnitudes. It is very finely tuned to an extent that it is capable of resolving, or distinguishing, frequencies with remarkable acuity. Finally, it is able to process acoustic signals varying in magnitude, or intensity range, in astonishing proportion.

Acoustic means pertaining to sound.

The physical processing of acoustic information occurs in three groups of structures, commonly known as the outer, middle, and inner ears. Physiological processing begins primarily in the inner ear and continues, via the VIIIth cranial nerve, to the central auditory nervous system. Psychological processing begins primarily in the brainstem and pons and continues to the auditory cortex and beyond. A useful diagrammatic representation of the auditory system is shown in Figure 2–13.

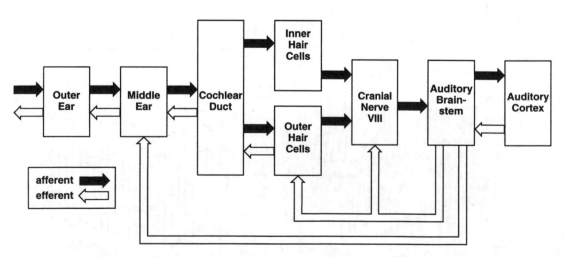

Figure 2-13 Schematic representation of structures and function of the auditory system, showing both afferent and efferent pathways. (Adapted from "Cochlear Neurobiology: Revolutionary Developments," by P. Dallos, 1988, *Asha, 30*, p. 55.)

Outer Ear

The **outer ear** serves to collect and resonate sound, assist in sound localization, and function as a protective mechanism for the middle ear. The outer ear has three main components: the auricle, the ear canal or meatus, and the outer layer of the eardrum or tympanic membrane.

The **auricle** is the visible portion of the ear, consisting of skin-covered cartilage. It is also known as the **pinna**. Some of the landmarks of the auricle are shown in the drawing of the anatomy of the ear in Figure 2–14. The upper rim of the ear is often referred to as the **helix** and the lower flabby portion as the **lobule**. The bowl at the entrance to the external auditory meatus is known as the **concha**.

The auricles serve mainly to collect sound waves and funnel them to the external auditory canal. In humans, the auricles serve a more minor role in sound collection than in other animals. The auricles are important for sound localization in the vertical plane (ability to locate sound above and below) and for protection of the ear canal. The **auricles** also serve as **resonators**, enhancing sounds around 4500 Hz.

The **external auditory meatus** is a narrow channel leading from an opening in the side of the head that measures 23–29 mm in length. The outer two thirds of the canal is composed of skin-covered cartilage. The inner one third is skin-covered bone. The canal is elliptical in shape and takes a downward bend as it approaches the tympanic membrane. The skin in the cartilaginous portion of the canal contains **glands** that secrete earwax or **cerumen**.

The **external auditory meatus** directs sound to the eardrum or tympanic membrane. It serves as a **resonator**, enhancing sounds around **2700 Hz**. It also serves to protect the tympanic membrane by its narrow opening. Cerumen in the canal also serves to protect the ear from intrusion by foreign objects, creatures, and so on.

The **tympanic membrane** lies at the end of the external auditory canal. It is a membrane made of several layers of skin embedded into the bony portion of the canal. The membrane is fairly taut, much like the head of a drum. Its shape is concave, curving slightly inward.

The **outer ear** includes the auricle, external auditory meatus, and lateral surface of the tympanic membrane.

The external cartilaginous portion of the ear is called the **auricle**.
Pinna = auricle

The **helix** is the prominent ridge of the auricle.
The **lobule** is another term for earlobe.
The **concha** is the bowl of the auricle.

A system that is set into vibration by another vibration is called a **resonator**. The action of this additional vibration is to enhance the sound energy at the vibratory frequency.

The **auricle** serves as a resonator, enhancing sound around 4500 Hz.

The **external auditory meatus** measures from 23 to 29 mm in length.

The **glands** in the outer ear that secrete wax are the **ceruminous** glands.

The **external auditory meatus** serves as a resonator, enhancing sound around **2700 Hz**.

Tympanic membrane = eardrum

ANATOMY OF THE HUMAN EAR

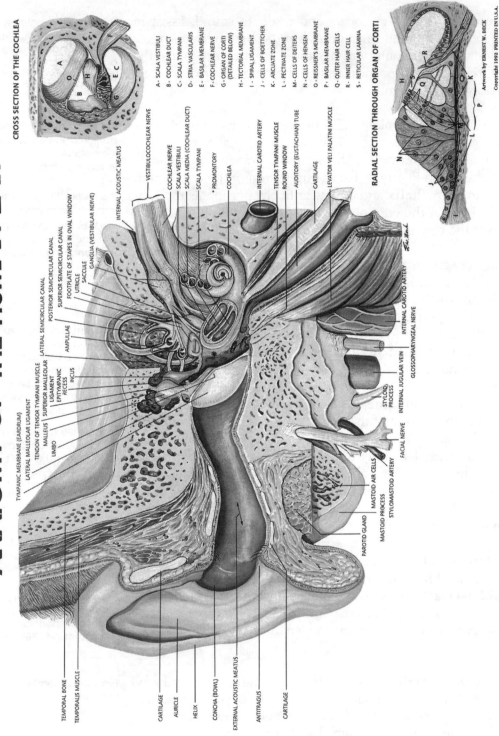

CROSS SECTION OF THE COCHLEA

A - SCALA VESTIBULI
B - COCHLEAR DUCT
C - SCALA TYMPANI
D - STRIA VASCULARIS
E - BASILAR MEMBRANE
F - COCHLEAR NERVE
G - ORGAN OF CORTI (DETAILED BELOW)
H - TECTORIAL MEMBRANE
I - SPIRAL LIGAMENT
J - CELLS OF BOETTCHER
K - ARCUATE ZONE
L - PECTINATE ZONE
M - CELLS OF DEITERS
N - CELLS OF HENSEN
O - REISSNER'S MEMBRANE
P - BASILAR MEMBRANE
Q - OUTER HAIR CELLS
R - INNER HAIR CELL
S - RETICULAR LAMINA

RADIAL SECTION THROUGH ORGAN OF CORTI

Artwork by ERNEST W. BECK
Copyright 1992 PRINTED IN U.S.A.

VESTIBULOCOCHLEAR NERVE
COCHLEAR NERVE
SCALA VESTIBULI
SCALA MEDIA (COCHLEAR DUCT)
SCALA TYMPANI
* PROMONTORY
COCHLEA
INTERNAL CAROTID ARTERY
TENSOR TYMPANI MUSCLE
ROUND WINDOW
AUDITORY (EUSTACHIAN) TUBE
CARTILAGE
LEVATOR VELI PALATINI MUSCLE

INTERNAL ACOUSTIC MEATUS
POSTERIOR SEMICIRCULAR CANAL
SUPERIOR SEMICIRCULAR CANAL
FOOTPLATE OF STAPES IN OVAL WINDOW
UTRICLE
SACCULE
GANGLIA (VESTIBULAR NERVE)

TYMPANIC MEMBRANE (EARDRUM)
LATERAL MALLEOLAR LIGAMENT
TENDON OF TENSOR TYMPANI MUSCLE
MALLEUS
UMBO
LATERAL SEMICIRCULAR CANAL
SUPERIOR MALLEOLAR LIGAMENT
EPITYMPANIC RECESS
INCUS
AMPULLAE

INTERNAL CAROTID ARTERY
INTERNAL JUGULAR VEIN
GLOSSOPHARYNGEAL NERVE

STYLOID PROCESS
FACIAL NERVE
MASTOID AIR CELLS
STYLOMASTOID ARTERY
MASTOID PROCESS
PAROTID GLAND

TEMPORAL BONE
TEMPORALIS MUSCLE

CARTILAGE
AURICLE
HELIX
CONCHA (BOWL)
EXTERNAL ACOUSTIC MEATUS
ANTITRAGUS
CARTILAGE

Figure 2–14. Anatomy of the ear. (From the American Academy of Audiology, by Ernest Beck. Reprinted with permission.)

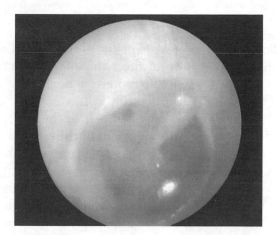

Figure 2–15. Photograph of the tympanic membrane. (From *The Human Ear Canal*, by B. Ballachanda, 1995, p. 66, San Diego: Singular Publishing Group. Reprinted with permission.)

A photograph of the tympanic membrane is shown in Figure 2–15. There are two main sections of the tympanic membrane, the **pars flaccida** and the **pars tensa**. The pars flaccida is the smaller and more compliant section of the drum, located superiorly and containing two layers of tissue. The pars tensa is the larger portion located inferiorly. It contains four membranous layers and is stiffer than the pars flaccida.

The superior, smaller, compliant portion of the tympanic membrane is called the **pars flaccida**.

The larger and stiffer portion of the tympanic membrane is called the **pars tensa**.

The tympanic membrane is set into motion by acoustic pressure waves striking its surface. The membrane vibrates with a magnitude proportional to the intensity of the sound wave at a speed proportional to its frequency.

Middle Ear

The *middle ear* is an air-filled space located within the temporal bone of the skull. It contains the **ossicular chain**, which consists of three contiguous bones suspended in space, linking the tympanic membrane to the oval window of the cochlea. The middle ear structures function as an impedance matching device, providing a bridge between the air-borne pressure waves striking the tympanic membrane and the fluid-borne traveling waves of the cochlea.

You may have learned the bones in the **ossicular chain** as the hammer, anvil, and stirrup.

Anatomy

The middle ear begins most laterally as the inner layers of the tympanic membrane. Beyond the tympanic membrane lies the middle ear cavity. A schematic representation of the middle ear cavity and its contents can be seen in the anatomy drawing in Figure 2–14. The cavity is air-filled. Air in the cavity is kept at atmospheric pressure via the **Eustachian tube**, which leads from the cavity to the back of the throat. If air pressure changes suddenly, such as it does when ascending or descending in an airplane, the cavity will have relatively more or less pressure than in the ear canal, and a feeling of fullness will result. Swallowing often opens the Eustachian tube, allowing the pressure to equalize.

The **Eustachian tube** is the passageway from the nasopharynx to the anterior wall of the middle ear.

Attached to the tympanic membrane is the ossicular chain (Figure 2–16). The ossicular chain is a series of three small bones or ossicles. The **ossicles**, called the malleus, incus, and stapes, transfer the vibration of the tympanic membrane to the inner ear or cochlea. The **malleus** consists of a long process called the **manubrium** that is attached to the tympanic membrane and a **head** that is attached to the body of the *incus.* A short process or **crus** (leg) of the incus is fitted into a recess in the wall of the tympanic cavity. The long crus of the incus attaches to the head of the stapes. The *stapes* consists of a head and two **crura** that attach to

The **ossicles** are the malleus, incus, and stapes.

The handle portion of the **malleus** is called the **manubrium.**

Crus = leg

Crura = legs

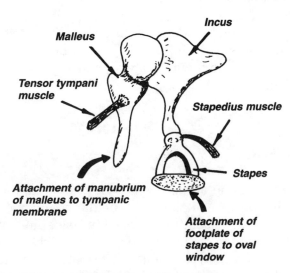

Figure 2–16. The ossicular chain. (From *The Speech Sciences,* by R. Kent, 1997, p. 215, San Diego: Singular Publishing Group. Reprinted with permission.)

a footplate. The *footplate* is fitted into the **oval window** of the cochlear wall, held in place by the **annular ligament**. The ossicular chain is suspended in the middle ear cavity by a number of ligaments, allowing it freedom to move in a predetermined manner. Thus, when the tympanic membrane vibrates, the malleus moves with it, which vibrates the incus and, in turn, the stapes. The stapes footplate is loosely attached to the bony wall of the fluid-filled cochlea and transmits the vibration to the fluid.

Physiology

Although it is by no means the entire story, the function of the middle ear can probably best be thought of as a means of matching the energy transfer from air to fluid. That is, the middle ear acts as an *impedance matching transformer.* Briefly, the ease (or difficulty) of energy flow is different through air than it is through fluid. Pressure waves propagating through air are substantively reflected by a fluid-filled space because of the difference in which energy flows through the two media. The different impedances of these two media need somehow to be matched or the functional gap between them bridged. The ossicular chain serves this purpose.

Air pressure waves vibrate the tympanic membrane, which vibrates the ossicles and sets the fluid of the cochlea into motion. If the middle ear did not exist, the air pressure waves would have to set the fluid of the cochlea into motion directly, and a substantial amount of energy would be lost in the process. Perhaps the best way to understand this is to understand that fish do not need a middle ear. Because the sounds that fish hear are propagated through water, the energy waves travel as fluid motion and set the inner-ear fluids into motion directly. Very little loss of energy results. But in humans, the energy waves are air-borne and need to be transformed into mechanical energy before being converted to hydraulic energy. The mechanical energy of the middle ear serves as an efficient energy converter from air to fluid.

The middle ear is designed to accomplish this in several ways. First, there is a substantial area difference between the tympanic membrane and the oval window. This area difference serves much the same purpose as the head of a nail. Pressure applied on the large end results in substantially greater pressure at the narrow end. The ossicles also act as a lever, pivoting around the **incudomalleolar joint**, which contributes to an increase in vibrational amplitude at the stapes.

The **oval window** leads into the scala vestibuli of the cochlea.

The **annular ligament** holds the footplate of the stapes in the oval window.

The two muscles of the middle ear are the **stapedius** muscle and the **tensor tympani** muscle.

The juncture of the incus and the malleus is called the **incudomalleolar joint**.

Inner Ear

The inner ear consists of the auditory and vestibular labyrinths. The term *labyrinth* is used to denote the intricate maze of connecting pathways in the **petrous** portion of each temporal bone. The *osseous labyrinth* is the channel in the bone; the *membranous labyrinth* is composed of soft-tissue fluid-filled channels within the osseous labyrinth that contain the end-organ structures of the hearing and vestibular systems. The auditory labyrinth is called the cochlea and is the sensory end-organ of hearing. It consists of fluid-filled membranous channels within a spiral canal that encircles a bony central core. Here the sound waves, transformed into mechanical energy by the middle ear, set the fluid of the cochlea into motion in a manner consistent with their intensity and frequency. Waves of fluid motion impinge on the membranous labyrinth and set off a chain of events that result in neural impulses being generated at the VIIIth cranial nerve.

Petrous means resembling stone.

Anatomy

The *cochlea* is a fluid-filled space within the temporal bone, which resembles the shape of a snail shell with 2.5 turns. An illustration of the bony labyrinth is shown in Figure 2–17. Suspended within this fluid-filled space, or *cochlear duct,* is the membranous labyrinth, which is another fluid-filled space often referred to as the *cochlear partition* or **scala media**. An illustration of the membranous labyrinth is shown in Figure 2–18.

The middle channel of the cochlear duct is called the **scala media** and is filled with endolymph.

The cochlear partition separates the **scala vestibuli** from the **scala tympani**, as shown in Figure 2–19. The scala vestibuli is the uppermost of two **perilymph-**filled channels of the cochlear duct and terminates basally at the *oval window.* The scala tympani is the lowermost channel and terminates basally at the *round window.* Both of these channels terminate at the apical end of the cochlea at the **helicotrema**.

The uppermost channel of the cochlear duct is called the **scala vestibuli** and is filled with perilymph.

The lowermost channel of the cochlear duct is called the **scala tympani** and is filled with perilymph.

The cochlear partition or scala media is an **endolymph**-filled channel that lies between the scala vestibuli and scala media. It is cordoned off by two membranes. *Reissner's membrane* serves as the cover of the partition, separating it from the scala vestibuli. The *basilar membrane* serves as the base of the partition, separating it from the scala tympani. Riding on the basilar membrane is the *organ of Corti,* which contains the sensory cells of hearing. Illustrations of the cochlear duct and organ of Corti are shown in

Perilymph is cochlear fluid that is high in sodium and calcium.

The passage connecting the scala tympani and the scala vestibuli is called the **helicotrema.**

Endolymph is cochlear fluid that is high in potassium and low in sodium.

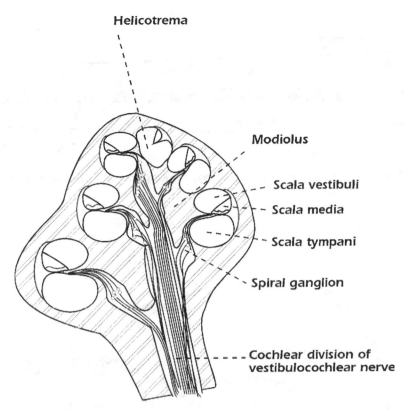

Helicotrema

Modiolus

Scala vestibuli

Scala media

Scala tympani

Spiral ganglion

Cochlear division of vestibulocochlear nerve

Figure 2-17. A section through the center of the cochlea, illustrating the bony labyrinth. (From *Neuroscience of Communication,* by D. Webster, 1995, p. 181, San Diego: Singular Publishing Group. Reprinted with permission.)

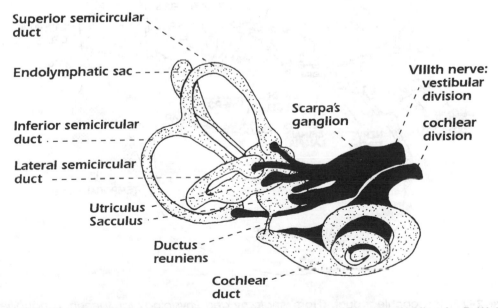

Superior semicircular duct

Endolymphatic sac

Inferior semicircular duct

Lateral semicircular duct

Utriculus
Sacculus

Ductus reuniens

Cochlear duct

Scarpa's ganglion

VIIIth nerve: vestibular division

cochlear division

Figure 2-18. The membranous labyrinth. (From *Neuroscience of Communication,* by D. Webster, 1995, p. 151, San Diego: Singular Publishing Group. Reprinted with permission.)

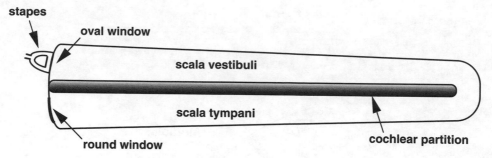

Figure 2-19. Schematic of an uncoiled cochlea, showing that the cochlear partition separates the scala vestibuli from the scala tympani.

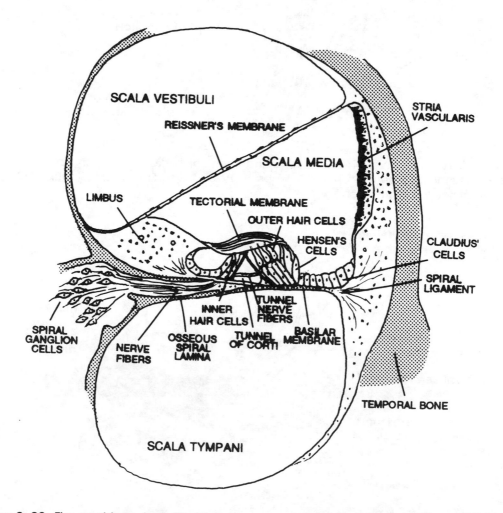

Figure 2-20. The cochlear duct. (From *Anatomy and Physiology for Speech, Language, and Hearing,* by J. A. Seikel, D. W. King, and D. G. Drumright, 1997, p. 554, San Diego: Singular Publishing Group. Reprinted with permission.)

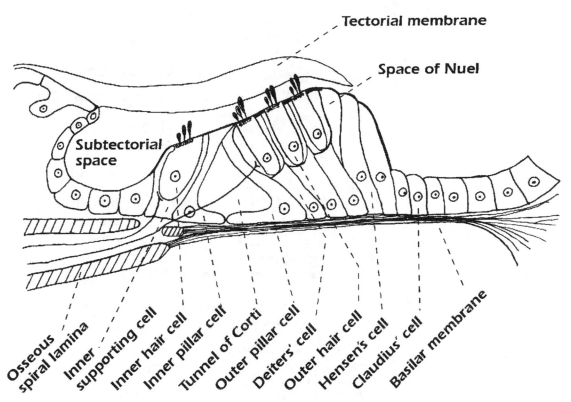

Figure 2-21. The organ of Corti. (From *Neuroscience of Communication,* by D. Webster, 1995, p. 185, San Diego: Singular Publishing Group. Reprinted with permission.)

Figures 2–20 and 2–21. It is obvious from this illustration that the microstructure of the organ of Corti is complex, containing numerous nutrient, supporting, and sensory cells.

There are two types of sensory cells, both of which are unique and very important to the function of hearing. These are termed the **outer hair cells** and **inner hair cells**. Outer hair cells are elongated in shape and have small hairs, or cilia, attached to their top. These cilia are embedded into the *tectorial membrane,* which covers the organ of Corti. There are three rows of outer hair cells throughout most of the length of the cochlea. The outer hair cells are innervated mostly by efferent, or motor, fibers of the nervous system. There are about **13,000 outer hair cells** in the cochlea. Outer hair cells and their innervation are shown in Figure 2–22.

There are about **13,000 outer hair cells**, and about **3,500 inner hair cells**.

Inner hair cells are also elongated and have an array of cilia on top. Inner hair cells stand in a single row, and their cilia are in

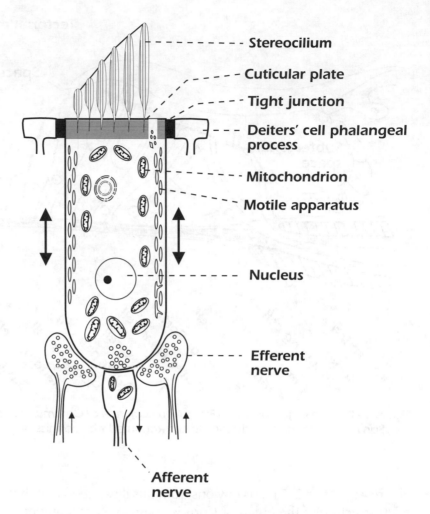

- - - - - - Stereocilium

- - - - Cuticular plate

- - - - Tight junction

- - - - Deiters' cell phalangeal process

- - - - Mitochondrion

- - - Motile apparatus

- - - - Nucleus

- - - - Efferent nerve

Afferent nerve

Figure 2-22. Diagram of a single outer hair cell. (From *Neuroscience of Communication*, by D. Webster, 1995, p. 190, San Diego: Singular Publishing Group. Reprinted with permission.)

The **saccule** and **utricle** are responsive to linear acceleration.

The **superior, lateral**, and **posterior semicircular canals** are three canals in the osseous labyrinth of the vestibular (balance) apparatus containing sensory epithelia that respond to angular motion.

proximity to, but not in direct contact with, the tectorial membrane. The inner hair cells are innervated mostly by afferent, or sensory, fibers of the nervous system. There are about **3,500 inner hair cells** in the cochlea. An illustration of inner hair cells is shown in Figure 2–23.

The vestibular portion of the inner ear also consists of a membranous labyrinth within a fluid-filled bony labyrinth. The labyrinth consists of two sacs, the **saccule** and **utricle**, and three circular canals, the **superior, lateral**, and **posterior semicircular canals**.

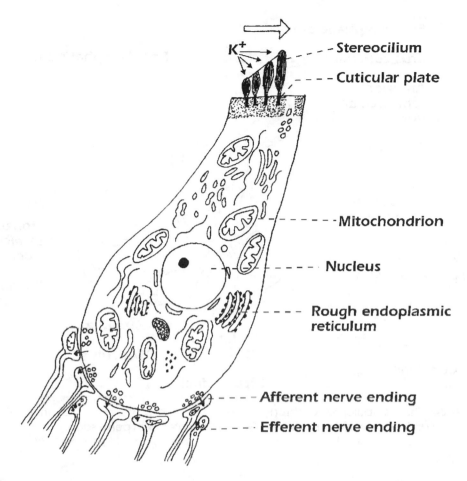

K$^+$
Stereocilium
Cuticular plate
Mitochondrion
Nucleus
Rough endoplasmic reticulum
Afferent nerve ending
Efferent nerve ending

Figure 2–23. Diagram of a single inner hair cell. (From *Neuroscience of Communication*, by D. Webster, 1995, p. 192, San Diego: Singular Publishing Group. Reprinted with permission.)

The vestibular labyrinth is shown in Figure 2–24. Both the saccule and utricle contain specialized **sensory epithelia**, as does the **ampulla** of each semicircular canal. The ampullae are enlarged portions of the tubes located at the entrance to each canal.

Physiology

Vibration of the stapes in and out of the oval window creates fluid motion in the cochlea, causing the structures of the membranous labyrinth to move, resulting in stimulation of the sensory cells and generation of neural impulses.

As the stapes vibrates in and out of the oval window, the fluid in the cochlea is set into a wavelike motion. This motion is referred

Sensory epithelia are groups of sensory and supporting cells.
The bulbous portion at the end of each of the three semicircular canals is called the **ampulla**.

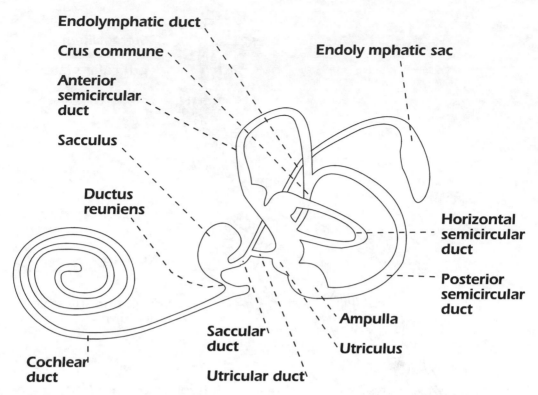

Endolymphatic duct

Crus commune

Anterior
semicircular
duct

Sacculus

Ductus
reuniens

Cochlear
duct

Saccular
duct

Utricular duct

Endoly mphatic sac

Horizontal
semicircular
duct

Posterior
semicircular
duct

Ampulla

Utriculus

Figure 2–24. The vestibular labyrinth. (From *Neuroscience of Communication,* by D. Webster, 1995, p.192, San Diego: Singular Publishing Group. Reprinted with permission.)

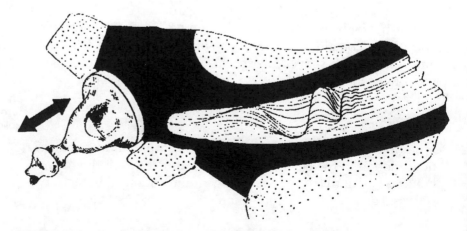

Figure 2–25. Schematic drawing of the traveling wave along the cochlear partition. (From "Cochlear Neurobiology: Revolutionary Developments," by P. Dallos, 1988, *Asha, 30,* p. 51. Reprinted with permission.)

to as the *traveling wave* and is depicted in Figure 2–25. This so-called traveling wave proceeds down the course of the cochlear partition, growing in magnitude, until it reaches a certain point of maximum displacement. For higher frequencies, this occurs closer to the oval window, nearer the basal end of the cochlea. For lower frequencies, it occurs farther from the oval window, at the apical end of the cochlea.

When the traveling wave reaches its point of maximum energy, the basilar membrane is displaced. At the point of basilar membrane displacement, the inner hair cells are stimulated, sending neural impulses to the auditory nerve.

The traveling wave by itself does not explain the extraordinary sensitivity and frequency selectivity of the cochlea. This concept is illustrated in Figure 2–26. This figure shows the "tuning" of an inner hair cell versus the tuning that can be explained by the traveling wave. Clearly some factors must be intervening to turn the basilar membrane displacement by the traveling wave into a sensitive, sharply tuned response at the inner hair cell.

The probable mechanism for this active process has only been revealed in the latter part of this century. Discovery of (a) the exquisite tuning of cochlear nerve fibers, (b) the existence of otoacoustic emissions, and (c) the **motility** of outer hair cells has led to the very compelling implication of outer hair cell contribution to hearing sensitivity. In brief, it appears that the sensitivity of the inner hair cells is controlled to some extent by the outer hair cells. Recall that the outer hair cells are embedded in the tectorial membrane and that they receive most of their innervation from efferent fibers of the brain. It appears that low-intensity sounds trigger the excitation or inhibition of outer hair cells, causing them to change shape and, likely, to influence position of the tectorial membrane in a manner that affects the inner hair cells, enhancing their sensitivity.

Motility of outer hair cells refers to their property of changing shape when stimulated.

Regardless, when the traveling wave reaches its maximum displacement, the inner hair cells are stimulated, resulting in the secretion of neurotransmitters that stimulate the nerve endings of the cochlear branch of the VIIIth nerve.

The vestibular system acts as a motion detector. The utricle and saccule are responsive to linear acceleration, and the ampullae of the semicircular canals are responsive to angular acceleration. As the head turns or body moves, the fluid in these structures flows in a direction opposite to the movement, resulting in stimulation

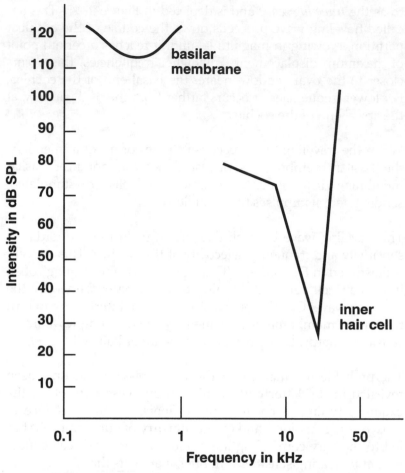

Figure 2-26 Generalized drawing of the "tuning" of an inner hair cell versus the tuning that can be explained by the traveling wave along the basilar membrane.

of the sensory epithelium and increased neural activity of the vestibular branch of the VIIIth nerve.

Auditory Nervous System

The auditory nervous system is a primarily afferent system that transmits neural signals from the cochlea to the auditory cortex. Like other nervous system activity, the auditory mechanism is functionally crossed, so that information from the right ear is transmitted primarily to the left cortex and information from the left ear primarily to the right cortex.

The auditory system also has an efferent component, which probably has multiple functions, including regulation of the outer hair cells and general inhibitory action throughout the central auditory nervous system.

Neurons leave the cochlea in a rather orderly manner and **synapse** in the lower brain stem. From that point on, the system becomes richly complex, with multiple crossing pathways and plenty of potential for efferent and intersensory interaction.

Neurons are the basic unit of the nervous system containing axons, cell bodies, and dendrites.

A **synapse** is the point of communication between neurons.

The VIIIth Cranial Nerve

Nerve fibers from the inner hair cells exit the organ of Corti through the **osseous spiral lamina** beyond which their cell bodies cluster to form the **spiral ganglion** in the **modiolus**. The nerve fibers exit the modiolus in an orderly manner, with fibers from the most apical turn of the cochlea in the middle of the nerve bundle and fibers from the basal end joining on the outside of the bundle. In this way, the frequency arrangement of the cochlea is preserved anatomically, with low frequencies from the apex in the middle and high frequencies from the base on the outside. This so-called **tonotopic** arrangement is preserved throughout the primary auditory pathways all the way to the cortex.

The bony shelf in the cochlea onto which the inner margin of the membranous labyrinth attaches and through which the nerve fibers of the hair cells course is called the **osseous spiral lamina**.

The **spiral ganglion** is a collection of cell bodies of the auditory nerve fibers, clustered in the modiolus.

The **modiolus** is the central bony pillar of the cochlea through which the blood vessels and nerve fibers of the labyrinth course.

Tonotopic means arranged according to frequency.

The cochlear branch of the VIIIth cranial nerve exits the modiolus, joins the vestibular branch, and leaves the cochlea through the *internal auditory canal* of the temporal bone. The cochlear branch of the nerve consists of some 30,000 nerve fibers, which carry information to the brain stem.

The VIIIth nerve codes auditory information in several ways. In general, intensity is coded as the rate of neural discharge. Frequency is coded as the place of neural discharge by fibers that are arranged tonotopically. Frequency may be additionally coded by temporal aspects of the discharge patterns of neuronal firing.

The Central Auditory Nervous System

The central auditory nervous system is best described by its various nuclei. Nuclei are bundles of cell bodies where nerve fibers synapse. Each nucleus serves as a relay station for neural information from the cochlea and VIIIth nerve to other nuclei in the auditory nervous system and to nuclei of other sensory and motor

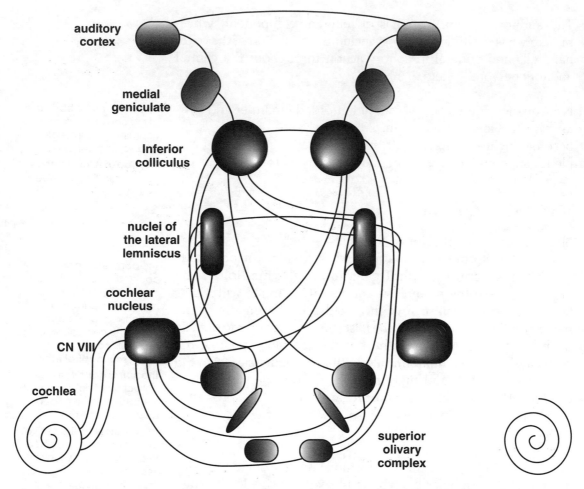

auditory
cortex

medial
geniculate

Inferior
colliculus

nuclei of
the lateral
lemniscus

cochlear
nucleus

CN VIII

cochlea

superior
olivary
complex

Figure 2-27. The central auditory nervous system. (Adapted from Structure and Function of the Central Auditory System, by G. Thompson, 1983, p. 91. *Seminars in Hearing, 4*(2)).

systems. The nuclei involved in the primary auditory pathway of the central auditory nervous system are:

- cochlear nucleus
- superior olivary complex
- lateral lemniscus
- inferior colliculus
- medial geniculate

A schematic representation of these various way stations in the brain is shown in Figure 2–27.

Ipsilateral pertains to the same side.

All VIIIth-nerve fibers have an obligatory synapse at the *cochlear nucleus* on the same, or **ipsilateral**, side of the brain. Fibers entering the cochlear nucleus **bifurcate**, with one fiber synapsing in the primary auditory portion of the nucleus and the other synapsing in portions of the nucleus that spawn secondary or parallel pathways.

Bifurcate means to divide into two branches.

From the cochlear nucleus, approximately 75% of the nerve fibers cross over to the **contralateral** side of the brain. Some fibers terminate on the *media nucleus of the trapezoid body* and some on the *medial superior olive.* Others proceed to nuclei beyond the superior olivary complex. Of the 25% that travel on the ipsilateral side of the brain, some terminate at the media superior olive, some at the *lateral superior olive,* and others at higher level nuclei.

Contralateral pertains to the opposite side.

From the superior olivary complex, neurons proceed to the *lateral lemniscus,* the *inferior colliculus,* and the *medial geniculate.* Nerve fibers may synapse on any of these nuclei or proceed beyond. Also, at each of these nuclei, some fibers cross over from the contralateral side of the brain. From the media geniculate, nerve fibers proceed in a tract called the *auditory radiations* to the *auditory cortex* in the temporal lobe.

This simplified explanation of the central auditory nervous system belies its rich complexity. For example, sound that is processed through the right cochlea has multiple, redundant pathways to both the right and left cortices. What begins as a pressure wave striking the tympanic membrane sets into motion a complex series of neural responses spread throughout the auditory system.

Much of the rudimentary processing of sound begins in the lower brain stem. For example, initial processing for sound localization occurs at the superior olive complex where small differences between sound reaching the two ears are detected. As another example, a simple reflex arc that triggers a contraction of the *stapedius muscle* occurs at the levels of the cochlear nucleus. This *acoustic reflex* occurs when sound reaches a certain loudness and causes the stapedius muscle to contract, resulting in a stiffening of the ossicular chain.

Processing of speech information occurs throughout the central auditory system. Its primary location for processing, however, occurs in the **left temporal lobe** of most humans. Speech that is detected by the right ear proceeds through the dominant contralateral auditory channels to the left temporal lobe. Speech

Processing of speech information occurs in the **left temporal lobe** in most people.

The **corpus callosum** is the white matter that connects the left and right hemispheres of the brain.

that is detected by the left ear proceeds through the dominant contralateral channel to the right cortex and then, via the **corpus callosum** to the left auditory cortex. Thus, in most humans, the right ear is dominant for the processing of speech information.

Our ability to hear relies on this very sophisticated series of structures that process sound. The pressure waves of sound are collected by the pinna and funneled to the tympanic membrane by the external auditory canal. The tympanic membrane vibrates in response to the sound, which sets the ossicular chain into motion. The mechanical movement of the ossicular chain then sets the fluids of the cochlea in motion, causing the hair cells on the basilar membrane to be stimulated. These hair cells send neural impulses through the VIIIth cranial nerve to the auditory brain stem. From the brain stem, networks of neurons act on the neural stimulation, sending signals to the auditory cortex.

The range between the threshold of sensitivity and the threshold of discomfort is called the **dynamic range**.

Although the complexity of these structures is remarkable, so too is the complexity of their function. All of this processing is obligatory and occurs constantly. The system is very sensitive in its ability to detect very soft sounds, is very sensitive in its ability to detect very small changes in sound characteristics, and has a very large **dynamic range**. And when we call on our auditory system to do the complicated tasks of listening to speech, it does so even under extremely adverse acoustic conditions.

HOW WE HEAR

As mentioned previously, the auditory system is an obligatory one. We simply cannot turn it off. In simpler life forms, the main function of the auditory system is protection. Because it is obligatory, it serves to constantly assess the surroundings for danger, as prey, and opportunity, as predator. In more evolved life forms, it takes on an increasingly important communication function, whether that be for mating calls or for talking on the telephone.

As you have seen the auditory system is highly complex. It is a sensitive system that can detect the smallest of pressure waves. In addition, it is a precise system that can effectively discriminate very small changes in the nature of sound. It is also a system with a large dynamic range. Remember that the difference in the magnitude of sound that can just barely be detected and the magnitude of sound that causes pain is on the order of 100 million to one.

Describing the function of such a rich, complex system is an academic discipline in and of itself, called **psychoacoustics**. Psychoacoustics is a branch of psychophysics concerned with the quantification of auditory sensation and the measurement of the psychological correlates of the physical characteristics of sound. The knowledge base of this field is broad and well beyond the scope of this text. However, there are some fundamentals that are necessary for you to understand as you pursue the study of clinical audiology. Much in the way of quantification of disordered systems stems from our knowledge of the response of normal systems and the techniques designed to measure those responses.

> **Psychoacoustics** is the branch of psychophysics concerned with the quantification of auditory sensations and the measurement of the psychological correlates of the physical characteristics of sound.

Absolute Sensitivity of Hearing

As you will learn later in this textbook, one of the hallmarks of audiology is the assessment of hearing sensitivity. Sensitivity is defined as the capacity of a sense organ to detect a stimulus and is quantified by the determination of threshold of audibility or threshold of detection of change. There are at least two kinds of sensitivity, absolute and differential. **Absolute sensitivity** pertains to the capacity of the auditory system to detect faint sound. **Differential sensitivity** pertains to the capacity of the auditory system to detect differences or changes in intensity, frequency, or some other dimension of a sound.

> **Absolute sensitivity** is the ability to detect faint sound.
>
> **Differential sensitivity** is the ability to detect differences or changes in intensity, frequency, or other dimensions of sound.

Hearing sensitivity most commonly refers to absolute sensitivity to faint sound. In contrast, *hearing acuity* most accurately refers to the differential sensitivity, usually to the ability to detect differences in signals that differ in the frequency domain.

Inherent in the description of hearing sensitivity is the notion of **threshold**. A threshold is the level at which a stimulus or change in stimulus is just sufficient to produce a sensation or an effect. Here again, it is useful to differentiate between absolute and differential threshold. In hearing, **absolute threshold** is the threshold of audibility, or the lowest intensity level at which an acoustic signal can be detected. It is usually defined as the level at which a sound can be heard 50% of the times that it is presented. **Differential threshold**, or *difference limen,* is the smallest difference that can be detected between two signals that vary in some physical dimension.

> **Threshold** is the level at which a stimulus is just sufficient to produce a sensation.
>
> **Absolute threshold** is the lowest level at which a sound can be detected.
>
> **Differential threshold** is the smallest difference that can be detected between two signals.

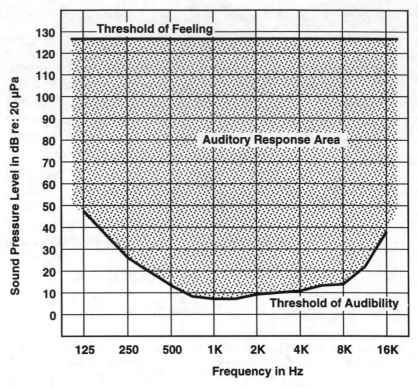

Figure 2–28. Auditory response area from the threshold of audibility to the threshold of feeling across the frequency range that encompasses most of human hearing.

The Nature of Hearing Sensitivity

Absolute sensitivity of hearing for humans varies as a function of numerous factors, including psychophysical technique, whether ears are tested separately or together, whether testing is done under earphones or in a sound field, the type of earphone that is used, the type of cushion on that earphone, and so on. Once these variables are defined and controlled, a consistent picture of hearing sensitivity emerges.

Figure 2–28 shows a graph of hearing sensitivity, defined as the threshold of audibility of pure tone signals, graphed in sound pressure level (SPL) across a frequency range that encompasses most of human hearing. This curve representing hearing sensitivity is often referred to as the *minimum audibility curve*. The minimum audibility curve is clearly not a straight line, indicating that hearing sensitivity varies as a function of signal frequency. That is, it takes more sound pressure at some frequencies to reach threshold than at others. You can see that hearing in the low-frequency and high-frequency ranges is not as sensitive as it is in the mid-frequency range. It should probably be no surprise that human audibility thresholds are best at frequencies corresponding to the most important components of speech.

The minimum audibility curve will vary as a function of measurement parameters. If it is determined by delivering signals to one ear via an earphone, it is referred to as the *minimum auditory pressure* response. If it is determined by delivering signals to both ears via loudspeaker, it is called the *minimum audible field* response.

Also shown on Figure 2–28 is the threshold of feeling, at which a tactile response will occur if the subject can tolerate sounds of this magnitude. This is the upper limit of hearing and has a clearly flatter profile across the frequency range. The area between the threshold of audibility and the threshold of feeling is known as the *auditory response area* and represents the range of human hearing. You will notice that the range varies as a function of frequency, so that the number of decibels of difference between audibility and feeling is substantially less at the low frequencies than at the high frequencies.

The minimum audible pressure curve serves as the basis for puretone audiometry, in which a patient's threshold of audibility is measured and compared to this normal curve. For clinical purposes, this curve is converted into a graph known as the audiogram.

The Audiogram

The audiogram is a graphic representation of the threshold of audibility across the audiometric frequency range. It is a plot of absolute threshold, designated in dB *hearing level* (HL), at octave or mid-octave intervals from 125 to 8000 Hz.

The designation of intensity in dB HL is an important one to understand. Recall from the minimum audibility curve that hearing sensitivity varies as a function of frequency. For clinical purposes, this curve is simply converted into a straight line and called **audiometric zero**. Audiometric zero is the sound pressure level at which the threshold of audibility occurs in average normal listeners. We know from the minimum audibility curve that the SPL required to reach threshold will vary as a function of frequency. If a standard SPL level is applied at each frequency, and threshold for the average normal listener is designated as 0 dB HL for

Audiometric zero is the sound pressure level at which the threshold of audibility occurs for normal listeners.

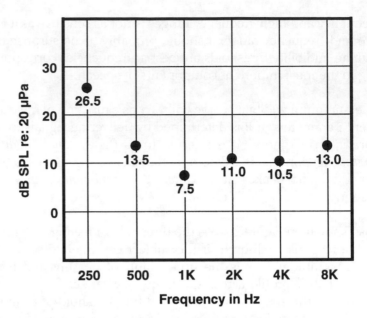

Figure 2–29. The designation of audiometric zero as different sound pressure levels across the frequency range.

each frequency, then we have effectively flattened out the curve and represented average normal hearing sensitivity as a flat line of 0 dB.

The concept of designating audiometric zero as different sound pressure levels across the frequency range is shown in Figure 2–29. Here you see the average normal threshold values, or audiometric zero plotted in SPL. When this curve is flattened by designating each of these levels as 0 dB HL and then the entire graph is flipped over, an audiogram results. The conversion is shown in Figure 2–30.

Abscissa indicates the horizontal or X axis on a graph.

Ordinate indicates the vertical or Y axis on a graph.

The **American National Standards Institute (ANSI)** is an association of specialists, manufacturers, and consumers that determines standards for measuring instruments, including audiometers.

Figure 2–31 is an audiogram. The **abscissa** on the graph is frequency in Hz. It is divided into octave intervals, ranging from 250 Hz to 8000 Hz. The **ordinate** on the graph is signal intensity in dB HL. It is divided into 10 dB segments, usually ranging from −10 dB to 120 dB HL. Typically on an audiogram, the HL will be further referenced to a standard, such as ANSI 1996. This standard, from the **American National Standards Institute (ANSI)**, relates to the SPL assigned to 0 dB HL, depending on the type of earphone and cushion used.

An audiogram will usually also have a shaded area, designating the range of normal hearing. You will learn in the next section

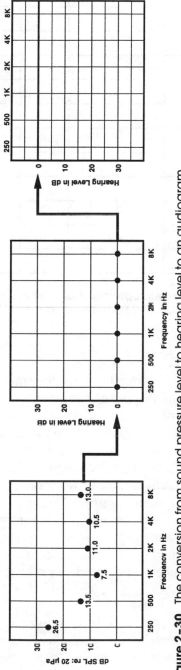

Figure 2–30. The conversion from sound pressure level to hearing level to an audiogram.

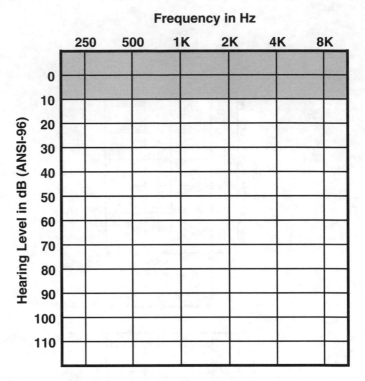

Figure 2-31. An audiogram with intensity, expressed in hearing level, plotted as a function of frequency, expressed in Hertz.

that there is some variability in determining hearing threshold and that normal responses can vary by as many as 10 decibels around audiometric zero. It is not uncommon then to have a shaded range from −10 to +10 dB to designate the normal range of hearing. On some audiograms, that range will be extended to 25 dB or so. This idea defines the normal range not in statistical terms, but in some notion of functional terms. The assumption here would be that, for example, 20 dB is not enough of a hearing loss to be considered meaningful, therefore it should be classified as normal. As you will learn in subsequent chapters, impairment cannot be defined by the audiogram alone, and increasingly the shaded range is either being defined by a statistical approach or being eliminated.

An audiogram is obtained by carrying out pure-tone audiometry to determine threshold of audibility. The techniques used to do this are described in detail in Chapter 6. Basically, signals are presented and the patient responds to those that are audible. The level at which the patient can just barely detect the presence of a pure-tone signal 50% of the time is determined. That level is then

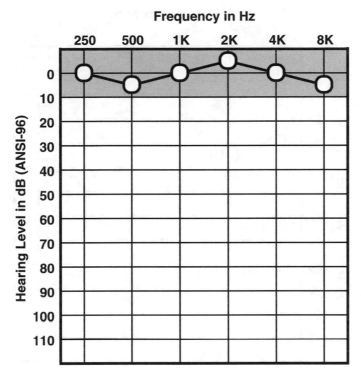

Figure 2-32. An audiogram depicting normal hearing.

marked on the audiogram. Figure 2–32 shows the audiogram of someone with normal hearing. Note that all of the symbols fall within the normal range. Figure 2–33 shows the audiogram of someone with a hearing loss. Note that, at each frequency, the intensity of the signal had to be increased significantly before it became audible. This represents a hearing sensitivity loss as a function of the normal, audiometric zero range.

There are two main ways to deliver signals to the ear, and they are plotted separately on the audiogram. One way is by the use of earphones. Here signals are presented through the air to the tympanic membrane and middle ear to the cochlea. Signals presented in this manner are considered air-conducted, and thresholds are called *air-conduction* thresholds. The other way is by use of a bone vibrator. Signals are delivered via a vibrator, usually placed on the forehead or on the **mastoid process** behind the ear, through the bones of the skull directly to the cochlea. Signals presented in this manner are considered bone-conducted, and thresholds are called *bone-conduction* thresholds. Because bone-conducted signals bypass the outer and middle ear, thresholds determined by bone conduction represent sensitivity of the coch-

The part of the temporal bone that creates a protuberance behind and below the auricle is called the **mastoid process**.

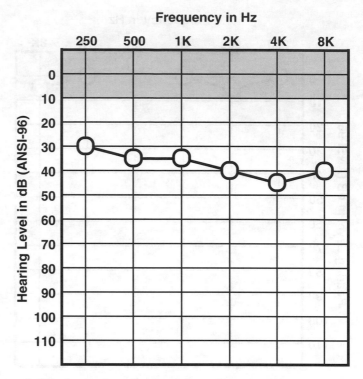

Figure 2–33. An audiogram depicting a hearing loss.

Sensorineural hearing loss is of cochlear origin.

Conductive hearing loss is of outer or middle ear origin.

lea. When the outer and middle ears are functioning normally, air-conduction and bone-conduction thresholds are the same, as shown in Figure 2–34. If there is a hearing loss of cochlear origin, a so-called **sensorineural hearing loss**, then both air and bone conduction thresholds will be affected similarly, as shown in Figure 2–35. When the outer or middle ears are not functioning normally, the intensity of the air conducted signals must be raised before threshold is reached, although the bone-conduction thresholds will remain normal, as shown in Figure 2–36. You will learn more about this type of **conductive hearing loss** in the next chapter.

Differential Sensitivity

Differential sensitivity is the capacity of the auditory system to detect change in intensity, frequency, or some other dimension of sound. It is usually measured as the differential threshold or difference limen (DL), defined as the smallest change in a stimulus that is detectable. When we measure absolute threshold, we are trying to determine the presence or absence of a stimulus.

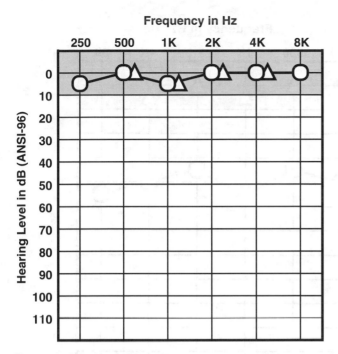

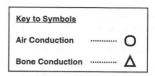

Figure 2–34. An audiogram showing that when the outer and middle ears are functioning normally, air-conduction and bone-conduction thresholds are the same.

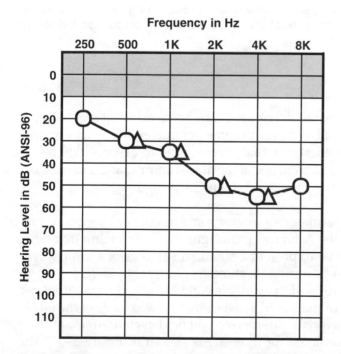

Figure 2–35. An audiogram demonstrating that when a hearing loss is of cochlear origin, resulting in a sensorineural hearing loss, both air and bone conduction thresholds are affected similarly.

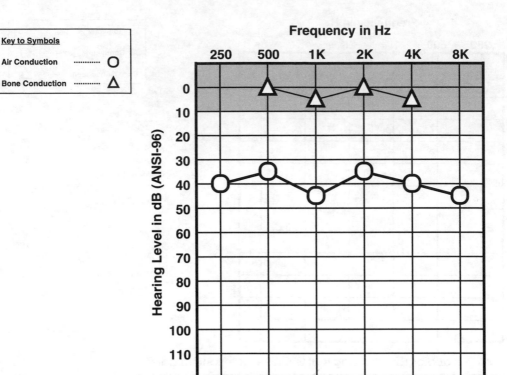

Figure 2–36. An audiogram demonstrating that when the outer or middle ears are not functioning normally, resulting in a conductive hearing loss, the intensity of the air-conducted signals must be raised before threshold is reached, while the bone-conduction thresholds remain normal.

When we measure differential threshold, we are trying to determine how small a change in some parameter of the signal can be detected. Another term that is often used to describe differential threshold is *just noticeable difference,* a term that accurately describes the perception that is being measured.

A **paradigm** is an example or model.

The difference limens for intensity and frequency have been studied extensively. A typical **paradigm** for determining difference limen would be to present a standard stimulus of a given intensity, followed by a variable stimulus of a slightly different intensity. The intensity of the variable stimulus would be manipulated over a series of trials until a determination was made of the intensity level at which a difference could be detected. An example of the difference limen for intensity is shown in Figure 2–37. The difference limen for intensity varies little across frequency. However, it is significantly poorer at levels near absolute threshold than at higher intensity levels.

An example of the difference limen for frequency is shown in Figure 2–38. In general, the difference limen for frequency increases with increasing frequency, so that a larger change in Hz is required at higher frequencies than at lower frequencies. As with intensity, the ability to detect changes becomes significantly poorer at intensity levels near absolute threshold.

Properties of Pitch and Loudness

The threshold of hearing sensitivity is just one way to describe hearing ability. It can also be described in terms of **suprathreshold** hearing perception.

An intensity level that is above threshold is considered **suprathreshold**.

Earlier you learned about the physical properties of intensity and frequency of an acoustic signal. The psychological correlates of these physical measures of sound are loudness and pitch, respectively.

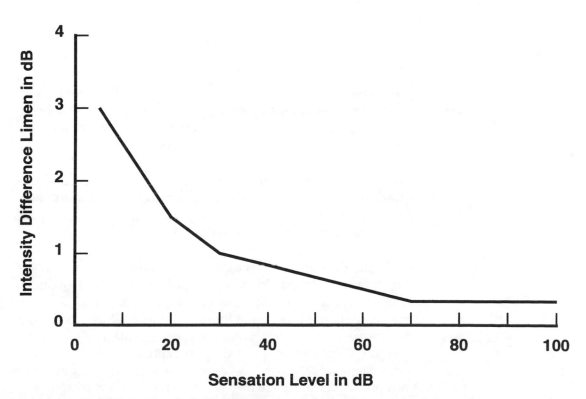

Figure 2–37. Generalized drawing of the relationship between intensity of a signal and difference limen for intensity.

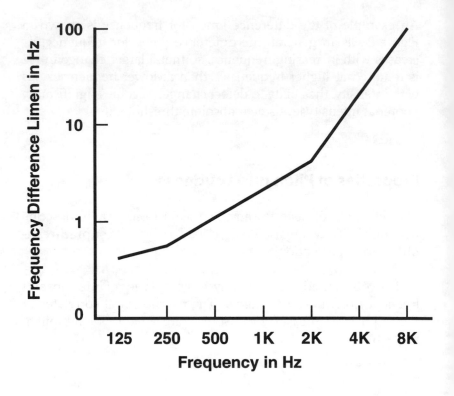

Intensity translates to the
perception of **loudness**;
frequency translates to
pitch.

Loudness refers to the perception that occurs at different sound intensities. Low **intensity** sounds are perceived as soft sounds, while high intensity sounds are perceived as loud sounds. As intensity increases, so too does the perception of loudness.

Pitch refers to the perception that occurs at different sound **frequencies**. Low-frequency sounds are perceived as low in pitch, and high-frequency sounds as high in pitch. As frequency increases, so does the perception of pitch.

Understanding of these basic aspects of hearing, absolute threshold, differential threshold, and perception of pitch and loudness, is, of course, only the beginning of understanding the full nature of how we hear. Once sound is audible, the auditory mechanism is capable of processing complex speech signals, often in the presence of similar, yet competing, background noise. The auditory system's ability to process changes in intensity and frequency in rapid sequence to perceive speech is truly a remarkable processing accomplishment.

Measurement of Sound

The accurate measurement of sound is an important component of hearing assessment. The standard audiogram is a plot of frequency versus intensity. The intensity level is referenced to a standard sound pressure level. Specifications for this sound pressure level are based on internationally accepted standards. To meet those standards, the instrumentation that produces the signals, the **audiometer**, must do so in an accurate and consistent manner.

The output of any audiometer is periodically checked to ensure that it meets *calibration* standards. An audiometer is considered to be calibrated if the pure tones and other signals emanating from the earphones are equal to the standard levels set by the American National Standards Institute or the International Organization for Standardization (ISO). To ensure calibration, the output must be measured. The instrument used to measure the output is called a *sound level meter.*

A sound level meter is an electronic instrument designed specifically for the measurement of acoustic signals. For audiometric purposes, the components of a sound level meter include:

- a standard coupler to which an earphone can be attached,
- a sensitive microphone to convert sound from acoustical to electrical energy,
- an amplifier to boost the low level signal from the microphone,
- adjustable attenuators to focus in on the intensity range of the signal,
- filtering networks to focus in on the frequency range of the signal,
- and a meter to display the measured sound pressure level.

As you might expect, all of these components must meet certain specifications as well to ensure that the sound level meter maintains its accuracy. Sound level meters are used for purposes other than audiometric calibration. Importantly, sound level meters are used to measure noise in the environment and are an important component of industrial noise measurement and control. A photograph of a coupler and sound level meter is shown in Figure 2–39.

An **audiometer** is an electronic instrument used to measure hearing sensitivity.

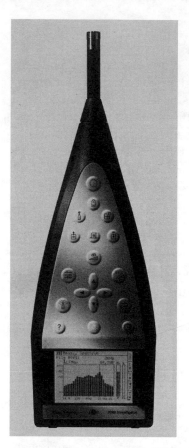
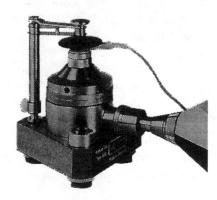

Figure 2–39. Photograph of a sound level meter and earphone coupler. (Courtesy of Brüel & Kjaer).

For audiometric calibration purposes, the sound level meter is used to measure the accuracy of the output of the audiometer through its transducers, either earphones or a bone-conduction vibrator. The process is one of placing the earphone or vibrator onto the standard coupler and turning on the pure tone or other signal at a specified level. The sound level meter is set to an intensity and frequency range, and the output level of the earphone is read from the meter. The output is expressed in dB SPL. Standard output levels for audiometric zero have been established for the earphones that are commonly used in audiometric testing. If the output measured by the sound level meter is equal to the standard output, then the audiometer is in calibration. If it is not in calibration, the output of the audiometer must be adjusted. The following measurements are typically made during a calibration assessment:

■ output in dB SPL to be compared to a standard for audiometric zero for a given transducer,

Table 2-2. Reference equivalent threshold sound pressure levels (re: 20 μPa) for supra-aural earphones on the NBS 9-A coupler and insert earphones on a HA-1 acoustic coupler.

Frequency (Hz)	Supra-aural (TDH-49, TDH-50)	Insert (ER-3A)
125	47.5	26.0
250	26.5	14.0
500	13.5	5.5
1000	7.5	0.0
2000	11.0	3.0
3000	9.5	3.5
4000	10.5	5.5
6000	13.5	2.0
8000	13.0	0.0

Note: Based on American National Standards Institute 1996 standards

■ attenuator linearity to assure that a change of 5 or 10 dB on the audiometer's attenuator dial is indeed that much change in intensity of the output,

■ frequency in Hz to ensure that it is accurate to within standardized tolerances,

■ **distortion** of the output to make sure that a pure tone is relatively pure or undistorted, and

■ rise-fall time to assure that the onset and offset of a tone are sufficiently slow to avoid **transient distortion** of a pure-tone signal.

The standard output levels for audiometric zero, known as *reference equivalent threshold sound pressure levels* (RETSPL), are shown in Table 2–2 for two common types of earphones, supra-aural and insert earphones. You will learn more about the audiometer and earphones in Chapter 6.

Distortion is the inexact reproduction of sound. **Transient distortion** occurs when the electrical signal applied to the earphone is changed too abruptly, resulting in a **transient**, or click, response of the earphone.

SUMMARY

■ Sound is a common type of energy that occurs as a result of pressure waves that emanate from some force being applied to a sound source. A sine wave is a graphic way of representing the pressure waves of sound.

■ The magnitude of a sound is described as its intensity. Intensity is related to the perception of loudness. Intensity is expressed in decibels sound pressure level, or SPL. One of the most common referents for decibels in audiometry is known as hearing level (HL), which represents decibels according to average normal hearing.

■ Frequency is the speed of vibration and is related to the perception of pitch. Frequency is usually expressed in cycles-per-second or Hertz (Hz).

■ The physical processing of acoustic information occurs in three groups of structures, commonly known as the outer, middle, and inner ears.

■ The outer ear has three main components: the auricle, the ear canal or meatus, and the outer layer of the ear-drum or tympanic membrane. The outer ear serves to collect and resonate sound, assist in sound localization, and function as a protective mechanism for the middle ear.

■ The middle ear is an air-filled space located within the temporal bone of the skull. It contains the ossicular chain, which consists of three contiguous bones suspended in space, linking the tympanic membrane to the oval window of the cochlea. The middle ear structures function as an impedance matching device, providing a bridge between the air-borne pressure waves striking the tympanic membrane and the fluid-borne traveling waves of the cochlea.

■ The inner ear contains the cochlea, which is the sensory end-organ of hearing. The cochlea consists of fluid-filled membranous channels within a spiral canal that encircles a bony central core. Here the sound waves, transformed into mechanical energy by the middle ear, set the fluid of the cochlea into motion in a manner consistent with their intensity and frequency. Waves of fluid motion impinge on the membranous labyrinth and set off a chain of events that result in neural impulses being generated at the VIIIth cranial nerve.

■ The auditory nervous system is primarily an afferent system that transmits neural signals from the cochlea to the auditory cortex. Neurons leave the cochlea via the VIIIth nerve in an orderly manner and synapse in the lower brain stem. From that point on, the system becomes richly complex, with multiple crossing pathways and plenty of opportunity for efferent and intersensory interaction.

■ Absolute threshold of hearing is the threshold of audibility, or the lowest intensity level at which an acoustic signal can be detected.

■ The standard audiogram is a plot of absolute threshold, designated in dB HL, at octave or mid-octave intervals from 125 to 8000 Hz. The intensity level is referenced to a standard sound pressure level. Specifications for this sound pressure level are based on internationally accepted standards.

SUGGESTED READINGS

Durrant, J. D., & Lovrinic, J. H. (1995). *Bases of hearing science* (3rd ed.). Baltimore: Williams & Wilkins

Seikel, J. A., King, D. W., & Drumright, D. G. (1996). *Anatomy and physiology for speech, language, and hearing* (exp. ed.). San Diego: Singular Publishing Group.

Speaks, C. E. (1992). *Introduction to sound.* San Diego: Singular Publishing Group.

Zemlin, W. R. (1988). *Speech and hearing science. Anatomy and physiology* (3rd ed.). Englewood Cliffs, NJ: Prentice-Hall.

3

The Nature of Hearing Impairment

Hearing impairment results from a number of causes and is usually characterized by the type and degree of hearing loss. Type of hearing loss is related to the site of the disorder within the auditory system, and degree of loss is related to the extent that the disorder is infringing on normal function. Defining both the type and degree of hearing loss is a cornerstone of audiology. This chapter covers types of hearing impairment and their functional consequences.

TYPES OF HEARING IMPAIRMENT

Hearing impairments are of two major types:

- hearing sensitivity loss
- auditory nervous system disorders.

Hearing sensitivity loss is the most common form of hearing loss. It is characterized by a reduction in the sensitivity of the auditory mechanism so that sounds need to be of higher intensity than normal before they are perceived by the listener. *Auditory nervous system disorders* are less common, may or may not include hearing sensitivity loss, and often result in reduced ability to hear suprathreshold sounds properly. A third type of impairment is known as *functional hearing loss.* Functional hearing loss is the exaggeration or fabrication of a hearing loss.

In addition to type of loss, a hearing impairment can be described in terms of time of onset, time course of the disorder or impairment, and whether one or both ears is involved.

A hearing loss can be described by the time of onset:

congenital:	present at birth
acquired:	obtained after birth
adventitious:	not congenital; acquired after birth

Hearing loss or auditory disorder can also be described by its time course:

acute:	of sudden onset and short duration
chronic:	of long duration
sudden:	having a rapid onset
gradual:	occurring in small degrees

temporary: of limited duration

permanent: irreversible

progressive: advancing in degree

fluctuating: aperiodic change in degree

In addition, hearing loss can be described by the number of ears involved:

unilateral: pertaining to one ear only

bilateral: pertaining to both ears

Hearing Sensitivity Loss

The major cause of hearing impairment is a loss of hearing sensitivity. A loss of hearing sensitivity means that the ear is not as sensitive as normal in detecting sound. Stated another way, sounds must be of a higher intensity than normal to be perceived.

Hearing sensitivity loss is caused by an abnormal reduction of sound being delivered to the brain by a disordered ear. This reduction of sound can result from a number of factors that affect the outer, middle, or inner ears. When sound is not *conducted* well through a disordered outer or middle ear, the result is a **conductive hearing loss**. When the *sensory* or *neural* cells or their connections within the cochlea are absent or not functioning, the result is a **sensorineural hearing loss**. When structures of both the conductive mechanism and the cochlea are disordered, the result is a **mixed hearing loss**.

A sensorineural hearing loss can also be caused by a disorder of the VIIIth nerve or auditory brain stem. That is, a tumor on the VIIIth nerve or a space-occupying **lesion** in the brainstem can result in a loss of hearing sensitivity that will be classified as sensorineural, rather than conductive or mixed. Generally, however, such disorders are treated separately as **retrocochlear disorders,** because their diagnosis, treatment, and impact on hearing ability can differ substantially from a sensorineural hearing loss of cochlear origin.

A **conductive hearing loss** is a reduction in hearing sensitivity due to a disorder of the outer or middle ear.

A **sensorineural hearing loss** is a reduction in hearing sensitivity due to a disorder of the cochlea.

A **mixed hearing loss** is a reduction in hearing sensitivity due to a combination of a disordered outer or middle and inner ear.

A **lesion** is the structural or functional pathologic change in body tissue.

A **retrocochlear** lesion pertains to damage to the neural structures of the auditory system beyond the cochlea.

Conductive Hearing Loss

A conductive hearing loss is caused by an abnormal reduction or attenuation of sound as it travels from the outer ear to the cochlea. You will recall that the outer ear serves to collect, direct, and enhance sound to be delivered to the tympanic membrane. The tympanic membrane and other structures of the middle ear transform acoustic energy into mechanical energy in order to serve as a bridge from the air pressure waves in the ear canal to the motion of fluid in the cochlea. This outer and middle ear systems can be thought of collectively as a *conductive mechanism,* or one that conducts sound from the atmosphere to the cochlea.

Attenuation means a decrease in magnitude.

If a structure of the conductive mechanism is in some way impaired, its ability to conduct sound is reduced, resulting in less sound being delivered to the cochlea. Thus, the effect of any disorder of the outer or middle ear is to reduce or **attenuate** the energy that reaches the cochlea. In this way, a soft sound that is perceptible by a normal ear might not be of sufficient magnitude to overcome the conductive deficit and reach the cochlea. Only when the intensity of this sound is increased can it overcome the conductive barrier.

Perhaps the simplest way to think of a conductive hearing loss is by placing earplugs into your ear canals. Sounds that would normally enter the ear canal are attenuated by the earplugs, resulting in reduced hearing sensitivity. The only way to hear the sound normally is to get closer to its source or to raise its volume.

Audiometric zero is the lowest level at which normal hearers can detect a sound.

A conductive hearing loss or the *conductive component* of a hearing loss is best measured by comparing air- and bone-conduction thresholds on an audiogram. Air conduction thresholds represent hearing sensitivity as measured through the outer, middle, and inner ears. Bone conduction thresholds represent hearing sensitivity as measured primarily through the inner ear. Thus, if air-conduction thresholds are poorer than bone conduction thresholds, it can be assumed that the attenuation of sound is occurring at the level of the outer or middle ears. An example of a conductive hearing loss is shown in Figure 3–1. Note that bone conduction thresholds are at or near **audiometric zero**, but air conduction thresholds require higher intensity levels before threshold is reached. The ear is acting as if the sound that you are delivering has been attenuated by, in this case, 30 dB. The size of the conductive component, often referred to as the *air-bone gap,* is described as the difference between the air- and bone-conduction thresholds. In this case, the conductive component to the hearing loss is 30 dB.

A conductive hearing loss is often described by its degree and audiometric configuration. The degree is the size of the conduc-

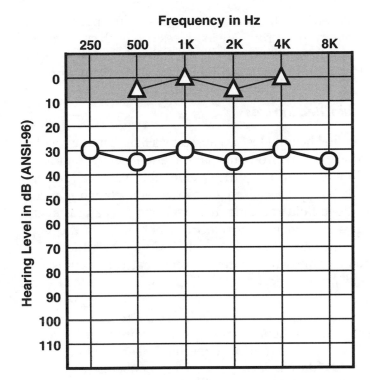

Figure 3–1. Audiogram showing a conductive hearing loss.

tive component and relates to the extent or severity of the disorder causing the hearing loss. As you will learn in Chapter 4, a number of disorders of the outer and middle ears can cause conductive hearing loss. Whether the disorder causes a conductive hearing loss and the degree of the loss that it causes is based on many factors related to the impact of the disorder on the functioning of the various parts of the conductive mechanism.

Audiometric configuration of a conductive hearing loss varies from low frequency to flat to high frequency depending on the physical obstruction of the structures of the conductive mechanism. In general, any disorder that adds mass to the conductive system will differentially affect the higher audiometric frequencies. Any disorder that adds or reduces stiffness to the system will affect the lower audiometric frequencies. Any disorder that changes both mass and stiffness will affect a broad range of audiometric frequencies.

Because a conductive hearing loss acts primarily as an **attenuator** of sound, it has little or no impact on *suprathreshold* hearing. That is, once sound is of a sufficient intensity, the ear acts as it nor-

An **attenuator** is something that reduces or decreases the magnitude.

mally would at suprathreshold intensities. Thus, perception of loudness, ability to discriminate loudness and pitch changes, and speech-recognition ability are all normal once the conductive hearing loss is overcome by raising the intensity of the signal.

Sensorineural Hearing Loss

A sensorineural hearing loss is caused by a failure in the cochlear transduction of sound from mechanical energy in the middle ear to neural impulses in the VIIIth nerve. You will recall that the cochlea is a highly specialized sensory receptor organ that converts hydraulic fluid movement, caused by mechanical energy from stapes movement, into electrical potentials in the nerve endings on the hair cells of the organ of Corti. The intricate sensory system composed of receptor cells that convert this fluid movement into electrical potentials contains both sensory and neural elements.

When a structure of this sensorineural mechanism is in some way damaged, its ability to transduce mechanical energy into electrical energy is reduced. This results in a number of changes in cochlear processing, including:

1. a reduction in the sensitivity of the cochlear receptor cells,
2. a reduction in the frequency-resolving ability of the cochlea, and
3. a reduction in the dynamic range of the hearing mechanism.

A sensorineural hearing loss is most often characterized clinically by its effect on cochlear sensitivity and, thus, the audiogram. If the outer and middle ears are functioning properly, then air-conduction thresholds accurately represent the sensitivity of the cochlea and are equal to bone-conduction thresholds. An example of a sensorineural hearing loss is shown in Figure 3–2. Note that air-conduction thresholds match bone-conduction thresholds and both require higher intensity levels than normal before threshold is reached.

A sensorineural hearing loss is often described by its degree and audiometric configuration. The degree is based on the range of decibel loss and relates to the extent or severity of the disorder causing the hearing loss. As you will learn in Chapter 4, a number of disorders of the cochlea and peripheral auditory nervous system can cause sensorineural hearing loss. Whether the disorder causes a sensorineural hearing loss and the degree of the loss that it causes is based on many factors related to the impact of

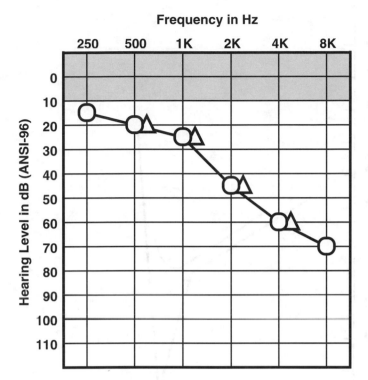

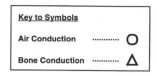

Figure 3-2. Audiogram showing a sensorineural hearing loss.

the disorder on the functioning of the various components of the sensorineural mechanism.

Audiometric configuration of a sensorineural hearing loss varies from low frequency to flat to high frequency depending on the location along the basilar membrane of hair cell loss or other damage. Various causes of sensorineural hearing loss have characteristic configurations, which will be shown later in this section.

The complexity of a sensorineural hearing loss tends to be greater than that of a conductive hearing loss because of its effects on frequency resolution and dynamic range. Recall that one important processing component of cochlear function is to provide fine tuning of the auditory system in the frequency domain. The broadly tuned traveling wave of cochlear fluid is converted into finely tuned neural processing of the VIIIth nerve by the active processes of the outer hair cells of the organ of Corti. One effect of the loss of these hair cells is a reduction in the sensitivity of the system. Another is broadening of the frequency-resolving ability. An example is shown in Figure 3–3.

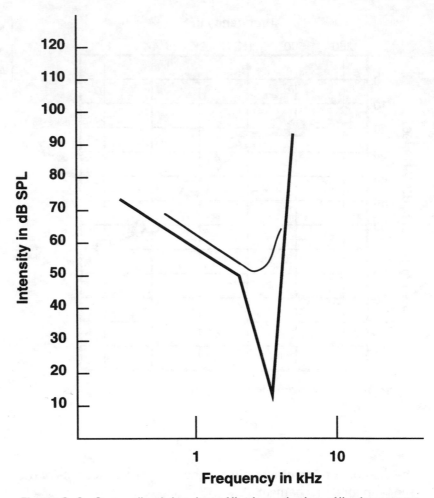

Figure 3-3. Generalized drawing of the broadening of the frequency resolving ability of the auditory system following outer hair cell loss. The thick line represents normal tuning; the thin line represents reduced tuning capacity.

Another important effect of cochlear hearing loss is that it reduces the dynamic range of cochlear function. Recall that the auditory system's range of perception from threshold of sensitivity to pain is quite wide. Unlike a conductive hearing loss, a sensorineural hearing loss reduces sensitivity to low intensity sounds but has little effect on perception of high intensity sounds. The relationship is shown in Figure 3–4. A normal dynamic range may exceed 100 dB; the dynamic range of an ear with sensorineural hearing loss can be considerably smaller.

Because of these complex changes in cochlear processing, a sensorineural hearing loss can have a significant impact on supra-

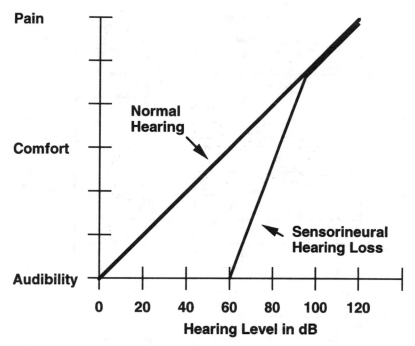

Figure 3-4. Generalized drawing of the relationship of loudness and intensity level in normal hearing and in sensorineural hearing loss.

threshold hearing. That is, even when sound is of a sufficient intensity, the ear does not necessarily act as it normally would at suprathreshold intensities. Thus, for example, speech recognition ability does not necessarily return to normal at intensity levels sufficient to overcome the sensitivity loss.

Mixed Hearing Loss

A hearing loss that has both a sensorineural component and a conductive component is considered a mixed hearing loss. A mixed hearing loss results when sound being delivered to an impaired cochlea is attenuated by a disordered outer or middle ear.

Figure 3–5 shows an example of a mixed hearing loss. Bone-conduction thresholds reflect the degree and configuration of the sensorineural component of the hearing loss. Air-conduction thresholds reflect both the sensorineural loss and an additional conductive component.

The causes of mixed hearing loss are numerous and varied. In some cases, a mixed loss is simply the addition of a conductive

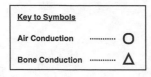

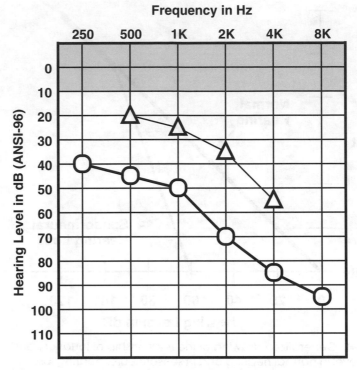

Figure 3–5. Audiogram showing a mixed hearing loss.

When you want to know the **etiology** of a hearing loss, you want to know the **cause**.

hearing loss, due for example to active middle-ear disease, to a longstanding sensorineural hearing loss of unrelated **etiology**. In other cases, the disease process causing middle ear disorder can also cause cochlear disorder and results in a mixed hearing loss of common origin. The **causes** of mixed hearing loss will be described in more detail later in Chapter 4.

Auditory Nervous System Impairments

Although there is a tendency to think of hearing impairment as the sensitivity loss that can be measured on an audiogram, there are other types of hearing impairment that may or may not be accompanied by sensitivity loss. These other impairments result from disease or damage to the central auditory nervous system in adults or delayed or disordered auditory nervous system development in children.

A disordered auditory nervous system, regardless of cause, will have functional consequences that can vary from subclinical to a substantial, easily measurable auditory deficit. Although the functional consequences may be similar, we tend to divide auditory nervous system impairments into two groups, depending on the nature of the underlying disorder.

1. When an impairment is caused by an active, measurable disease process, such as a tumor or other space-occupying lesion, or from damage due to trauma or stroke, it is often referred to as a retrocochlear disorder. That is, retrocochlear disorders result from structural lesions of the nervous system.
2. When an impairment is due to developmental disorder or delay or from diffuse changes such as the aging process, it is often referred to as a **central auditory processing disorder**. That is, central auditory processing disorders results from "functional lesions" of the nervous system.

Central auditory processing disorder (CAPD) is an auditory disorder that results from deficits in central auditory nervous system function.

The consequences of both types of disorder can be remarkably similar from a hearing perspective, but the disorders are treated differently because of the consequences of diagnosis and the likelihood of a significant residual communication disorder.

Retrocochlear Hearing Disorder

A retrocochlear disorder is caused by a change in neural structure and function of some component of the peripheral or central auditory nervous system. As a general rule, the more peripheral a lesion, the greater its impact will be on auditory function. Conversely, the more central the lesion, the more subtle its impact will be. One might conceptualize this by thinking of the nervous system as a large oak tree. If you were to damage one of its many branches, overall growth of the tree would be affected only subtly. Damage its trunk, however, and the impact on the entire tree could be significant. A well placed tumor on the auditory nerve can substantially impact hearing, whereas a lesion in the mid brain is likely to have more subtle effects.

A retrocochlear lesion may or may not affect auditory sensitivity. This will depend on many factors, including lesion size, location, and impact. A tumor on the VIIIth cranial nerve can cause a substantial sensorineural hearing loss, depending on how much pressure it places on the nerve, the damage that it causes to the nerve, or the extent to which it interrupts blood supply to the cochlea. A tumor in the temporal lobe, however, is quite unlikely to result in any change in hearing sensitivity. This relationship is shown in Figure 3–6.

More subtle hearing disorders from retrocochlear disease are often noted in measures of suprathreshold function such as **speech recognition** ability. Using various measures that stress the audi-

Speech recognition is the ability to perceive and identify speech.

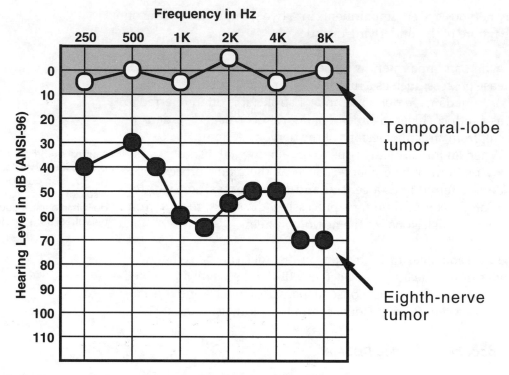

Figure 3–6. Representative audiometric outcomes resulting from temporal-lobe and VIIIth-nerve tumors.

tory system, the audiologist can detect some of the more subtle changes resulting from retrocochlear lesions.

Central Auditory Processing Disorder

Disorders of central auditory nervous system function occur primarily in two populations,

1. young children and
2. the aging population.

CAPD in Children. The vast majority of childhood central auditory disorders do not result from documented **neuropathologic** conditions. Rather, they present as communication disorders that resemble hearing impairment. The specific hearing impairment is related to an **idiopathic** dysfunction of the central auditory nervous system and is commonly referred to as *central auditory processing disorder.* Although the auditory symptoms and clinical findings in children with CAPD may mimic those of children with auditory disorders due to discrete pathology in the central audi-

Neuropathologic conditions are those that involve the peripheral or central nervous systems.

When a hearing loss is **idiopathic**, it is of an **unknown** cause.

tory nervous system, they result from no obvious pathological condition that requires medical intervention.

CAPD can be thought of as a hearing disorder that occurs as a result of dysfunction of the central auditory nervous system. Although some children may be **genetically predisposed** to CAPD, it is more likely to be a developmental delay or disorder, resulting from inconsistent or degraded auditory input during the critical period for auditory perceptual development. CAPD is **symptomatic** in nature and is often confused with an impairment of hearing sensitivity. It can be an isolated disorder, or it can co-exist with **attention deficit disorders, learning disabilities**, and language disorders. Functionally, children with CAPD act as if they have hearing-sensitivity deficits, although they are usually capable of hearing faint sounds. In particular, they exhibit difficulty in perceiving spoken language or other sounds in **hostile acoustic environments**. Thus, CAPD is commonly identified early in children's academic lives, when they enter a conventional classroom situation and are unable to understand instructions from the teacher.

When a person is **genetically predisposed** he or she is susceptible to a heredity condition.

When a person is **symptomatic**, he or she is exhibiting a condition that indicates the existence of a particular disease.

An **attention deficit disorder** results in reduced ability to focus on an activity, task, or sensory stimulus.

A **learning disability** is the lack of skill in one or more areas of learning that is inconsistent with the person's intellectual capacity.

A **hostile acoustic environment** is a difficult listening environment, such as a room with a significant amount of background noise.

As our understanding of CAPD has progressed, we have begun to better define its true nature and to agree on clinical, operational definitions of the disorder. Consensus is beginning to emerge on a definition of CAPD that distinguishes it from language processing disorders and other neuropsychological disorders. One useful classification scheme for categorizing disorder types is shown in Table 3–1. Under this scheme,

- ■ *CAPD* is defined as an auditory disorder that results from deficits in central auditory nervous system function.
- ■ *Receptive language processing disorders* are defined as deficits in linguistic-processing skills and may affect language comprehension and vocabulary development.
- ■ *Neuropsychological disorders,* such as auditory attention and auditory memory, are defined as deficits in cognitive ability.

Clearly, overlap exists among these disorders, they may co-exist, and they are often difficult to separate. For example, the change from perception to comprehension must occur on a continuum, and deciding where one ends and the other begins can only be defined operationally. Similarly, the relation of memory and attention to either perception or comprehension is difficult to separate. Nevertheless, distinguishing among these classes of

Table 3-1. Classification system for describing types of disorders that can affect the ability to turn sound into meaning.

Disorder Type	Nature of Deficit
Central auditory processing disorders — speech-in-noise problems — dichotic deficits — temporal processing disorders	Auditory
Receptive language processing disorders — linguistically dependent problems — deficits in analysis, synthesis, closure	Linguistic
Neuropsychological disorders — auditory attention — auditory memory	Cognitive

Sequelae refer to diseases following or occurring as a consequence of another disease.

disorders is important clinically because they tend to have different **sequelae** and to be treated differently.

CAPD, then, can be thought of as an auditory disorder that occurs as a result of dysfunction in the manipulation and utilization of acoustic signals by the central auditory nervous system. It is broadly defined as an impaired ability to process acoustic information that cannot be attributed to impaired hearing sensitivity, impaired language, or impaired intellectual function.

Reduced redundancy means less information is available.

To **lateralize** sound means to determine its perceived location in the head or ears.

Dichotic stimuli are different signals presented simultaneously to each ear.

Temporal cues are timing cues.

Central auditory processing disorders have been characterized based on models of deficits in children and adults with acquired lesions of the central auditory nervous system. Such deficits include reduced ability to understand in background noise, to understand speech of **reduced redundancy**, to localize and **lateralize** sound, to separate **dichotic stimuli**, and to process normal or altered **temporal cues**. Children with CAPD exhibit deficits similar to those with acquired lesions, although they may be less pronounced in severity and are more likely to be generalized than ear-specific.

CAPD in the Elderly. Changes in structure and function occur throughout the peripheral and central auditory nervous systems as a result of the aging process. Structural degeneration occurs as a result of the aging process in the cochlea and in the central auditory nervous system pathways. Evidence of **neural degeneration** has been found in the auditory nerve, brain stem, and cortex.

Neural degeneration occurs when the anatomic structure degrades.

Whereas the effect of structural change in the auditory periphery is to attenuate and distort incoming sounds, the major effect of structural change in the central auditory nervous system is the degradation of auditory processing. Hearing impairment in the elderly, then, can be quite complex, consisting of attenuation of acoustic information, distortion of that information, and/or disordered processing of neural information. In its simplest form, this complex disorder can be thought of as a combination of peripheral cochlear effects (attenuation and distortion) and central nervous system effects (auditory processing disorder). The consequences of peripheral sensitivity loss in the elderly are similar to those of younger hearing-impaired individuals. The functional consequence of structural changes in the central auditory nervous system is central auditory processing disorder.

Auditory processing ability is usually defined operationally on the basis of behavioral measures of speech understanding. Degradation in auditory processing has been demonstrated most convincingly by the use of **"sensitized"** speech audiometric measures. Age-related changes have been found on degraded speech tests that use both frequency and **temporal alteration**. Tests of dichotic performance have also been found to be adversely affected by aging. In addition, aging listeners do not perform as well as younger listeners on tasks that involve the understanding of speech in the presence of background noise.

Sensitized speech audiometric measures are measures in which speech targets are altered in various ways to reduce their informational content in an effort to more effectively challenge the auditory system.

Temporal alteration refers to changing the speed or timing of speech signals.

Functional Hearing Loss

Functional hearing loss is the exaggeration or feigning of hearing impairment. Many terms have been used to describe this type of hearing "impairment," including nonorganic hearing loss, pseudohypacusis, malingering, factitious hearing loss, and so on. Since there may be some organicity to the hearing loss, it is probably best considered as an exaggerated hearing loss or a functional overlay to an organic loss. The term functional hearing loss is the term most commonly used to describe such outcomes.

In many cases of functional hearing loss, particularly in adults, an organic hearing sensitivity loss exists but is willfully exaggerated, usually for compensatory purposes. In other cases, often secondary to trauma of some kind, the entire hearing loss will be willfully feigned.

Adults and children feign hearing loss for different reasons. Adults are usually seeking secondary or financial gain. That is, an employee may be applying for worker's compensation for hearing loss secondary to exposure to excessive sound in the workplace. Or someone discharged from the military may be seeking compensation for hearing loss from excessive noise exposure. Although most patients have legitimate concerns and provide honest results, a small percentage tries to exaggerate hearing loss in the mistaken notion that they will receive greater compensation. There are also those who have had an accident or altercation and are involved in a lawsuit against an insurance company or someone else. Occasionally such a person will think that feigning a hearing loss will lead to greater monetary award.

Children with functional hearing loss are often using hearing impairment as an excuse for poor performance in school or to gain attention. The idea may have emerged from watching a classmate or sibling getting special treatment for having a hearing impairment. It may also be secondary to a bout of otitis media and the consequent parental attention paid to the episode.

IMPACT OF HEARING IMPAIRMENT

Defining the impact of a hearing impairment is complicated by the many factors involved in the hearing loss itself and in the patient who has the hearing loss. Hearing sensitivity loss varies in degree from minimal to profound. Similarly, speech perception deficits vary from mild to severe. The extent to which these problems cause a communication disorder depends on a number of factors, including:

- degree of sensitivity loss,
- audiometric configuration,
- type of hearing loss, and
- degree and nature of a speech perception deficit.

Confounding this issue further are individual patient factors that are inter-related to these auditory factors, including:

- age of onset of loss,
- whether the loss was sudden or gradual, and
- communication demands on the patient.

Patient Factors

Congenital means present at birth.

One of the most important factors determining the impact of hearing impairment in children is the age of onset of a hearing loss. When a hearing loss is **congenital**, it obviously occurs before linguistic development. If the degree of loss is severe enough and intervention is not implemented early enough, the **prognosis** for developing adequate spoken language is diminished. Conversely, when a hearing loss is acquired after spoken language development, or **postlinguistically**, the prognosis for continued speech and language development is significantly better.

An important factor in the impact of hearing loss on adults is the speed with which a hearing loss occurs. Sudden hearing loss has a significantly greater impact on communication than a gradual hearing loss. Those who develop hearing loss slowly over many years tend to develop **compensatory strategies**, such as **speechreading** and **environmental alteration**. This concept seems to hold even for mild hearing loss. The gradual development of a mild hearing loss has little impact on most patients, and many will not seek treatment for a mild disorder. However, the same mild hearing loss of sudden onset can cause significant communication disorder for a patient.

Another patient factor that influences the impact of hearing loss is the communication demands a patient faces in everyday life. Two patients with the same type, degree, and configuration of hearing loss will have significantly different perceptions of the impact of the hearing loss if their communication demands are substantially different. The active businesswoman who spends most of her days in meetings and on the telephone will find the impact of a moderate hearing loss to be much greater than the retired person who lives alone.

Although these patient factors will influence the extent of impairment, there are, nevertheless, some general rules about the impact of degree, configuration, and type of hearing loss on communication ability.

Prognosis is a prediction of the course or outcome of a disease or treatment.

Postlinguistic means occurring after the time of speech and language development.

Compensatory skills are skills that a person learns in order to compensate for the loss or reduction of auditory ability.

Speechreading is the ability to understand speech by watching the movements of the lips and face; also known as lipreading.

Environmental alteration refers to the manipulation of physical characteristics of a room or a person's location within that room to provide an easier listening situation (e.g., rooms can be acoustically altered with carpet, drapes, and acoustic tile to absorb sound).

Degree and Configuration of Hearing Sensitivity Loss

Degree of hearing sensitivity loss is commonly defined on the basis of the audiogram. Following is a general guideline for describing degree of hearing loss. Normal hearing is defined as audiometric zero, plus or minus two standard deviations of the mean. Thus, normal sensitivity ranges from −10 to +10 dB HL. All other classifications are based on generally accepted terminology.

Degree of loss	Range in dB HL
Normal	−10 to 10
Minimal	11 to 25
Mild	25 to 40
Moderate	40 to 55
Moderately severe	55 to 70
Severe	70 to 90
Profound	90

These terms might be used to describe the pure-tone thresholds at specific frequencies, or they might be used to describe the pure-tone average or threshold for speech recognition. In this way, the audiogram in Figure 3–7 might be described as a mild hearing loss through 1000 Hz and a moderate hearing loss above 1000 Hz, or, based on the pure-tone average, a moderate hearing loss for the **speech frequencies**. It is important to remember that

The term **speech frequencies** generally refers to 500, 1000, and 2000 Hz.

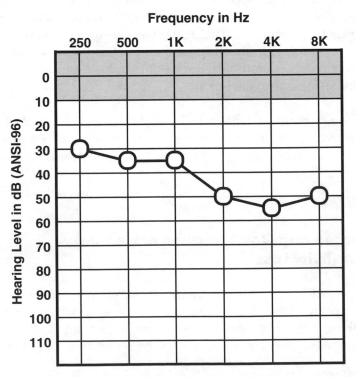

Figure 3–7. Audiogram showing a mild hearing loss through 1000 Hz and a moderate hearing loss above 1000 Hz.

these descriptions are just words and that "mild is in the ear of the listener." What might truly be a mild problem to one individual with a mild loss can be a severe communication problem for another patient with the same mild degree of sensitivity loss. Nevertheless, these terms serve as a means for consistently describing the degree of sensitivity loss across patients.

In terms of communication, the degree of hearing loss might be considered as follows:

Minimal	difficulty hearing faint speech in noise
Mild	difficulty hearing faint or distant speech, even in quiet
Moderate	hears conversational speech only at a close distance
Moderately severe	hears loud conversational speech
Severe	cannot hear conversational speech
Profound	may hear loud sounds; hearing is not the primary communication channel

Another important aspect of the audiogram is the shape of the audiometric configuration. In general, shape of the audiogram can be defined in the following terms:

Flat	thresholds are within 20 dB of each other across the frequency range
Rising	thresholds for low frequencies are at least 20 dB poorer than for high frequencies
Sloping	thresholds for high frequencies are at least 20 dB poorer than for low frequencies
Low-frequency	hearing loss is restricted to the low-frequency region of the audiogram
High-frequency	hearing loss is restricted to the high-frequency region of the audiogram
Precipitous	steeply sloping high frequency hearing loss of at least 20 dB per octave

Examples of these various configurations are shown in Figure 3–8.

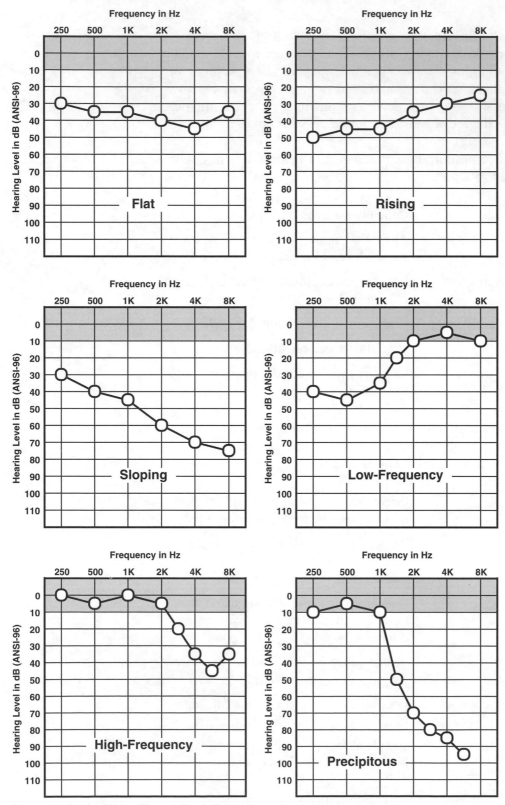

Figure 3-8. Audiometric configurations.

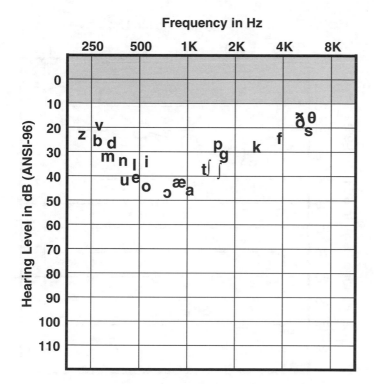

Figure 3-9. Generalized phonetic representations of speech sounds occurring at normal conversational levels plotted on an audiogram.

The shape of the audiogram combined with the degree of the loss provides a useful description of hearing sensitivity. How a particular hearing loss might affect communication can begin to be understood by assessing the relationship of the pure-tone audiogram to the intensity and frequency areas of speech sounds during normal conversations. Figure 3–9 shows an example. Here, **phonetic** representations of speech sounds spoken at normal conversational levels are plotted as a function of frequency and intensity on an audiogram. Next, three examples of audiograms are superimposed on these symbols.

Phonetic refers to an individual speech sound.

Figure 3–10 shows a mild, low-frequency hearing loss. In this case, nearly all the speech sounds would be **audible** to the listener. Some of the lower frequency sounds, such as the vowels, may be less audible, but because they do not carry nearly as much meaning as consonant sounds, suprathreshold speech perception should not be affected.

Audible is "hearable."

Figure 3–11 shows a moderately severe, flat hearing loss. In this example, none of the speech signals of normal conversational

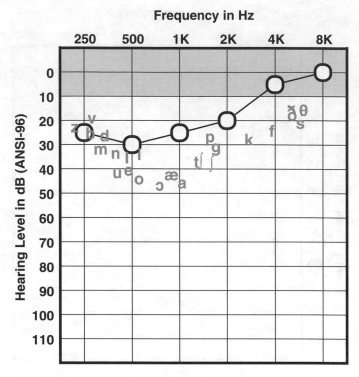

Figure 3-10. The audibility of speech sounds in the presence of a mild, rising audiometric configuration.

speech would be perceived. In order for perception of speech sounds to occur, the intensity of the speech sounds would have to be increased by moving closer to the sound source or by amplifying the sound.

Figure 3–12 shows a moderate high-frequency hearing loss. In this case, low-frequency sounds are perceived adequately, but high-frequency sounds are imperceptible. Again, because the high-frequency sounds are consonant sounds, and because consonant sounds carry much of the meaning in the English language, this patient would be at a disadvantage for perceiving speech adequately.

It is not quite this simple of course. Perception of speech in the real world is made easier by built-in redundancy of information. For example, **co-articulation** from one sound to the other can provide enough information about the next sound that the listener does not even need to hear it to accurately perceive what was being said. As another example, many consonant sounds are visible on the speaker's lips, so that the combination of hearing

Co-articulation refers to the influence of one speech sound on the next.

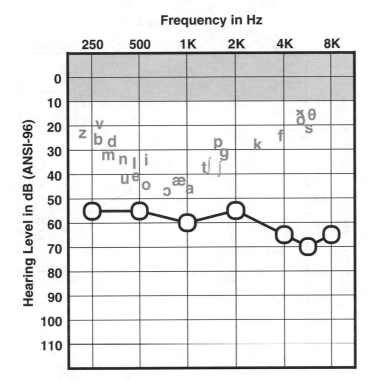

Figure 3–11. The inaudibility of speech sounds in the presence of a moderately severe, flat audiometric configuration.

some frequencies of speech and seeing others can provide enough information for adequate understanding.

Although redundancy in the communication process makes perception easier, noise and **reverberation** make it more difficult. Those important high-frequency consonant sounds have the least acoustic energy of any speech sounds. As a consequence, noise of any kind is likely to cover up or mask those signals first. Add a high-frequency sensitivity loss to the mix, and the most important speech sounds are the least likely to be perceived.

Reverberation is the prolongation of a sound by multiple reflections, more commonly termed an echo.

Type of Hearing Loss

The type of hearing loss is also a factor in the impact that a hearing loss has on communication ability. For example, the simple attenuation created by a conductive hearing loss has a significantly different impact than the more complex impairment that can result from a retrocochlear disorder.

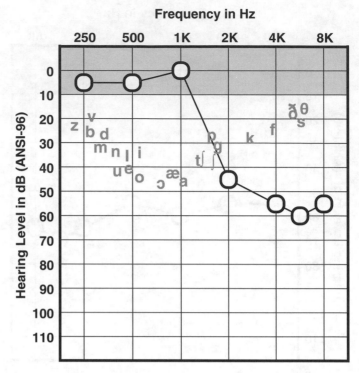

Figure 3–12. The selective audibility of speech sounds in the presence of a moderate, high-frequency audiometric configuration.

Conductive Hearing Loss

A **conductive hearing loss** has a maximum limit of approximately 60 dB HL.

The effects of **conductive hearing loss** are probably the easiest to understand. The configuration of a conductive hearing loss is generally either flat or low-frequency in nature. In addition, conductive hearing loss has a maximum limit of approximately 60 dB HL. This represents the loss due both to the lack of impedance-matching function of the middle ear and additional mass and stiffness components related to the nature of the disorder.

As a general rule, a conductive hearing loss simply reduces the volume of the incoming signal. Although too much attenuation makes the hearing of speech difficult, it can be fairly easily overcome by increasing the intensity level of the speech. At suprathreshold level, the ear with a conductive hearing loss acts quite normally. As long as sound can be made sufficiently loud, hearing will be normal.

Most conductive hearing loss results from auditory disorders that can be treated medically. As a result, conductive loss is seldom of a longstanding duration. Thus, its impact on communication is usually **transient**. Under some circumstances, however, conductive hearing loss can have a more long-term effect. Occasionally, a patient will have chronic middle-ear disorder that has gone untreated. In some cases, this will lead to permanent conductive hearing loss that can only be treated with hearing aid amplification.

In this context, **transient** means short-lived or not long term.

But there is also a more **insidious** effect of conductive hearing loss. Some children have chronic middle ear disorder that results in fluctuating conductive hearing loss throughout much of their early lives. Evidence suggests that some children who experience this type of inconsistent auditory input during their formative years will not develop appropriate auditory and listening skills. Such children may be at risk for later learning and achievement problems.

When something is more dangerous than seems evident, it is **insidious**.

Sensorineural Hearing Loss

As you learned earlier, a sensorineural hearing loss has at least three fundamentally important effects on hearing: a reduction in the cochlear sensitivity, a reduction in frequency resolution, and a reduction in the dynamic range of the hearing mechanism. In many ways, the reduction in hearing sensitivity can be thought of as having the same effects as a conductive hearing loss in terms of reducing the audibility of speech. That is, a conductive hearing loss and a sensorineural hearing loss of the same degree and configuration will have the same effect on audibility of speech sounds. The difference between the two types of hearing loss occurs at suprathreshold levels.

One of the consequences of sensorineural hearing loss is *recruitment,* or abnormal loudness growth. Recall from Figure 3–4 that loudness grows more rapidly than normal at intensity levels just above threshold in an ear with sensorineural hearing loss. This recruitment results in a reduced dynamic range from the threshold level to the discomfort level.

Reduction in frequency resolution and in dynamic range affect the perception of speech. In most sensorineural hearing loss, this effect on speech understanding is predictable from the audiogram and is poorer than would be expected from a conductive hearing loss of similar magnitude. At the extreme end of the audiogram the reduction in frequency resolution and dynamic range can severely limit the usefulness of **residual hearing**.

Residual hearing refers to the remaining hearing ability in a person with a hearing loss.

Retrocochlear Hearing Loss

In general, hearing loss from retrocochlear disorder is distinguishable from cochlear or conductive hearing loss by the extent to which it can adversely affect speech perception. Conductive loss impacts speech perception only by attenuating it. Cochlear hearing loss adds distortion, but it is reasonably minimal and predictable. Retrocochlear disorder can cause severe distortion of incoming speech signals in a manner that limits the usefulness of hearing.

In addition to speech-recognition deficits, other suprathreshold abnormalities can occur. Loudness growth can be abnormal in patients with retrocochlear disorder. Instead of the abnormally rapid growth of loudness characteristic of cochlear hearing loss, retrocochlear disorder will usually show no recruitment or *decruitment,* an abnormally slow growth in loudness with increasing intensity. Another abnormality that can occur as a result of retrocochlear disorder is abnormal *auditory adaptation.* The normal auditory system tends to adapt to ongoing sound, especially at near-threshold levels, so that, as adaptation occurs, an audible signal becomes inaudible. At higher intensity levels, ongoing sound tends to remain audible without adaptation. However, in an ear with retrocochlear disorder, the audibility may diminish rapidly due to excessive auditory adaptation, even at higher intensity levels.

The impact of retrocochlear disorder often depends on the level in the auditory nervous system at which the disorder is occurring. A disorder of the VIIIth nerve is likely to have a significant impact on the audiogram and on speech perception. A disorder of the brain stem may spare the audiogram and negatively influence only hearing of speech in noisy or other complex listening environments.

Central Auditory Processing Disorder

Consequences of CAPD can range from mild difficulty understanding a teacher in a noisy classroom to substantial difficulty understanding speech in everyday listening situations at home and school. One of the most important deficits in children with CAPD is difficulty understanding in background noise. In an acoustic environment that would be adequate for other children, a child with CAPD may have substantial difficulty understanding what is being said. Thus, parents will often complain that the child cannot understand them when the television is on, while riding in the car, or when the parents are speaking from another room. The teacher will complain of the child's inability to follow directions, distractibility, and general unruliness. In effect, the complaints will be similar to those expressed by parents or teachers of children with impairments of hearing sensitivity. In a quiet environment, with one-on-one instruction, a child with CAPD may thrive in a manner consistent with his or her academic potential. In a more adverse acoustic environment, a child with CAPD will struggle.

In general, children with CAPD will act as if they have a hearing sensitivity loss, even though most will have normal audiograms. They will ask for repetition, fail to follow instructions, and so on, particularly in the presence of background noise or other factors that reduce the redundancy of the acoustic signal. To the extent that such difficulties result in frustration, secondary problems may develop related to their behavior and motivation in the classroom. Some children with CAPD will have **concomitant** speech and language deficits, learning disabilities, and attention deficit disorders. Thus, CAPD may be accompanied by distractibility, attention problems, memory deficits, language comprehension deficits, restricted vocabulary, and reading and spelling problems.

In this context **concomitant** means together with or accompanying.

In general, elderly patients with CAPD will experience substantially greater difficulty hearing than would be expected from their degree and configuration of hearing loss. This difficulty will be exacerbated in the presence of background noise or competition. As a result, disorders in central auditory processing may adversely impact benefit from conventional hearing aid use.

SUMMARY

- Hearing impairments are of two major types: hearing sensitivity loss and auditory nervous system disorders.
- The major cause of hearing impairment is a loss of hearing sensitivity. A loss of hearing sensitivity means that the ear is not as sensitive as normal in detecting sound. Hearing sensitivity losses are of three types: conductive, sensorineural, and mixed.
- A conductive hearing loss is caused by an abnormal reduction or attenuation of sound as it travels from the outer ear to the cochlea. A sensorineural hearing loss is caused by a failure in the cochlear transduction of sound from mechanical energy in the middle ear to neural impulses in the VIIIth nerve. A mixed hearing loss results

when sound being delivered to an impaired cochlea is attenuated by a disordered outer or middle ear.

■ Auditory nervous system impairments are of two types, depending on the nature of the underlying disorder: retrocochlear disorders and central auditory processing disorders.

■ Retrocochlear disorders result from structural lesions of the nervous system, such as a tumor or other space-occupying lesions or damage due to trauma or stroke.

■ Central auditory processing disorders result from "functional lesions" of the nervous system, such as developmental disorder or delay or diffuse changes such as those related to the aging process.

■ Functional hearing loss is the exaggeration or feigning of hearing impairment. In many cases of functional hearing loss, particularly in adults, an organic hearing sensitivity loss exists but is willfully exaggerated.

■ The impact of hearing impairment on communication depends on factors such as age of onset of loss, whether the loss was sudden or gradual, and communication demands on the patient.

■ The impact of hearing impairment on communication also depends on hearing-loss factors, including degree of sensitivity loss, audiometric configuration, type of hearing loss, and degree and nature of speech perception deficits.

SUGGESTED READINGS

Chermak, G. D., & Musiek, F. E. (1997). *Perspectives in central auditory processing.* San Diego: Singular Publishing Group.

Jacobson, J. T., & Northern, J. L. (1991). *Diagnostic audiology.* Austin, TX: Pro-Ed.

Northern, J. L. (1996). *Hearing disorders* (3rd ed.). Boston: Allyn and Bacon.

Task Force on Central Auditory Processing Consensus Development, American Speech-Language Hearing Association. (1996). *American Journal of Audiology, 5*(2), 41–54.

4

Causes of Hearing Impairment

■ **Auditory Pathology**

■ **Outer and Middle Ear Disorders**
Microtia and Atresia
Impacted Cerumen
Tympanic-Membrane Perforation
Other Outer Ear Disorders
Otitis Media
Otosclerosis
Cholesteatoma
Other Middle Ear Disorders

■ **Sensorineural Hearing Loss From Cochlear Disorder**
Syndromes and Inherited Disorders
Acoustic Trauma
Other Trauma

Infections
Congenital Infections
Acquired Infections
Ototoxicity
Ménière's Disease
Presbyacusis
Other Causes

■ **Central Auditory Nervous System Disorders**
VIIIth Nerve Tumors
Neural Disorders
Brain Stem Disorders
Temporal Lobe Disorder
Other Nervous System Disorder

■ **Summary**

■ **Suggested Readings**

There are a number of causes of hearing impairment, some affecting the growing embryo, some the newborn and young child, others adults and the elderly. Some of the causes affect the outer ear or middle ear. Others affect only the cochlea or the auditory nervous system. Still others can affect the entire auditory mechanism. This section provides a brief overview of the various pathologies that can cause auditory disorder.

AUDITORY PATHOLOGY

Toxins are poisonous substances.

Vascular disorders are disorders of blood vessels.

Neoplastic pertains to a mass of newly formed tissue or tumor.

If only one gene of a pair is needed to carry a genetic characteristic or mutation, the gene is **dominant**.

If both genes of a pair are needed to carry a genetic characteristic or mutation, the gene is **recessive**.

Maternal prenatal infections are infections such as rubella that a pregnant mother contracts that can cause abnormalities in her unborn fetus.

Teratogenic drugs are drugs that if ingested by the mother during pregnancy can cause abnormal embryologic development.

A **genetic syndrome** is a syndrome obtained due to a heredity factor.

Meningitis is a bacterial or viral inflammation of the membranes covering the brain and spinal cord that can cause significant hearing loss.

Cochlear labyrinth is another term for inner ear.

There are several major categories of pathology or noxious influences that can adversely affect the auditory system, including developmental defects, infections, **toxins**, trauma, **vascular disorders**, neural disorders, immune-system disorders, bone disorders, aging disorder, tumors and other **neoplastic** growths, and disorders of unknown or multiple causes.

Potential developmental defects are numerous, and many of them are inherited. Hereditary disorders, both **dominant** and **recessive**, are a significant cause of sensorineural hearing loss. Many inherited disorders result in congenital hearing loss; others result in progressive hearing loss later in life. Other developmental defects result from certain **maternal prenatal infections**, such as maternal rubella, or from maternal ingestion of **teratogenic drugs**, such as thalidomide or accutane. A number of other outer, middle, and inner ear defects can occur in isolation during embryologic development or as part of a **genetic syndrome**.

Infections are a common cause of outer and middle ear disorder and, in some cases, can result in significant sensorineural hearing loss. Bacterial infections of the external ear and tympanic membrane are not uncommon, though usually treatable and of little consequence to hearing. Infections of the middle ear are quite common. Although treatable, chronic middle ear infections can have a long-lasting impact on hearing ability. Bacterial infections of the brain lining, or **meningitis**, can affect the **cochlear labyrinth**, resulting in severe sensorineural hearing loss. Viral and other infections, resulting in measles, mumps, cytomegalovirus, and syphilis can all result in substantial and permanent sensorineural hearing loss.

Certain drugs and environmental toxins can cause temporary or permanent sensorineural hearing loss. A group of antibiotics known as aminoglycosides are ototoxic, or toxic to the ear. Other drugs including aspirin, quinine, and lasix are associated with ototoxicity. Certain solvents used for industrial purposes and additives used in commercial products can be toxic to the ear of a person exposed to high levels. In addition, certain components of the drugs used in chemotherapy treatment of cancer are ototoxic.

Trauma to the auditory system, both physical and acoustic, can cause temporary or permanent damage to hearing. Physical trauma can cause tympanic membrane perforation, ossicular disruption, and fracture of the temporal bone. Acoustic trauma, or trauma due to excessive noise, is a common cause of permanent sensorineural hearing loss. Trauma to the hearing mechanism can also occur because of changes in air pressure that occur when rapidly ascending or descending during diving or flying. Hearing can also be affected by radiation trauma used in the treatment of cancer.

Hearing loss can occur from vascular disorders. Interruption or diminution of blood supply to the cochlea can cause a loss of hair cell function, resulting in permanent sensorineural hearing loss. Causes of blood supply disruption include stroke, **embolism**, other occlusion, or diabetes mellitus.

An **embolism** is an occlusion or obstruction of a blood vessel by a transported clot or other mass.

Neural disorders can affect the auditory system. **Neuritis**, or inflammation of the auditory nerve, can cause temporary or permanent hearing disorder. Other disorders, such as **multiple sclerosis** and **brain stem gliomas**, can affect hearing function. Neoplastic growth, including carcinoma, glomus tumors, and meningiomas, can affect the auditory system. One of the more common neoplasms of the auditory system, the cochleovestibular schwannoma or acoustic tumor, is an important cause of retrocochlear hearing disorder.

Neuritis is inflammation of a nerve with corresponding sensory or motor dysfunction.

Multiple sclerosis (MS) is a demyelinating disease in which plaques form throughout the white matter of the brain, resulting in diffuse neurologic symptoms, including hearing loss and speech recognition deficits.

A **brain stem glioma** is any neoplasm derived from neuroglia (non-neuronal supporting tissues of the nervous system) located in the brain stem.

Immune-system disorders have been associated with hearing loss. Hearing disorder due specifically to autoimmune disease has been described. Other hearing disorders that occur secondarily to systemic autoimmunity, such as AIDS, have also been described.

Certain types of bone disorders commonly affect the auditory system. **Otosclerosis** is a common cause of middle ear disorder and may also cause sensorineural hearing loss. Other bone defects, both developmental and progressive, can impact on auditory function.

Otosclerosis is a disorder characterized by new bone formation around the stapes and oval window, resulting in stapes fixation and related conductive hearing loss.

Other hearing disorders are of unknown origin. Idiopathic endolymphatic hydrops, or an excessive collection of endolymph in the cochlea of unknown origin, also known as Ménière's disease,

When a hearing loss is **idiopathic**, it is of an **unknown** cause.

can result in permanent sensorineural hearing loss. Other **idiopathic** disorder, particularly sudden hearing loss, is not an uncommon finding clinically.

OUTER AND MIDDLE EAR DISORDERS

Disorders of the outer and middle ear are commonly of two types, either structural defects due to embryologic malformations or structural changes secondary to infection or trauma. Another common abnormality, otosclerosis, is a bone disorder.

Microtia and Atresia

Auricular pertains to the outer ear or auricle.

Microtia and atresia are congenital malformations of the auricle and external auditory canal. *Microtia* is an abnormal smallness of the auricle. It is one of a variety of auricular malformations. Others that fall into the general category of congenital **auricular** malformations include:

accessory auricle:	an additional auricle or additional auricular tissue
anotia:	congenital absence of an auricle
auricular aplasia:	anotia
cleft pinna:	congenital fissure of the auricle
coloboma lobuli:	congenital fissure of the earlobe
macrotia:	congenital excessive enlargement of the auricle
melotia:	congenital displacement of the auricle
low-set ears:	congenitally displaced auricles
polyotia:	presence of an additional auricle on one or both sides
preauricular pits:	small hole of variable depth lying anterior to the auricle
preauricular tags:	small appendage lying anterior to the auricle
scroll ear:	auricular deformity in which the rim is rolled forward and inward

Microtia in and of itself may not affect hearing in any substantial way. The auricle serves an important purpose in horizontal sound localization and in providing certain acoustic alterations to incoming signals. But the absence of auricles, or the presence of auricles that are deformed, does not in itself create a significant communication disorder for patients. Ears with microtia or other deformities will often be surgically corrected at an early age.

Atresia is the absence of an opening of the external auditory meatus. An ear is said to be atretic if the ear canal is closed at any point. Atresia is a congenital disorder and may involve one or both ears. *Bony atresia* is the congenital absence of the ear canal due to a wall of bone separating the external auditory meatus from the middle ear. *Membranous atresia* is the condition in which a dense soft tissue plug is obstructing the ear canal.

Atresia is the congenital absence or pathologic closure of a normal anatomical opening.

Atresia can occur in isolation. However, the underlying embryologic cause of this malformation can also affect surrounding structures. So it is not unusual for atresia to be accompanied by microtia or other auricular deformity. Atresia can also be accompanied by a malformed middle-ear mechanism, such as ossicular malformation, and/or malformed cochlea, again depending on its cause.

Atresia causes a significant conductive hearing loss, which can be as great as 60 dB. An example of an audiogram obtained from an atretic ear is shown in Figure 4–1. The additional bone or membranous plug adds mass and stiffness to the outer ear system, resulting in a relatively flat conductive hearing loss.

There are a number of causes of microtia, atresia, and other malformations of the outer and middle ears. Many of these are genetic syndromes, associations, or anomalies that are inherited. A list of some of the syndromes and other inherited disorders is presented in Table 4–1.

Impacted Cerumen

One common cause of transient hearing disorder is the accumulation and impaction of cerumen in the external auditory canal. As you learned earlier, the ear canal naturally secretes cerumen as a mechanism for protecting the ear canal and tympanic membrane. Cerumen has a natural tendency to migrate out of the ear canal and, with proper aural hygiene, seldom interferes with hearing.

Ceruminosis is the excessive accumulation of cerumen (wax) in the external auditory meatus (ear canal).

In some individuals, however, cerumen is secreted excessively, a condition known as **ceruminosis**. In these patients, routine ear

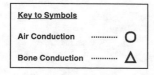

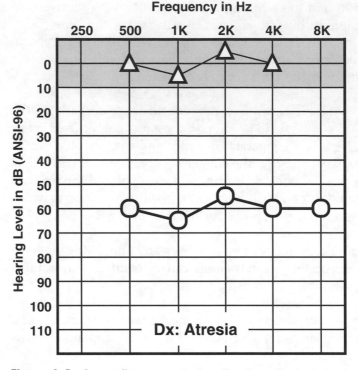

Figure 4-1. An audiogram representing the effect of atresia.

Table 4-1. Syndromes and inherited disorders associated with outer and middle ear malformation.

Syndromes and Inherited Disorders	
acrocephalosyndactyly, type I	long arm 18 deletion syndrome
acrodysostosis	Madelung deformity
acrofacial dysostosis	malformed low-set ears syndrome
Antley-Bixler syndrome	mandibulofacial dysostosis
Apert syndrome	Melnick-Fraser syndrome
Baller-Gerold syndrome	Mohr syndrome
Beckwith-Weidemann syndrome	Nager syndrome
Carpenter syndrome	oculoauricovertebral dysplasia
Cornelia de Lange syndrome	osteogenesis imperfecta
Crouzon syndrome	otopalatodigital syndrome
DiGeorge syndrome	Patau syndrome
ectodermal dysplasia	renal-genital syndrome
Goldenhar syndrome	symphalangism
hemifacial microsomia	Treacher Collins syndrome
lobster-claw syndrome	

canal cleaning may be required to forestall the effects of excessive cerumen accumulation.

Regardless of whether or not a patient experiences ceruminosis, occasionally excessive cerumen can accumulate in the ear canal and become impacted. The problem is usually somewhat **insidious**, and the impaction can become fairly significant before a patient will seek treatment.

When something is more dangerous than seems evident, it is **insidious**.

Figure 4–2 demonstrates the effect of impacted cerumen on hearing sensitivity. This case would represent a moderate level of impaction. Not unlike atresia, the effect is one of both mass and stiffness, resulting in **attenuation** across the frequency range, giving a flat audiogram.

Attenuation means to reduce or decrease in magnitude.

Although impacted cerumen often results in only a mild conductive hearing loss, the loss can have a significant impact on children in a classroom or on patients with pre-existing hearing loss.

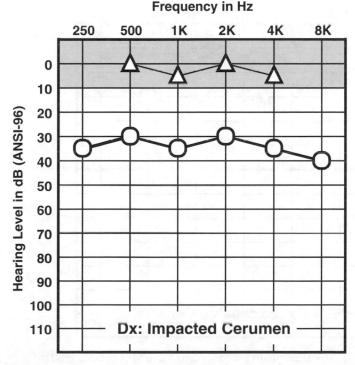

Figure 4-2. An audiogram representing the effect of impacted cerumen.

When something is **occluding**, it is blocking or obstructing.

Sometimes cerumen is pushed down into the ear canal and onto the tympanic membrane without **occluding** the ear canal. This results in an increase in the mass of the tympanic membrane, resulting in a high-frequency conductive hearing loss, as shown in Figure 4–3.

Impacted cerumen is often managed first by a course of eardrops to soften the impaction, followed by irrigation of the ear canal to remove it.

Tympanic-Membrane Perforation

Otitis media = middle ear inflammation.

The tympanic membrane can be perforated in one of two ways, either by trauma or secondary to a middle ear infection, or **otitis media**. *Traumatic perforation* can occur when a foreign object is placed into the ear canal in an unwise effort to remove cerumen. It can also occur with a substantial blow to the side of the head.

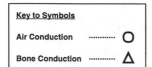

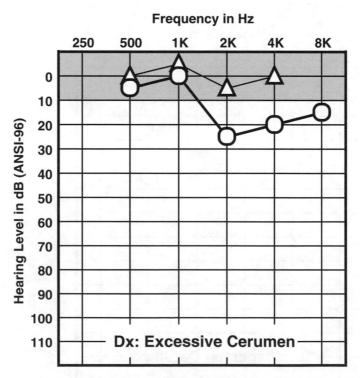

Figure 4–3. An audiogram representing the effect of cerumen resting on the tympanic membrane, increasing its mass and resulting in a high-frequency conductive hearing loss.

Perforation of the tympanic membrane can occur secondary to a middle ear infection. Sometimes, in the later stages of an acute attack of otitis media, the fluid trapped in the middle ear space is so excessive that the membrane ruptures to relieve the pressure. In other cases, chronic middle ear infections erode portions of the tympanic membrane, weakening it to the point that a perforation forms.

Perforations of the tympanic membrane are of three types, depending on location. A *central perforation* is one of the **pars tensa** portion of the tympanic membrane, with a rim of the membrane remaining at all borders. An *attic perforation* is one of the **pars flaccida** portion. A *marginal perforation* is one located at the edge or the margin of the membrane.

The **pars tensa** is the larger and stiffer portion of the tympanic membrane.

The **pars flaccida** is the smaller and more compliant portion of the tympanic membrane, located superiorly.

A perforation in the tympanic membrane may or may not result in hearing loss, depending on its location and size. In general, if a perforation causes a hearing loss, it will be a mild, conductive hearing loss. An example of an audiogram from an ear with a perforation is shown in Figure 4–4.

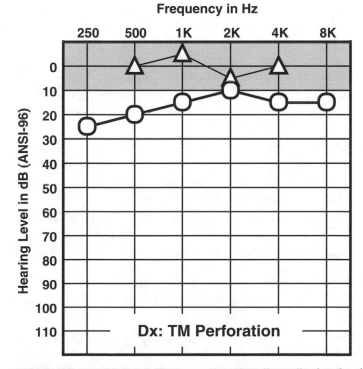

Frequency in Hz

Key to Symbols

Air Conduction ·········· O

Bone Conduction ·········· △

Dx: TM Perforation

Figure 4-4. An audiogram representing the effects of a tympanic membrane perforation.

Regardless of type, most perforations heal spontaneously. Those that do not are usually too large or are sustained by recurrent infection. In such cases, surgery may be necessary to repair or replace the membrane.

Other Outer Ear Disorders

Other disorders of the outer ear are caused by infections, cancer, and other neoplastic growths. In general, outer ear disorders do not impact hearing ability unless they result in ear canal **stenosis** or blockage.

Stenosis is a narrowing of the diameter of an opening or canal.

Infections of the ear canal or auricle, are referred to collectively as **otitis externa**, or inflammation of the external ear. They are often caused by bacteria, virus, or fungus cultivated in the external ear canal. One common type is known as *swimmer's ear*, or acute diffuse **external otitis**, and is characterized by diffuse reddened pustular lesions surrounding hair follicles in the ear canal due to a gram-negative bacterial infection during hot, humid weather and often initiated by swimming.

External otitis is an inflammation of the external auditory meatus, also called otitis externa.

Carcinoma of the auricle is not uncommon. **Basal-cell, epidermoid**, and **squamous-cell carcinoma** can all occur around the auricle and external auditory meatus.

Basal-cell carcinoma is a slow-growing malignant skin cancer which can occur on the auricle and external auditory meatus.

Epidermoid carcinoma is a cancerous tumor of the auricle, external auditory canal, middle ear, and/or mastoid.

Tumors of various types can proliferate around the external auditory meatus and auricle, including adenoma, ceruminoma, granuloma, hemangioma, osteoma, and cutaneous tuberculosis.

Squamous-cell carcinoma is the most common malignant (cancerous) tumor of the auricle.

Otitis Media

The most common cause of transient conductive hearing loss in children is *otitis media* with **effusion**. Otitis media is inflammation of the middle ear. It is caused primarily by Eustachian tube dysfunction. When it is accompanied by middle ear effusion, otitis media often causes conductive hearing loss.

Effusion is the escape of fluid into tissue or a cavity.

Recall that the Eustachian tube is a normally closed passageway that permits pressure equalization between the middle ear and the atmosphere. Sometimes the Eustachian tube is restricted from opening by, for example, an upper respiratory infection that causes **edema** of the **mucosa** of the nasopharynx. When this occurs, oxygen that is trapped in the middle ear space begins to be absorbed by the mucosa of the middle ear cavity. This creates

Edema = swelling

Mucosa is any epithelial lining of an organ or structure, such as the tympanic cavity, that secretes mucus; also called the mucous membrane.

a relative vacuum in the cavity and results in significant negative pressure in the middle ear. The lining of the middle ear then becomes inflamed. If allowed to persist, the inflamed tissue begins the process of **transudation** of fluid through the mucosal walls into the middle ear cavity. Once this fluid is sufficient to impede normal movement of the tympanic membrane and ossicles, a conductive hearing loss results.

The passage of a body fluid through a membrane or tissue surface is called **transudation.**

Eustachian tube dysfunction is a common problem in young children. The opening to the Eustachian tube is surrounded by the large adenoid tissue in the nasopharynx. An upper respiratory infection or inflammation causes swelling of this tissue and can block Eustachian tube function. The inflammation can also travel across the mucosal lining of the tube. Children seem to be particularly at risk because their Eustachian tubes are shorter, more horizontal, and more compliant.

There are a number of ways to classify otitis media, including by type, effusion type, and duration. Various descriptions are provided in Table 4–2.

There are several classifications of otitis media types. *Otitis media without effusion* is just that, inflammation that does not result in exudation of fluid from the mucosa. *Adhesive otitis media* refers to inflammation of the middle ear caused by prolonged Eustachian tube dysfunction, resulting in severe retraction of the tympanic membrane and obliteration of the middle ear space. *Otitis media with effusion* has already been described, although there are a number of types of effusion.

Serous effusion is a common form of effusion and is characterized as thin, watery, sterile fluid. *Purulent* effusion contains pus. *Suppurative* is a synonym of purulent. *Nonsuppurative* refers to serous fluid or mucoid fluid. *Mucoid* refers to fluid that is thick, viscid, and mucuslike. *Sanguineous* fluid contains blood.

Otitis media is also classified by its duration. Although definitions vary, the following may be used as a general guideline. *Acute* otitis media is a single bout lasting fewer than 21 days. *Chronic* otitis media refers to that which persists beyond 8 weeks or results in permanent damage to the middle ear mechanism. *Subacute* refers to an episode of otitis media that lasts from 22 days to 8 weeks. Otitis media is considered *unresponsive* if it fails to resolve after 48 hours of antibiotic therapy and *persistent* if it fails to resolve after 6 weeks. *Recurrent* otitis media is often defined as three or more acute episodes within a 6-month period. Finally, someone

Table 4-2. Various descriptions of otitis media, based on type, effusion type, and duration.

Description	Definition
otitis media	inflammation of the middle ear, resulting predominantly from Eustachian tube dysfunction
otitis media, acute	inflammation of the middle ear having a duration of fewer than 21 days
otitis media, acute serous	acute inflammation of middle ear mucosa with serous effusion
otitis media, acute suppurative	acute inflammation of the middle ear with infected effusion containing pus
otitis media, adhesive	inflammation of the middle ear caused by prolonged Eustachian tube dysfunction resulting in severe retraction of the tympanic membrane and obliteration of the middle ear space
otitis media, catarrhal	middle ear inflammation resulting from catarrh of the nasopharynx with congestion of the Eustachian tube
otitis media, chronic	persistent inflammation of the middle ear having a duration of greater than 8 weeks
otitis media, chronic adhesive	longstanding inflammation of the middle ear caused by prolonged Eustachian tube dysfunction resulting in severe retraction of the tympanic membrane and obliteration of the middle ear space
otitis media, chronic atticoantral suppurative	persistent, purulent inflammation of the attic and mastoid antrum of the middle ear
otitis media, chronic suppurative	persistent inflammation of the middle ear with infected effusion containing pus
otitis media, mucoid	inflammation of the middle ear, with mucoid effusion
otitis media, mucosanguinous	inflammation of the middle ear with effusion consisting of blood and mucus
otitis media, necrotizing	persistent inflammation of the middle ear that results in tissue necrosis
otitis media, nonsuppurative	inflammation of the middle ear with effusion that is not infected, including serous and mucoid otitis media
otitis media, persistent	middle-ear inflammation with effusion for 6 weeks or longer following initiation of antibiotic therapy

is said to be *otitis prone* if otitis media occurs before the age of 1 year or if six bouts occur before the age of 6 years.

76–95% of all children have one episode of **otitis media** by 6 years of age.

Otitis media is a common middle-ear disorder in children. Estimates are that from **76 to 95% of all children** have one episode of **otitis media** by 6 years of age. The prevalence of otitis media is

Table 4–2. *(continued)*

Description	Definition
otitis media, purulent	inflammation of the middle ear with infected effusion containing pus; synonym: suppurative otitis media
otitis media, recurrent	middle ear inflammation that occurs 3 or more times in a 6-month period
otitis media, reflux	inflammation of the middle ear mucosa resulting from the passage of nasopharyngeal secretions through the Eustachian tube
otitis media, sanguinous	inflammation of the middle ear, accompanied by bloody effusion
otitis media, secretory	otitis media with effusion, usually referring to serous or mucoid effusion
otitis media, seromucinous	inflammation of the middle ear with an accumulation of fluid of varying viscosity in the middle ear cavity and other pneumatized spaces of the temporal bone
otitis media, serous	inflammation of middle ear mucosa, with serous effusion
otitis media, subacute	inflammation of the middle ear ranging in duration from 22 days to 8 weeks
otitis media, suppurative	inflammation of the middle ear with infected effusion containing pus
otitis media, tuberculous	chronic inflammation of the middle ear and mastoid secondary to tuberculosis, resulting in early perforation and suppurative otorrhea
otitis media, unresponsive	middle ear inflammation that persists after 48 hours of initial antibiotic therapy, occurring more frequently in children with recurrent otitis media
otitis media with effusion	inflammation of the middle ear with an accumulation of fluid of varying viscosity in the middle ear cavity and other pneumatized spaces of the temporal bone; synonym: seromucinous otitis media
otitis media with perforation	inflammation of the middle ear, with secondary perforation of the tympanic membrane
otitis media without effusion	inflammation of the middle ear

Source: From *Comprehensive Dictionary of Audiology,* by B. A. Stach, 1997. Baltimore: Williams and Wilkins. Reprinted with permission.

highest during the first 2 years and declines with age. Approximately 50% of those children who have otitis media before the age of 1 year will have 6 or more bouts within the ensuing 2 years. Otitis media is more common in males, and its highest occurrence is during the winter and spring months. Certain groups appear to be more at risk for otitis media than others,

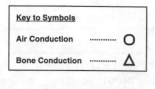

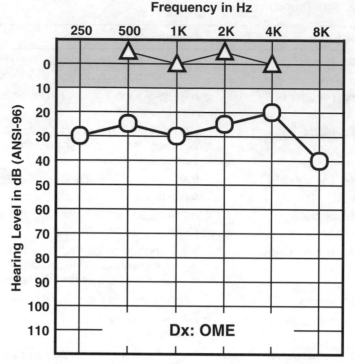

Figure 4–5. An audiogram representing the effects of otitis media with effusion.

including children with cleft palate or other craniofacial anomalies, children with Down syndrome, children with learning disabilities, Native populations, children who live in the inner city, those who attend day-care centers, and those who are passively exposed to cigarette smoking.

One of the consequences of otitis media with effusion is conductive hearing loss. An illustrative example of an audiogram is shown in Figure 4–5. The degree and configuration of the loss depends on the amount and type of fluid and its influence on functioning of the tympanic membrane and ossicles. This hearing loss is transient and resolves along with the otitis media. In cases of chronic otitis media, damage to the middle ear structures can occur, resulting in more permanent conductive and/or sensorineural hearing loss.

Recurrent or chronic otitis media can also have a far reaching impact on communication ability. For example, in studies of children with central auditory processing disorders or children with learning disabilities, there is evidence of a higher prevalence of chronic otitis media. It appears likely that children who have

aperiodic disruption in auditory input during the critical period for auditory development may be at risk for developing central auditory processing disorder or language and psychoeducational delays.

Aperiodic means occurring at irregular intervals.

Otitis media is usually treated with antibiotic therapy. If it is unresponsive to such treatment, then surgical **myringotomy** and **pressure-equalization tube** placement is a likely course of action. In myringotomy, a needle is passed through the tympanic membrane to remove the effusion. A tube is then placed through the opening to serve as a temporary replacement of the Eustachian tube in its role as middle-ear pressure equalizer.

Myringotomy involves the passage of a needle through the tympanic membrane to remove fluid from the middle ear.
PE tube, or pressure equalization tube, is a small tube inserted in the tympanic membrane following myringotomy to provide equalization of air pressure within the middle ear space as a substitute for a nonfunctional Eustachian tube.

Otosclerosis

Otosclerosis is a disorder of bone growth that affects the stapes and the bony labyrinth of the cochlea. The disease process is characterized by resorption of bone and new spongy formation around the stapes and oval window. Gradually, the stapes becomes fixed within the oval window, resulting in conductive hearing loss.

Otosclerosis is a common cause of middle-ear disorder. A family history of the disease occurs in over half of the cases. Women are more likely to be diagnosed with otosclerosis than men, and its onset is often related to pregnancy.

Otosclerosis usually occurs **bilaterally**, although the time course of its effect on hearing may differ between ears. The primary symptom of otosclerosis is hearing loss and the degree of loss appears to be directly related to the amount of fixation.

When a disorder involves both ears it is **bilateral**; when it involves one ear it is **unilateral**.

An audiogram characteristic of otosclerosis is shown in Figure 4–6. The degree of the conductive hearing loss varies with the progression of fixation, but the configuration of the bone-conduction thresholds is almost a signature of the disease. Note that the bone conduction threshold dips slightly at 2000 Hz, reflecting the elimination of factors that normally contribute to bone-conducted hearing due to the fixation of the stapes into the wall of the cochlea. This 2000 Hz notch is often referred to as "Carhart's notch," named after Raymond Carhart who first described this characteristic pattern.

Otosclerosis is usually treated surgically. The surgical process frees the stapes and replaces it with some form of prosthesis to allow the ossicular chain to function adequately again.

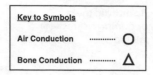

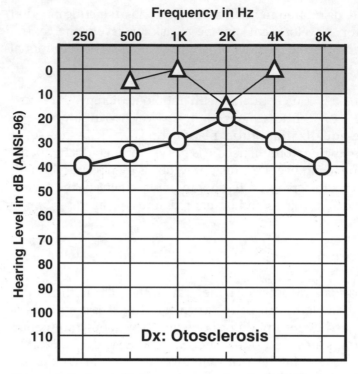

Figure 4–6. An audiogram representing the effects of otosclerosis.

Cholesteatoma

The attic of the middle ear cavity is called the **epitympanum**.

Following chronic otitis media, a common pathologic occurrence is the formation of a *cholesteatoma*. A cholesteatoma is an epithelial pocket that forms, usually in the **epitympanum**, as a consequence of epidermal invasion through a perforation or a retraction of the pars flaccida. Once this occurs, the normal exfoliation (shedding) of epithelium results in growth of the cholesteatoma, which is capable of resorption of adjacent bone. The result can be substantial erosion of the ossicles and even invasion of the bony labyrinth.

Depending on the location of cholesteatoma growth, the magnitude of conductive hearing loss can vary from nonexistent to substantial. Typically, the cholesteatoma will impede the ossicles, resulting in a significant conductive hearing loss. An illustrative example of a hearing loss caused by cholesteatoma is shown in Figure 4–7.

Cholesteatoma, once detected, is removed surgically, with or without ossicular replacement, depending on the disease process.

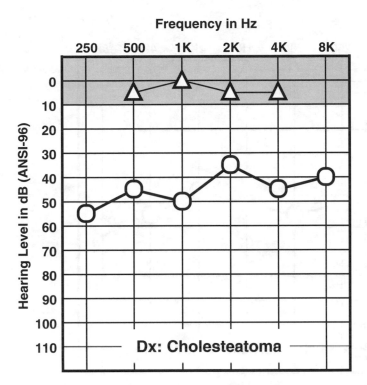

Figure 4–7. An audiogram representing the effects of cholesteatoma.

Other Middle Ear Disorders

Physical *trauma* can result in middle ear disorder. One consequence of trauma is a partial or total disarticulation of the ossicular chain, with or without *longitudinal fracture* of the temporal bone. The most common forms of *ossicular discontinuity* are partial fracture of the incus with separation of the **incudostapedial joint**, complete fracture of the **incus**, fracture of the **crura** of the stapes, and fracture of the **malleus**. Any of these types of ossicular disruptions can result in substantial conductive hearing loss. An example of an audiogram from an ear with a disarticulated ossicular chain is shown in Figure 4–8. A complete disarticulation terminates the impedance-matching capabilities of the middle ear by eliminating the stiffness component. In addition, the remaining unattached ossicles add mass to the system, resulting in a maximum, flat conductive hearing loss.

Another form of insult to the middle ear results from **barotrauma**, or trauma related to a sudden, marked change in atmospheric pressure. This often occurs when an airplane descends from altitude too fast without proper airplane cabin pressure equaliza-

The point of articulation of the incus and stapes is called the **incudostapedial joint**.
The point of articulation of the incus and malleus is called the **incudomalleolar joint**.

Barotrauma is a traumatic injury caused by a rapid marked change in atmospheric pressure resulting in a significant mismatch in air pressure in the pneumatized spaces of the body.

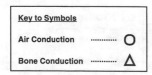

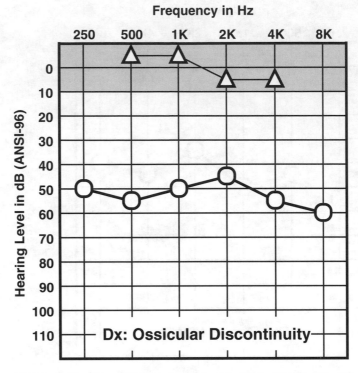

Figure 4–8. An audiogram representing the effects of a disarticulated ossicular chain.

tion or when a diver ascends too rapidly in the water. It can also occur under more normal ascending and descending conditions if a person's Eustachian tube is not providing adequate pressure equalization. Under both circumstances, a severe negative air pressure is created in the middle ear space due to failure of the Eustachian tube to open adequately. If air pressure changes are sudden and intense, the tympanic membrane may rupture. If not, it is stretched medially, followed by increased blood flow, swelling, and bruising of the mucosal lining of the middle ear. Effusion then forms within the middle ear from the traumatized tissue.

Glomus tumors are small neoplasms of paraganglionic tissue with a rich vascular supply located near or within the jugular bulb.

Vascular pertains to blood vessels.

Pulsatile tinnitus is the perception of a pulsing sound in the ear that results from vascular abnormalities.

Tumors may also occur within the middle ear. One neoplasm commonly found in the middle ear is a **glomus tumor**, or glomus tympanicum. A glomus tumor is a mass of cells with a rich **vascular** supply. It arises from the middle ear and can result in significant conductive hearing loss. One distinctive symptom of this tumor is that it often causes **pulsatile tinnitus**. An untreated glomus tumor can encroach on the cochlea, resulting in mixed hearing loss.

Middle ear disorder can also result from changes in structure and function that occur secondarily to chronic otitis media. One example is tympanosclerosis. *Tympanosclerosis* is the formation of whitish plaques on the tympanic membrane, with **nodular** deposits in the mucosal lining of the middle ear. These plaques can cause an increased stiffening of the ossicles and even fixation of the ossicular chain. Conductive hearing loss can occur, depending on the severity and location of the deposits.

Nodular means a small knot or rounded lump.

SENSORINEURAL HEARING LOSS FROM COCHLEAR DISORDERS

Cochlear disorders result from many causes. In newborns, structural defects due to embryologic malformations or structural changes secondary to infection are a common cause of sensorineural hearing loss. Inherited hearing loss can be present at birth or can manifest in adulthood. Cochlear disorders that can occur at any age include acoustic trauma, infections, **endolymphatic hydrops**, ototoxicity, and others. Another common cause is presbyacusis, or hearing loss related to the aging process.

Endolymphatic hydrops, the underlying cause of **Ménière's disease**, is an excessive accumulation of endolymph within the cochlear and vestibular labyrinths, resulting in fluctuating sensorineural hearing loss, vertigo, tinnitus, and a sensation of fullness.

Syndromes and Inherited Disorders

Hereditary factors are common causes of sensorineural hearing loss. Hearing loss of this nature is one of two types. *Syndromic hearing disorder* occurs as part of a constellation of other medical and physical disorders that occur together commonly enough to constitute a distinct clinical entity. *Nonsyndromic hearing disorder* is an autosomal recessive or dominant genetic condition in which there is no other significant feature besides hearing loss.

Genetic inheritance is either related to non-sex-linked (autosomal) chromosomes or is linked to the X-chromosome. In *autosomal dominant* inheritance, only one gene of a pair must carry a genetic characteristic or mutation in order for it to be expressed; in *autosomal recessive* inheritance, both genes of a pair must share the characteristic. *X-linked hearing disorder* is a genetic condition that occurs due to a faulty gene located on the X chromosome.

Some of the more common *syndromic disorders* that can result in hearing loss in children are:

- *Alport syndrome:* genetic syndrome characterized by progressive kidney disease and sensorineural hearing loss,

Collagen is the main protein of connective tissue, cartilage, and bone, the age-related loss of which can reduce auricular cartilage strength and result in collapsed ear canals.

Branchial clefts are a series of openings between the embryonic branchial arches. Branchial arches are a series of five pairs of arched structures in the embryo that play an important role in the formation of head and neck structures.

An abnormal passage or hole formed within the body by disease, surgery, injury, or other defect is called a **fistula**.

Renal pertains to the kidneys.

A **coloboma** is a congenital fissure (cleft or slit).

Hypoplasia is the incomplete development or underdevelopment of tissue or an organ.

Retinitis pigmentosa is a chronic progressive disease characterized by retinal-tissue degeneration and optic-nerve atrophy.

probably resulting from X-linked inheritance through a gene that codes for **collagen**;

■ *Branchio-oto-renal syndrome:* autosomal dominant disorder consisting of **branchial clefts, fistulas**, and cysts, **renal** malformation, and conductive, sensorineural, or mixed hearing loss;

■ *Cervico-oculo-acoustic syndrome:* congenital branchial arch syndrome, occurring primarily in females, characterized by fusion of two or more cervical vertebrae, similar to Klippel-Feil syndrome, with retraction of eyeballs, lateral gaze weakness, and hearing loss;

■ *CHARGE association:* genetic association featuring **coloboma**, *h*ea*r*t disease, *a*tresia choanae (nasal cavity), *r*etarded growth and development, *g*enital **hypoplasia**, and *e*ar anomalies and/or hearing loss that can be conductive, sensorineural, or mixed;

■ *Jervell and Lange-Nielsen syndrome:* autosomal recessive cardiovascular disorder accompanied by congenital bilateral profound sensorineural hearing loss;

■ *Pendred syndrome:* autosomal recessive endocrine metabolism disorder resulting in goiter and congenital, symmetric, moderate-to-profound sensorineural hearing loss;

■ *Usher syndrome:* autosomal recessive disorder characterized by congenital sensorineural hearing loss and progressive loss of vision due to **retinitis pigmentosa**;

■ *Waardenburg syndrome:* autosomal dominant disorder characterized by lateral displacement of the medial canthi, increased width of the root of the nose, multicolored iris, white forelock, and mild-to-severe sensorineural hearing loss.

A list of other syndromes associated with sensorineural hearing loss is included in Table 4–3.

Some of the more common *nonsyndromic disorders* that can result in hearing loss are:

■ *Dominant hereditary hearing loss:* hearing loss due to transmission of a genetic characteristic or mutation in which only one gene of a pair must carry the characteristic in order to be expressed, and both sexes have an equal chance of being affected;

■ *Dominant progressive hearing loss:* genetic condition in which sensorineural hearing loss gradually worsens over a period of years, caused by dominant inheritance;

Table 4-3. Syndromes and inherited disorders associated with sensorineural hearing loss.

Syndromes and Inherited Disorders	
Abruzzo-Erickson syndrome	Klippel-Feil syndrome
Albers-Schönberg disease	Krabbe disease
albinism syndrome	large vestibular aqueduct syndrome
Albrecht syndrome	Laurence-Moon-Biedl-Bardet syndrome
Alstrom syndrome	Marshall syndrome
ataxia-hypogonadism syndrome	Melnick-Fraser syndrome
Björnstad syndrome	Mondini dysplasia
branchio-oto-renal syndrome	Muckle-Wells syndrome
chondrodystrophia fetalis	multiple lentigines syndrome
cleidocranial dysostosis	myopia and congenital deafness
Cockayne syndrome	Norrie syndrome
craniocervical dysplasia	onychodystrophy
diastrophic dwarfism	opticocochleodentate degeneration
Duane retraction syndrome	oto-spondylo-megaepiphyseal dysplasia
Edward syndrome	Pelizaeus-Merzbacher disease
Fehr corneal dystrophy	piebaldness
Friedrich ataxia	Pierre Robin syndrome
Hallgren syndrome	Ramsay Hunt syndrome
hand-hearing syndrome	Refsum syndrome
Harboyan syndrome	Richards-Rundle syndrome
Herrmann syndrome	Scheibe dysplasia
Hunter syndrome	Tietze syndrome
Hurler syndrome	Townes-Brocks syndrome
hyperprolinemia II	trisomy 13–15 syndrome
Kearns-Sayre syndrome	trisomy 18 syndrome
keratopachyderma and digital constrictions	Turner syndrome

- *Progressive adult-onset hearing loss:* autosomal dominant nonsyndromic hearing loss with onset in adulthood, characterized by progressive, symmetric sensorineural hearing loss;
- *Recessive hereditary sensorineural hearing loss:* most common inherited hearing loss, in which both parents are carriers of the gene but only 25% of offspring are affected, occurring in either nonsyndromic or syndromic form;
- *X-linked hearing disorder:* hereditary hearing disorder due to a faulty gene located on the X chromosome, such as that found in Alport syndrome and Hunter syndrome.

Acoustic Trauma

Acoustic trauma is the most common cause of sensorineural hearing loss other than **presbyacusis**. The term *acoustic trauma* is

Presbyacusis is age-related hearing impairment. An alternative spelling is **presbycusis**.

generally used in one of two ways: (a) to describe the effect of a single exposure to a transient, high-intensity sound; or (b) to refer generically to the effects of excessive acoustic exposure, whether it be by trauma from a single high-intensity blast or by long-term insult to the cochlea from prolonged exposure to excessive noise. Regardless, the result of acoustic trauma is noise-induced sensorineural hearing loss.

Noise induced hearing loss (NIHL) can be temporary or permanent. Exposure to excessive sound results in a change in the threshold of hearing sensitivity or a threshold shift. Thus, if a noise-induced hearing loss is temporary, it is often referred to as *temporary threshold shift* or TTS. If the hearing loss is permanent, it is often called a *permanent threshold shift* or PTS.

Permanent hearing loss caused by acoustic trauma from a single exposure results from mechanical destruction of the organ of Corti by excessive pressure waves. Gradual hearing loss that occurs from repeated exposure to excessive sound occurs first from outer hair cell loss in the cochlea due to metabolic changes from repeated exhaustion of the cells. Continued exposure following outer hair cell loss can result eventually in inner hair cell damage.

You have probably experienced TTS. It is a common occurrence following exposure to loud music at a concert or following exposure to nearby firing of a gun or explosion of fireworks. The experience is usually one of sound seeming to be muffled, often accompanied by tinnitus. If you listen to your radio or CD player while you have TTS, you may notice that it just does not sound right.

If the loud sounds to which you were exposed were not of sufficient intensity, or the duration of your exposure was not excessive, your hearing loss will be temporary, and hearing sensitivity will return to normal over time. However, if the signal intensity and the duration of exposure were of a sufficient magnitude, your hearing loss will be permanent. Repeated exposure will result in a progression of the hearing loss.

There are several important acoustic factors that make sound potentially damaging to the cochlea:

- the intensity of the sound,
- the frequency composition of the sound, and
- the duration of exposure to the sound.

Table 4–4. Damage risk criteria expressed as the maximum permissible noise exposure for a given duration during a work day. Sound level is expressed in dBA, a weighted decibel scale that reduces lower frequencies from the overall decibel measurement.

Duration per Day (in hours)	Sound Level (in dBA)
8.0	90
6.0	92
4.0	95
3.0	97
2.0	100
1.5	102
1.0	105
0.5	110
0.25	115

Note: Criteria based on the U.S. Occupational Safety and Health Act 1983 regulations.

In general, higher frequency sounds are more damaging than lower frequency sounds. Whether or not a particular intensity of sound is damaging to an ear depends on the duration of exposure to that sound. That is, for example, a **broad-spectrum noise** with an intensity of 100 **dBA** is not considered dangerous if the duration of exposure is below 2 hours per day. However, exposure duration of greater than that can result in permanent damage to the ear.

Damage-risk criteria have been established as guidelines for this tradeoff between exposure duration and signal intensity. An example of commonly accepted damage-risk criteria for industry is shown in Table 4–4. Exposure above these levels over prolonged periods in the workplace will most likely result in significant PTS. Exposure to sound below these levels is considered safe by these standards.

Other factors also influence the risk of permanent noise-induced hearing loss. For example, some individuals are more susceptible than others, so that safe damage risk criteria for the population in general will not be safe levels for some individuals who are unusually susceptible. Also, the damaging effects of a given noise can be exacerbated by simultaneous exposure to certain ototoxic drugs and industrial chemicals.

The most common type of permanent hearing loss from acoustic trauma is a slowly progressive high-frequency hearing loss that

Broad-spectrum noise is a noise comprised of a broad band of frequencies.

dBA is decibels expressed in sound pressure level as measured on the A-weighted scale of a sound level meter filtering network.

occurs from repeated exposure over time. An example of a noise-induced hearing loss is shown in Figure 4–9. Typically, with TTS or with PTS in its early form, the configuration will have a notch that peaks in the 4000 to 6000 Hz region of the audiogram. This is sometimes referred to as a *noise notch* or a *4K notch,* consistent with exposure to excessive noise. As additional exposure occurs, the threshold in this region will worsen, followed by a shift in threshold at progressively lower frequencies. Figure 4–10 shows the progression of hearing loss from industrial noise exposure over a 4-decade period of time.

Hearing loss that occurs from acoustic trauma as a result of a single exposure to excessive sound may resemble the noise-induced hearing loss from prolonged exposure, or it may result in a flatter audiometric configuration. The audiogram shown in Figure 4–11 resulted from a single exposure to an early cordless telephone that rang as the user held the phone up to his ear. The level of the sound was estimated to be over 140 dB SPL, resulting in a relatively flat, moderate sensorineural hearing loss.

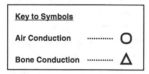

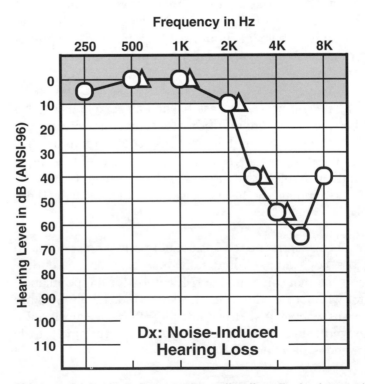

Figure 4–9. An audiogram representing the effects of excessive noise exposure.

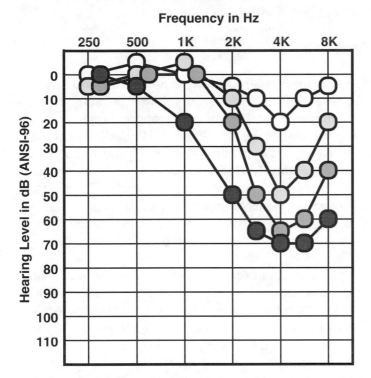

Figure 4-10. The progression of hearing loss from industrial noise exposure over a 4-decade period of time.

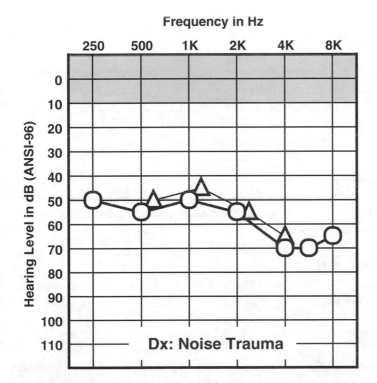

Key to Symbols

Air Conduction ·········· O

Bone Conduction ·········· △

Figure 4-11. An audiogram representing the effect of a single exposure to an early cordless telephone that rang in close proximity to the user's ear.

Other Trauma

In addition to acoustic trauma, other insults to the auditory system can cause significant hearing loss. Physical trauma that results in a **transverse fracture** of the temporal bone can cause extensive destruction of the membranous labyrinth. This type of trauma is often caused by a blow to the **occipital** region of the skull. Recall that a **longitudinal** fracture can result in damage to the middle ear structures, but seldom to the cochlea. Conversely, a transverse fracture tends to spare the middle ear and damage the cochlea. Depending on the extent of the labyrinthine destruction, the sensorineural hearing loss can be quite severe.

Another form of trauma occurs as a result of **radionecrosis**, or the death of tissue due to excessive exposure to radiation. Injury to the auditory system secondary to X-ray irradiation occurs as a result of **atrophy** of the spiral and annular ligaments causing degeneration of the organ of Corti. Hearing loss of this nature is sensorineural, progressive, and usually has a delayed onset. X-ray irradiation injury is increasingly common as "gamma knife" surgery is used in an effort to irradiate acoustic tumors.

Infections

Sensorineural hearing loss can result from acquired infections, the pathogens from which can directly insult the membranous labyrinth of children or adults. Sensorineural hearing loss can also result from teratogenic effects of congenital infection of a mother during embryologic development of a fetus.

Congenital Infections

Congenital infections most commonly associated with sensorineural hearing loss include:

- **cytomegalovirus** (CMV),
- human immunodeficiency virus (HIV),
- rubella,
- syphilis, and
- toxoplasmosis.

CMV is the leading cause of nongenetic congenital hearing loss in infants and young children. CMV is a type of herpes virus that can be transmitted in utero. Infants with congenital CMV infections are most often asymptomatic at birth. In those who de-

Transverse means a slice in the horizontal plane.
Occipital refers to the lobe of the brain located in the back of the head.
Longitudinal means lengthwise.

When tissue dies due to excessive exposure to radiation it is called **radionecrosis**, which in the auditory system may occur immediately following exposure or have a later onset.
Atrophy is the wasting away or shrinking of a normally developed organ or tissue.

Cytomegalovirus (CMV) is a viral infection usually transmitted in utero, which can cause central nervous system disorder, including brain damage, hearing loss, vision loss, and seizures.

velop hearing loss, the loss is usually of delayed onset, often **asymmetric**, progressive, and sensorineural. Other complications can include neurodevelopmental deficits such **microcephaly** and mental retardation.

HIV is the virus that causes *acquired immunodeficiency syndrome* (AIDS). Congenital HIV infections are increasingly common and can result in substantial neurodevelopmental deficits. Hearing is at risk mostly from opportunistic infections such as meningitis that are secondary to the disease or from ototoxic drugs used to treat the infections.

Rubella, or **German measles**, is a viral infection. Prior to vaccination against the disease, congenital infections resulted in tens of thousands of children born with congenital rubella syndrome, with characteristic features including cardiac defects, congenital cataracts, and sensorineural hearing loss. In the 1960s and 1970s, it was the leading nongenetic cause of hearing loss. In countries where vaccinations are routine, rubella has been nearly eliminated as a causative factor.

Syphilis is a venereal disease, caused by the **spirochete** Treponema pallidum, that can be transmitted from an infected mother to the fetus. Although most children with congenital syphilis will be asymptomatic at birth, a late form of the disease, occurring after 2 years of age, can result in progressive sensorineural hearing loss.

Toxoplasmosis is caused by a parasite infection, contracted mainly through contaminated food or close contact with domestic animals carrying the infection. Congenital toxoplasmosis can result in retinal disease, **hydrocephalus**, mental retardation, and sensorineural hearing loss.

Acquired Infections

Infections from bacteria, viruses, and fungi can result in sensorineural hearing loss. Bacterial infections can cause inflammation of the membranous labyrinth of the cochlea, or labyrinthitis, through several routes. Serous or toxic labyrinthitis is an inflammation of the labyrinth caused by bacterial contamination of the tissue and fluids, either by invasion through the middle ear *(otogenic)* or via the **meninges** *(meningogenic). Serous labyrinthitis* may be transient, resulting in mild hearing loss and dizziness. In more severe forms, however, it can be toxic to the sensory cells of the cochlea, causing substantial sensorineural hearing loss. Serous

If a person has a moderate hearing loss in one ear and a severe hearing loss in the other, the hearing is considered **asymmetric**. If the amount of hearing loss is the same in both ears it is considered **symmetric**. **Microcephaly** is an abnormal smallness of the head.

Measles is a highly contagious viral infection, characterized by fever, cough, conjunctivitis, and a rash, which can cause significant hearing loss.

A **spirochete** is a slender, spiral, motile microorganism that can cause infection.

Hydrocephalus is the excessive accumulation of cerebrospinal fluid in the subarachnoid or subdural space of the brain.

The three membranes of the brain and spinal cord, the arachnoid, dura mater, and pia mater, are called the **meninges**.

labyrinthitis sometimes occurs secondary to serous otitis media, presumably from the bacterial toxins traveling through the membranes of the oval or round windows. It may also occur secondary to meningitis, with the inflammation traveling along the brain's linings to the membranous labyrinth of the cochlea.

Bacterial infections can also cause otogenic *suppurative labyrinthitis.* In this type of infection, bacteria invade the cochlea from the temporal bone. The pus formation in the infection can cause permanent and severe damage to the cochlear labyrinth, resulting in substantial sensorineural hearing loss. Suppurative labyrinthitis can also be meningogenic in nature. That is, the cochlea can be invaded via the brain lining through the cochlear aqueduct or the internal auditory canal. Cochlear changes can be extreme, including total labyrinth obliteration.

Some of the more common acquired viral infections that can cause sensorineural hearing loss include herpes zoster oticus and mumps.

Herpes zoster oticus, or Ramsay Hunt syndrome, is caused by a virus that also causes chicken pox. The virus, often acquired during childhood, can lie dormant for years in the central nervous system. At some point in time, due to changes in the immune system or to the presence of systemic disease, the virus is reactivated, causing burning pain around the ear, skin eruptions in the external auditory meatus and concha, facial nerve paralysis, dizziness, and sensorineural hearing loss. Hearing loss is of varying degree and often has a high-frequency audiometric configuration.

Mumps is a contagious systemic viral disease, characterized by painful enlargement of the parotid glands, fever, headache, and malaise, that can cause sudden, permanent, profound unilateral sensorineural hearing loss.

Mumps, or epidemic parotitis, is an acute systemic viral disease, most often occurring in childhood after the age of 2 years. Depending on severity, it usually causes painful swelling of the **parotid glands** and can cause a number of complications related to **encephalitis**. Despite the systemic nature of the disease, hearing loss is peculiar in that it is almost always unilateral in nature. Because of this, it often goes undiagnosed until later in life. Mumps is probably the single most common cause of unilateral sensorineural hearing loss, and the loss is usually profound.

The **parotid glands** are the salivary glands near the ear.
Encephalitis is inflammation of the brain.

Syphilis is a congenital or acquired disease caused by a spirochete, which in its secondary and tertiary stages can cause auditory and vestibular disorders.

Another cause of hearing loss from acquired infection is **syphilis**, a venereal disease that can also cause congenital hearing loss. Syphilis is usually described in terms of clinical stages, from primary infection, through secondary involvement of other organs, to tertiary involvement of the cardiovascular and nervous sys-

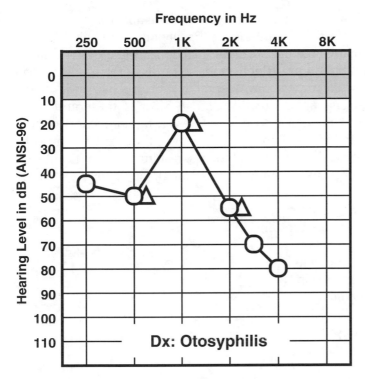

Figure 4–12. An audiogram representing the effects of otosyphilis.

tems. Hearing loss from *otosyphilis* occurs in the secondary or **tertiary** stages and results from membranous labyrinthitis associated with acute meningitis or **osteitis** of the temporal bone. Hearing loss from syphilis is not unlike that from Ménière's disease, characterized by fluctuation attacks and progression in severity. An example of a hearing loss from otosyphilis is shown in Figure 4–12. Besides the fluctuation and progression, another common finding is disproportionately poor speech recognition ability.

Tertiary means third in order.

Osteitis is inflammation of the bone.

Ototoxicity

Certain drugs and chemicals are toxic to the cochlea. Ototoxicity can be acquired or congenital. *Acquired ototoxicity* results from the ingestion of certain drugs that are administered for medical purposes, such as in the treatment of infections and cancer. Ototoxicity can also result from excessive exposure to certain environmental toxins. *Congenital ototoxicity* results from the teratogenic effects of drugs administered to the mother during pregnancy.

Several families of drugs are ototoxic. The *aminoglycosides* are a group of bacteriocidal antibiotics that are often ototoxic. They are used primarily against bacterial infections. Some of the amino-glycosides have a **predilection** for hair cells of the cochlea *(cochleotoxic)*, while others have a predilection for hair cells of the vestibular end-organs *(vestibulotoxic)*. Most of these antibiotics can be used in smaller doses to effectively fight infection without causing ototoxicity. Sometimes, however, the infections must be treated aggressively with high doses, resulting in significant sensorineural hearing loss. Ototoxic antibiotics include:

Predilection means a partiality or preference.

- amikacin
- dihydrostreptomycin
- garamycin
- gentamicin
- kanamycin
- neomycin
- netilmicin
- streptomycin
- tobramycin
- viomycin

Newer drugs that are ototoxic have been developed in the fight against cancer. *Carboplatin* and *cisplatin* are antimitotic and **antineoplastic** drugs often used in cancer treatment. It is not unusual for patients who undergo chemotherapy regimens that contain either or both of these drugs to develop permanent sensorineural hearing loss.

Antineoplastic refers to an agent that prevents the development, growth, or proliferation of tumor cells.

Hearing loss from ototoxicity is usually permanent, sensorineural, bilateral, and symmetric. The mechanism for damage varies depending on the drug, but, in general, hearing loss results initially from damage to the outer hair cells of the cochlea at its basal end. Thus, the hearing loss typically begins as a high-frequency loss and progresses to lower frequencies with additional drug exposure. An example of a hearing loss resulting from ototoxicity due to cisplatin chemotherapy is shown in Figure 4–13.

Quinine is an antimalarial drug that can have a teratogenic effect on the auditory system of the developing embryo.

Some drugs cause ototoxicity that is reversible. *Antimalarial drugs,* including chloroquine and **quinine**, have been associated with ototoxicity. Typically, the hearing loss from these drugs is temporary. However, in high doses the loss can be permanent.

Drugs known as *salicylates* can also be ototoxic. Salicylates such as acetylsalicylic acid and aspirin are used in large quantities as

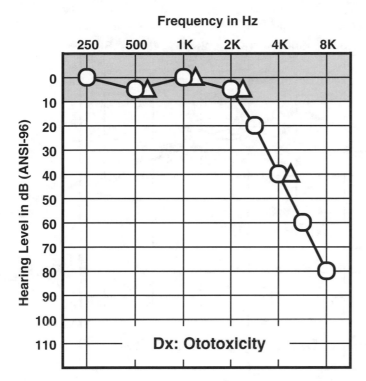

Figure 4-13. An audiogram representing the effects of ototoxicity.

therapeutic agents in the treatment of arthritis and other connective tissue disorders. Hearing loss is usually reversible and accompanied by tinnitus. In the case of salicylate intoxication, the hearing loss often has a flat rather than a steeply sloping configuration. An example is shown in Figure 4–14.

Loop diuretics, including ethacrynic acid, furosemide, and **lasix**, are used to promote the excretion of urine by inhibiting resorption of sodium and water in the kidneys. Hearing loss from loop diuretics may be reversible or permanent.

Other ototoxic substances include *industrial solvents,* such as styrene, toluene, and trichlorethylene, which can be ototoxic if inhaled in high concentrations over extended periods. Potassium bromate, a chemical neutralizer used in food preservatives and other commercial applications has also been associated with ototoxicity.

Some drugs have a *teratogenic effect* on the auditory system of the developing embryo when taken by the mother during pregnancy. Ingestion of these drugs, especially early in pregnancy, can result

Lasix is an ototoxic loop diuretic used in the treatment of edema (swelling) or hypertension, which can cause a sensorineural hearing loss secondary to degeneration of the stria vascularis.

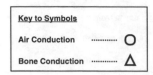

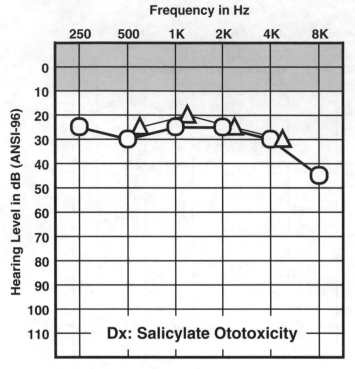

Figure 4–14. An audiogram representing the temporary effects of salicylate intoxication.

Accutane is a retinoic acid drug prescribed for cystic acne that can have a teratogenic effect on the auditory system of the developing embryo.

Thalidomide is a tranquilizing drug that can have a teratogenic effect on the auditory system of the developing embryo.

Ménière's Disease, named after Prosper Ménière, is idiopathic endolymphatic hydrops, characterized by fluctuating vertigo, hearing loss, tinnitus, and aural fullness.

Episodic vertigo is the repeated occurrence of dizziness.

in multiple developmental abnormalities, including profound sensorineural hearing loss. These drugs include **accutane**, dilantin, quinine, and **thalidomide**.

Ménière's Disease

A common disorder of the cochlea is *endolymphatic hydrops.* Endolymphatic hydrops is a condition resulting from excessive accumulation of endolymph in the cochlear and vestibular labyrinths. This excessive accumulation of endolymph often causes **Ménière's disease**, a constellation of symptoms of **episodic vertigo**, hearing loss, tinnitus, and aural fullness. The name of this syndrome is derived from the French scientist, Prosper Ménière, who in 1861 first attributed the diverse symptoms of dizziness, vomiting, and hearing loss to a disorder of the inner ear rather than the central nervous system.

The classic symptoms of Ménière's disease are an attack of vertigo with hearing loss, tinnitus, and pressure in the involved ear. The hearing loss is typically unilateral, fluctuating, progressive, and sensorineural. The feeling of pressure, the sensation of tinnitus, and hearing loss often build up before an attack of vertigo, which is often accompanied by nausea and vomiting. The spells can last from minutes to 2 or 3 hours and often include unsteadiness between spells. In the early stages of the disease, attacks are dominated by vertigo, and recovery can be complete. In the later stages, attacks are dominated by hearing loss and tinnitus, and permanent, severe hearing loss can occur.

The underlying cause of Ménière's disease is endolymphatic hydrops. The underlying cause of endolymphatic hydrops is most often unknown, although sometimes it can be attributed to allergy, vascular insult, physical trauma, syphilis, acoustic trauma, viral insult, or other causes. In the early stages of Ménière's disease, the buildup of endolymph occurs mainly within the cochlear duct and saccule. Essentially, these structures distend or dilate from an increase in fluid and cause ruptures of the membranous labyrinth.

Although Ménière's disease usually involves both the auditory and vestibular mechanisms, two variant forms exist, so-called *cochlear Ménière's disease* and *vestibular Ménière's disease.* In the cochlear form of the disease, only the auditory symptoms are present, without vertigo. In the vestibular form, only the vertiginous episodes are present, without hearing loss.

Hearing loss from Ménière's disease is most often unilateral, sensorineural, and fluctuating. In the early stages of the disease, the hearing loss configuration is often low frequency in nature. An example is shown in Figure 4–15. After repeated attacks, the loss usually progresses into a flat, moderate-to-severe hearing loss, as shown in Figure 4–16. One common feature of Ménière's disease is poor speech-recognition ability, much poorer than would be expected from the degree of hearing sensitivity loss.

Presbyacusis

Presbyacusis (or *presbycusis*) is a decline in hearing as a part of the aging process. As a collective cause, it is the leading contributor to hearing loss in adults. Estimates suggest that from **25 to 40% of those over the age of 65 years** have some degree of **hearing impairment**. The percentage increases to approximately 90% of those over the age of 90 years.

25–40% of all people over the age of 65 have some degree of **hearing impairment**.

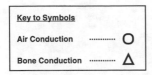

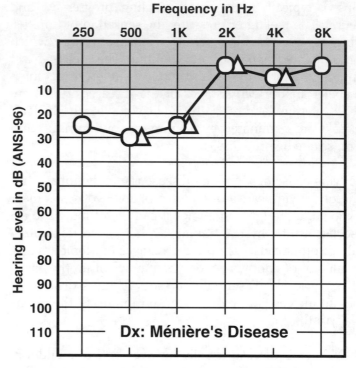

Figure 4-15. An audiogram representing the effects of the early stages of Ménière's disease.

All hearing loss that is present in aging individuals is not, of course, due to the aging process per se. During a lifetime, an individual can be exposed to excessive noise, vascular and systemic disease, dietary constraints, environmental toxins, ototoxic drugs, and so on. Add to these any genetic predisposition to hearing loss, and you may begin to wonder how anyone's hearing can be normal in older age. If you were able to restrict exposure to all of these factors, you would be able to study the specific effects of the aging process on the auditory structures. What you would likely find is that a portion of hearing loss is attributable to the aging process and a portion is attributable to the exposure of the ears to the world for the number of years it took to become old. How much is attributable to each can be estimated, although it will never be truly known in an individual. Regardless, if we think of living as a contributing factor to the aging process, then the hearing loss that occurs with the aging process, which cannot be attributed to other causative factors, can be considered presbyacusis.

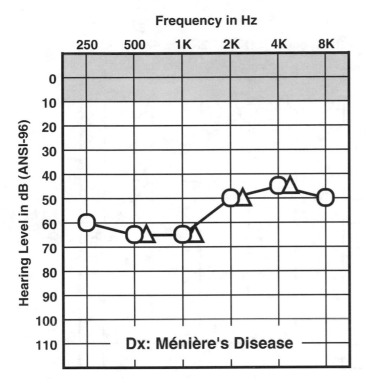

Figure 4-16. An audiogram representing the effects of Ménière's disease that has progressed.

Structures throughout the auditory system degenerate with age. Changes in cochlear hair cells, the **stria vascularis**, the **spiral ligament**, and the cochlear neurons all conspire to create sensorineural hearing loss. Changes in the auditory nerve, brain stem, and cortex conspire to create central auditory processing disorder.

Hearing sensitivity loss from presbyacusis is bilateral, usually symmetric, progressive, and sensorineural. An example of the effects of aging are shown in Figure 4–17. The systematic decline in the audiogram is greatest in the higher frequencies, but present across the frequency range. There are some interesting differences in the audiometric configurations of males and females attributable to aging. As shown in Figure 4–18, men tend to have more high frequency hearing loss, and women tend to have flatter audiometric configurations. When noise exposure is controlled, the amount of high-frequency hearing loss is similar in the two groups, but women tend to have more low-frequency hearing loss.

The **stria vascularis** is the highly vascularized band of cells on the internal surface of the spiral ligament, located within the scala media, extending from the spiral prominence to Reissner's membrane.

The **spiral ligament** is the band of connective tissue that affixes the basilar membrane to the outer bony wall, against which lies the stria vascularis within the scala media.

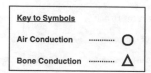

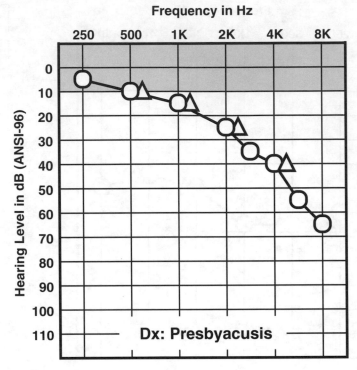

Figure 4-17. An audiogram representing the effects of presbyacusis.

Presbyacusis is also characterized by decline in the perception of speech that has been sensitized in some manner. Decline in understanding of speech in background competition or speech that has been temporally altered is consistent with aging changes in the central auditory nervous system. An example is shown in Figure 4–19.

Other Causes

There are a number of other causes of sensorineural hearing loss. A few of the more important ones include autoimmune hearing loss, cochlear otosclerosis, and sudden hearing loss.

Autoimmune refers to a disordered immunologic response in which the body produces antibodies against its own tissues.

Autoimmune hearing loss is an auditory disorder characterized by bilateral, asymmetric, progressive, sensorineural hearing sensitivity loss in patients who test positively for autoimmune disease. It tends to be diagnosed on the basis of exclusion of other causes, but it is increasingly attributed as the causative factor in progressive sensorineural hearing loss. An example of autoimmune

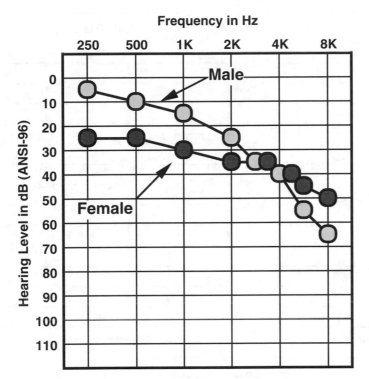

Figure 4-18. Generalized representation of the difference in the audiometric configurations of males and females as they age.

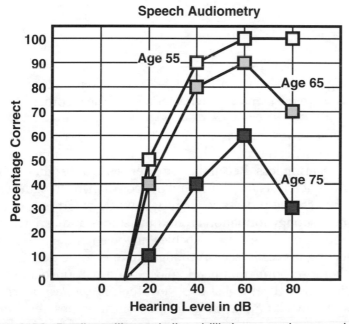

Figure 4-19. Decline with age in the ability to recognize speech in a background of competition.

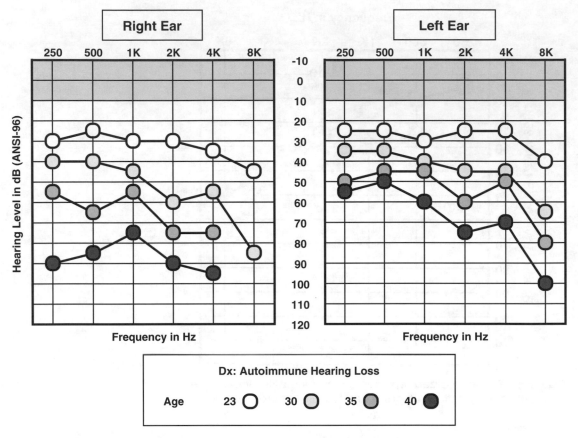

Figure 4–20. Illustrative example of the progression of autoimmune hearing loss.

hearing loss is shown in Figure 4–20. The asymmetry and progression are the signature characteristics of the disorder.

The same otosclerosis that can fix the stapes footplate into the oval window can occur within the cochlea and result in sensorineural hearing loss. Recall that otosclerosis is a disorder of bone growth that affects the stapes and the bony labyrinth of the cochlea. The disease process is characterized by resorption of bone and new spongy formation around the stapes and oval window. Depending on the extent of cochlear involvement, a sensorineural hearing loss can occur. Although there is some debate about whether a sensorineural hearing loss can occur in isolation, it is certainly theoretically possible. Nevertheless, *cochlear otosclerosis* is commonly accompanied by fixation of the stapes, resulting in a mixed hearing loss. An example of this type of hearing loss is shown in Figure 4–21.

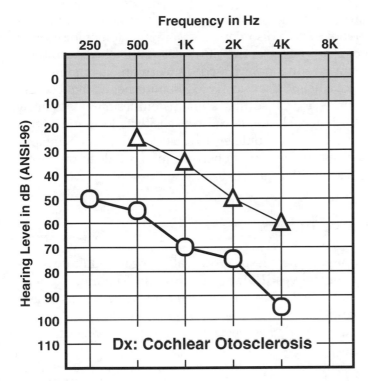

Figure 4–21. An audiogram representing the effects of cochlear otosclerosis.

Idiopathic *sudden hearing loss* is a term that is used to describe a sudden, often unilateral, sensorineural hearing loss. Idiopathic sudden hearing loss is often noticed upon awakening and is usually accompanied by tinnitus. The extent of the sensorineural hearing loss ranges from mild to profound. Partial or full recovery of hearing occurs in approximately 75% of patients. The term idiopathic is used because the cause is often unknown, although evidence favors a viral etiology.

Idiopathic is of an unknown cause.

CENTRAL AUDITORY NERVOUS SYSTEM DISORDERS

Any disease or disorder process that affects the peripheral and central nervous system can, of course, result in auditory disorder if the auditory nervous system is involved. Neoplastic growths on the VIIIth nerve or in the auditory brain stem, cranial nerve neuritis, multiple sclerosis, and brain **infarcts** can all result in some form of auditory disorder.

Infarcts are localized areas of ischemic necrosis.

An **infarction** is the sudden insufficiency of blood supply due to occlusion of arterial supply or venous drainage.

The nature of hearing impairment that accompanies central auditory nervous system disorder varies as a function of location of the disorder. A disorder of the VIIIth nerve is likely to result in a sensorineural hearing loss with poor speech understanding. The likelihood of a hearing sensitivity loss diminishes as the disorder becomes more central, so that a brain stem lesion is less likely than an VIIIth nerve lesion to cause a sensitivity loss, and a temporal lobe lesion is quite unlikely to cause a such a loss. Similarly, disorders of speech perception become more subtle as the disorder becomes more central.

VIIIth Nerve Tumors

The most common neoplastic growth affecting the auditory nerve is called a **cochleovestibular schwannoma**. The more generic terms *acoustic tumor* or *acoustic neuroma* are typically referring to a cochleovestibular schwannoma. Other terms used to describe this tumor are *acoustic neurinoma* and *acoustic neurilemoma*.

Cochleovestibular schwannoma is the proper term for acoustic neuroma.

A cochleovestibular schwannoma is a **benign**, encapsulated tumor composed of Schwann cells that arises from the VIIIth cranial nerve. Schwann cells serve to produce and maintain the **myelin** that ensheathes the **axons** of the VIIIth nerve. This tumor arising from the proliferation of Schwann cells is benign in that it is slow growing, is encapsulated thereby avoiding local invasion of tissue, and does not disseminate to other parts of the nervous system. Acoustic tumors are unilateral and most often arise from the vestibular branch of the VIIIth nerve. Thus, they are sometimes referred to as *vestibular schwannomas.*

When a tumor is **benign**, it is nonmalignant or noncancerous.

The tissue enveloping the axon of myelinated nerve fibers is called **myelin.**

Axons are the efferent processes of a neuron that conduct impulses away from the cell body and other cell processes.

The effects of a cochleovestibular schwannoma depend on its size, location, and the extent of the pressure it places on the VIIIth nerve and brain stem. Auditory symptoms may include tinnitus, hearing loss, and unsteadiness. Depending on the extent of the tumor's impact, it may cause headache, motor incoordination from cerebellar involvement, and involvement of adjacent cranial nerves. For example, involvement of the Vth cranial nerve can cause facial numbness, involvement of the VIIth cranial nerve can cause facial weakness, and involvement of the IVth cranial nerve can cause **diplopia**.

Diplopia means double vision.

Among the most common symptoms of cochleovestibular schwannoma are unilateral tinnitus and unilateral hearing loss. The hearing loss varies in degree depending on the location and size of the tumor. An example of a hearing loss resulting from an

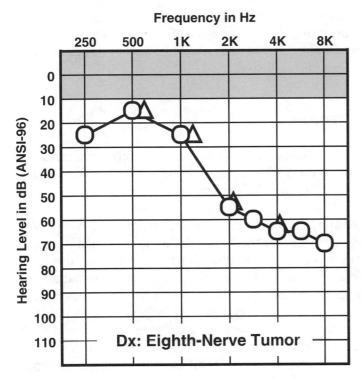

Figure 4–22. An audiogram representing the effects of an acoustic or VIIIth-nerve tumor.

acoustic tumor is shown in Figure 4–22. Speech understanding typically is disproportionately poor for the degree of hearing loss.

One other important form of schwannoma is *neurofibromatosis.* This tumor disorder has two distinct types. *Neurofibromatosis 1* (NF-1), also known as von Recklinghausen's disease, is an autosomal dominant disease characterized by **café-au-lait spots** and multiple **cutaneous tumors**, with associated optic gliomas, peripheral and spinal neurofibromas, and, rarely, acoustic neuromas. In contrast, *Neurofibromatosis 2* (NF-2) is characterized by bilateral cochleovestibular schwannomas. The schwannomas are faster growing and more virulent than the unilateral type. This is also an autosomal dominant disease and is associated with other intracranial tumors. Hearing loss in NF-2 is not particularly different from the unilateral type of schwannoma, except that it is bilateral and often progresses more rapidly.

In addition to cochleovestibular schwannoma, a number of other types of tumors, cysts, and aneurysms can affect the VIIIth nerve and the **cerebellopontine angle**, where the VIIIth nerve enters

Café-au-lait spots are brown birthmarklike spots that appear on the skin. Tumors on the skin are called **cutaneous tumors**.

Cerebellopontine angle is the anatomical angle formed by the proximity of the cerebellum and the pons from which the VIIIth cranial nerve exits into the brain stem.

Meningiomas are benign tumors that may encroach on the cerebellopontine angle, resulting in a retrocochlear disorder.

the brain stem. These other neoplastic growths, such as lipoma and **meningioma**, occur more rarely than cochleovestibular schwannoma. The effect of these various forms of tumor on hearing is usually indistinguishable.

Neural Disorders

In addition to acoustic tumors, other disease processes can affect the function of the VIIIth nerve. Two important neural disorders are *cochlear neuritis* and *diabetic cranial neuropathy.*

Not unlike any cranial nerve, the VIIIth nerve can develop neuritis, or inflammation of the nerve. Although rare, acute *cochlear neuritis* can occur as a result of a direct viral attack on the cochlear portion of the nerve. This results in degeneration of the cochlear neurons in the ear. Hearing loss is sensorineural and often sudden and severe. It is accompanied by poorer speech understanding than would be expected from the degree of hearing loss. One specific form of this disease occurs as a result of syphilis. *Meningo-neuro-labyrinthitis* is an inflammation of the membranous labyrinth and VIIIth nerve that occurs as a predominant lesion in early congenital syphilis or in acute attacks of secondary and tertiary syphilis.

Diabetes mellitus is a metabolic disorder caused by a deficiency of insulin, with chronic complications including neuropathy and generalized degenerative changes in blood vessels. Neuropathies can involve the central, peripheral, and autonomic nervous systems. When neuropathy from diabetes affects the auditory system, it usually results in vestibular disorder and hearing loss consistent with retrocochlear disorder.

Brain Stem Disorders

Ischemia results from a localized shortage of blood due to obstruction of blood supply.

Brain stem disorders that affect the auditory system include infarcts, gliomas, and multiple sclerosis. *Brain stem infarcts* are localized areas of **ischemia** produced by interruption of the blood supply. Auditory disorder varies depending on the site and extent of the disorder. Two syndromes related to vascular lesions that include hearing loss are *inferior pontine syndrome* and *lateral inferior pontine syndrome.* Inferior pontine syndrome results from a vascular lesion of the pons involving several cranial nerves. Symptoms include ipsilateral facial palsy, ipsilateral sensorineural hearing loss, loss of taste from the anterior two thirds of the tongue, and paralysis of lateral conjugate gaze movement of the eyes. Lateral inferior pontine syndrome results from a vascular lesion of the inferior pons, with symptoms that include facial palsy, loss of taste from the anterior two thirds of the tongue, **analgesia** of the face, paralysis of lateral conjugate gaze movements, and sensorineural hearing loss.

Analgesia means the reduction or abolition of sensitivity to pain.

A *glioma* is a tumor composed of neuroglia, or supporting cells of the brain. It comes in various forms, depending on the types of cells involved, including **astrocytomas, ependymomas, glioblastomas**, and **medulloblastomas**. Any of these can affect the auditory pathways of the brain stem, resulting in various forms of retrocochlear hearing disorder, including hearing sensitivity loss and speech perception deficits.

Astrocytoma is a central nervous system tumor consisting of astrocytes, which are star-shaped neuroglia cells.

Glioblastoma is a rapidly growing and malignant tumor composed of undifferentiated glial cells.

Medulloblastoma is a malignant tumor that often invades the meninges.

Multiple sclerosis is a **demyelinating disease**. It is caused by an autoimmune reaction of the nervous system that results in small scattered areas of demyelination and the development of demyelinated plaques. During the disease process, there is local swelling of tissue that exacerbates symptoms, followed by periods of remission. If the demyelination process affects structures of the auditory nervous system, hearing disorder can result. There is no characteristic hearing sensitivity loss that emerges as a consequence of the disorder, although all possible configurations have been described. Speech perception deficits are not uncommon in patients with multiple sclerosis.

A **demyelinating disease** is an autoimmune disease process that causes scattered patches of demyelination of white matter throughout the central nervous system, resulting in retrocochlear disorder when the auditory nervous system is affected.

Temporal-Lobe Disorder

Cerebrovascular accident, or stroke, is caused by an interruption of blood supply to the brain due to aneurysm, embolism, or clot. This results in sudden loss of function related to the damaged portion of the brain. When this occurs in the temporal lobe, audition may be affected, although more typically, receptive language processing is affected while hearing perception is relatively spared. Indeed, hearing ability is seldom impaired except in the case of bilateral temporal lobe lesions. In such cases, "cortical deafness" can occur, resulting in symptoms that resemble **auditory agnosia**.

Agnosia means the lack of sensory-perceptual ability to recognize stimuli.

Other Nervous System Disorders

Any other disease processes, lesions, or trauma that affect the central nervous system can affect the central auditory nervous system. For example, AIDS is a disease that compromises the efficacy of the immune system, resulting in **opportunistic infectious** diseases that can affect central auditory nervous system structures. When these structures are affected, auditory disorder occurs, usually resembling retrocochlear disorder or central auditory processing disorder.

Opportunistic infections are those that take advantage of the opportunity afforded by a weakened physiologic state of the host.

SUMMARY

■ There are several major categories of pathology or noxious influences that can adversely affect the auditory system, including developmental defects, infections, toxins, trauma, vascular disorders, neural disorders, immune-system disorders, bone disorders, aging disorder, tumors and other neoplastic growths, and disorders of unknown or multiple causes.

■ Disorders of the outer and middle ear are commonly of two types, either structural defects due to embryologic malformations or structural changes secondary to infection or trauma. Another common abnormality, otosclerosis, is a bone disorder.

■ Microtia and atresia are congenital malformations of the auricle and external auditory canal. Microtia is an abnormal smallness of the auricle. It is one of a variety of auricular malformations. Atresia is the absence of an opening of the external auditory meatus.

■ One common cause of transient hearing disorder is the accumulation and impaction of cerumen in the external auditory canal.

■ The most common cause of transient conductive hearing loss in children is otitis media with effusion. Otitis media is inflammation of the middle ear. It is caused primarily by Eustachian tube dysfunction.

■ Otosclerosis is a disorder of bone growth that affects the stapes and the bony labyrinth of the cochlea.

■ A cholesteatoma is a growth in the middle ear that forms as a consequence of epidermal invasion through a perforation or a retraction of the tympanic membrane.

■ Hereditary factors are common causes of sensorineural hearing loss.

■ Acoustic trauma is the most common cause of sensorineural hearing loss other than presbyacusis.

■ Congenital infections most commonly associated with sensorineural hearing loss include: cytomegalovirus

(CMV), human immunodeficiency virus (HIV), rubella, syphilis, and toxoplasmosis.

■ Acquired bacterial infections can cause inflammation of the membranous labyrinth of the cochlea, or labyrinthitis.

Some of the more common acquired viral infections that can cause sensorineural hearing loss include herpes zoster oticus and mumps.

Certain drugs and chemicals are toxic to the cochlea. Ototoxicity can be acquired or congenital.

■ A common disorder of the cochlea is endolymphatic hydrops, a condition resulting from excessive accumulation of endolymph in the cochlear and vestibular labyrinths, which often causes Ménière's disease, a constellation of symptoms of episodic vertigo, hearing loss, tinnitus, and aural fullness.

■ Presbyacusis is a decline in hearing as a part of the aging process. As a collective cause, it is the leading contributor to hearing loss in adults.

■ Other causes of sensorineural hearing loss include autoimmune hearing loss, cochlear otosclerosis, and sudden hearing loss.

Neoplastic growths on the VIIIth nerve or in the auditory brain stem, cranial nerve neuritis, multiple sclerosis, and brain infarcts can all result in some form of auditory disorder.

The most common neoplastic growth affecting the auditory nerve is called a cochleovestibular schwannoma.

SUGGESTED READINGS

Gilbert, P. (1996). *The A–Z reference book of syndromes and inherited disorders.* San Diego: Singular Publishing Group.

Hayes, D., & Northern, J. L. (1996). *Infants and hearing.* San Diego: Singular Publishing Group.

Northern, J. L. (1996). *Hearing disorders* (3rd ed.). Boston: Allyn and Bacon.

Schuknecht, H. F. (1993). *Pathology of the ear* (2nd ed.). Philadelphia: Lea & Febiger.

5

Introduction to Hearing Assessment

The main purpose of a hearing evaluation is to define the nature and extent of hearing impairment. The hearing evaluation serves as a first step in the rehabilitation of hearing handicap that results from the impairment. Toward this end, there are some common questions to be answered as a part of any audiologic evaluation. They include:

- Why is the patient being evaluated?
- Should the patient be referred for medical consultation?
- What is the patient's hearing sensitivity?
- How well does the patient understand speech?
- How well does the patient process auditory information?
- Does the hearing impairment cause a hearing handicap?

Patients have their hearing evaluated for a number of reasons. The focus of a particular hearing evaluation, as well as the types and nature of tests that are used, will vary as a function of the reason. For example, many patients seek the professional expertise of an audiologist because they feel that they have hearing impairment and may need hearing devices. In such cases, the audiologist seeks to define the nature and extent of the impairment, in a thorough manner, with an emphasis on factors that may indicate or contraindicate successful hearing-device use.

As another example, patients may be referred because they are seeking compensation for hearing loss that is allegedly caused by exposure to noise in the workplace, by an accident, or by other means that may be compensible. In these cases, the audiologist must focus on hearing sensitivity, with suspicion aroused for exaggeration of the hearing impairment. The audiologist must use acceptable cross-checks to verify the extent of identified hearing impairment.

Behavioral measures = pure tone audiometry, speech audiometry

Electroacoustic measures = immittance audiometry and otoacoustic emissions

Electrophysiologic measures = auditory brain stem response

Audiologists are often called upon to evaluate the hearing of young children. In many cases, children are evaluated at an age when they are not able to cooperate with behavioral hearing assessment. In these cases, the audiologist must use **behavioral, electroacoustic**, and **electrophysiologic measures** as cross-checks in identification of hearing sensitivity levels.

Other children are evaluated not because of suspicion of a hearing sensitivity loss, but because of concerns about problems in the processing of auditory information. Here the emphasis is not on careful quantification of hearing sensitivity but on careful quantification of speech understanding. Because time is often limited with younger children, the approach that is used by the audiologist is critical in terms of focusing on the nature of the concern.

Patients are often evaluated in consultation with otolaryngologists to determine the nature and extent of hearing impairment that results from active disease processes. In such cases, the otolaryngologist is likely to treat the disease process with drugs or surgery and is interested in evaluating hearing before and after treatment. Careful quantification of middle ear function and hearing sensitivity are often important features of the pre- and postsurgical assessment.

Some patients are evaluated simply to assure that they have normal hearing sensitivity. Newborns, children entering school, adults in noisy work environments, and a number of other individuals have their hearing sensitivity screened in an effort to rule out hearing impairment. The focus of the screening is on the rapid identification of those with normal hearing sensitivity, rather than the quantification of hearing impairment and handicap.

Thus, although the fundamental goal of an audiologic assessment is similar for most patients, the specific focus of the evaluation can vary considerably, depending on the nature of the patient and problem. As a result, a very important aspect of the audiologic evaluation is the first question, *Why is the patient being evaluated?*

THE FIRST QUESTION

Why is the patient being evaluated? It sounds like such a simple question. Yet the answer is a very important step in the assessment process because it guides the audiologist to an appropriate evaluative strategy. There are usually two main sources of information for answering this question. One source is the nature of the referral. This alone often provides sufficient information to understand what the expected outcome of the evaluation will be. The other is the case history.

Referral-Source Perspective

There are many reasons for evaluating hearing and several categories of referral sources from which patients come to be evaluated by audiologists. Referral sources include the patient, the patient's parents, the patient's children, the patient's spouse, oto-laryngologists, pediatricians, gerontologists, oncologists, neurologists, speech-language pathologists, other patients, attorneys, teachers, and nurses. The nature of the referral source is often a good indicator of why the patient is being evaluated.

Self-referrals or referrals from family members usually indicate that the patient has a significant communication disorder resulting from hearing impairment. If it is a self-referral, the patient probably has been concerned about a problem with hearing for some time and has conceded to the possibility of **hearing-device** use. If it is a family referral, it is likely that the family members have noticed a decline in communication function and have urged the patient to seek professional consultation. In all cases of direct referrals, the audiologic evaluation proceeds by first addressing the issue of whether the disorder is of a nature that can be treated medically. Once established, the evaluation proceeds with a focus on hearing assessment for the potential fitting of hearing devices.

Hearing device = hearing aid or assistive listening device

Referrals from physicians and other health-care professionals do not always have as clear a purpose. That may seem unusual, but few days pass by in a busy clinic without some patients expressing that they have no idea why their doctors wanted them to have a hearing evaluation. In these cases, the specialty of the physician making the referral is usually helpful in determining why the patient was referred. For example, an adult referred by a neurologist is likely to be under suspicion of having some type of brain disorder. The neurologist is seeking to determine whether a hearing sensitivity loss exists either for purposes of additional testing by **auditory evoked potentials** or to address whether the central auditory nervous system is involved in the dysfunction. As another example, a child referred by a speech-language pathologist has probably been referred either to rule out the presence of a hearing sensitivity loss as a contributing factor to a speech and language disorder or to assess central auditory processing status. As a final example, when an otolaryngologist refers a patient for a hearing consultation, it will be for one of several reasons including:

An **auditory evoked potential** is a measurable response of the electrical activity of the brain in response to acoustic stimulation.

- the patient has a hearing impairment and entered the health care system through the otolaryngologist;
- the patient is dizzy, and the physician is concerned about the possibility of a tumor on the VIIIth cranial nerve;
- the patient has ear disease, and the physician is interested in pretreatment assessment of hearing;

■ the patient is seeking compensation for trauma-related incident that has allegedly resulted in a hearing problem, and the physician is interested in the nature and degree of that problem; or

■ the physician has determined that the patient has a hearing problem that cannot be corrected medically or surgically and has sent the patient to the audiologist for evaluation and fitting of hearing aid amplification or other rehabilitation as necessary.

It is important to understand why the patient is being evaluated because it dictates the emphasis of the evaluative process. Occasionally, the interest of the referral source in the outcome of a hearing consultation is not altogether clear, and the audiologist must seek that information directly from the referral source prior to starting an evaluation.

Importance of the Case History

An important starting point of any audiologic evaluation is the case history. Sample adult and child case histories are shown in the Clinical Note on pages 168–171. An effective case history guides the experienced audiologist in a number of ways. It provides necessary information about the nature of auditory complaints, including whether it is in one ear or both; whether it is acute or chronic; and the duration of the problem. All of this information is important because it helps the audiologist to formulate clinical testing strategies.

Case histories are also important because they shed light on possible factors contributing to the hearing impairment. In adult case histories, questions are asked about exposure to excessive noise, family history of hearing loss, or the use of certain types of medication. This information serves at least three purposes. First, it begins to prepare the audiologist for what is likely to be found during the audiologic evaluation. Certain types of hearing loss configurations are typical of certain causative factors, and knowledge of the potential contribution of these factors is useful in preparing the clinician for testing. Second, knowledge about preventable factors in hearing loss, particularly noise exposure, will lead to appropriate recommendations about ear protection and other preventive measures. Third, some hearing loss is temporary in nature. Reversible hearing loss may result from recent noise exposure. It may also result from ingestion of high doses of certain drugs, such as aspirin. It is important to know whether

The Case History

Following are examples of a case history, one for adults and one for children. The adult form is for use by the patient; the pediatric form is for use by the parent. Regardless of which form is used, there are some commonalities of purpose:

- ■ to secure proper identifying information;
- ■ to provide information about the nature of auditory complaints; and
- ■ to shed light on possible factors contributing to the hearing impairment.

Adult case histories also include information about:

- ■ warning signs that may lead to medical referral;
- ■ whether and under what circumstances a hearing impairment is handicapping; and
- ■ whether consideration has been given to potential use of hearing aid amplification.

Case histories for children also include information about:

- ■ speech and language development;
- ■ general physical and psychosocial development; and
- ■ academic achievement.

In addition, if the child has a history of otitis media, an in depth case history into the nature of the disorder may be of interest to both the audiologist and the managing physician.

There are almost as many examples of case histories as there are clinics using them. Some important factors that you should keep in mind when considering a case history form:

- ■ keep it at a simple reading level,
- ■ keep it as concise as possible, and
- ■ translate it into other languages common to your region.

The case history form should be designed, not as an end in itself, but as a form that will lead you into a discussion of the reasons that the patient is in your office and the nature of the auditory complaint.

<u>**Adult Case History**</u>

Name: _____ Age: _____ Birthdate: _____

Referred by: _____

• Primary complaint: _____

• Do you have hearing problems?   Yes _____ No _____
     Which ear? Right _____ Left _____ Both _____
     Has the hearing loss been: Gradual? _____ Sudden? _____ Fluctuating? _____
     Do you presently use a hearing device? Yes _____ No _____ For how long? _____
     Are you interested in using a hearing device?   Yes _____ No _____

• Do you hear noises in your ears or head?   Yes _____ No _____
     Which ear?   Right _____ Left _____ Both _____
     How often do you hear noises? Constantly _____ Occasionally _____ Rarely _____

• Do you ever have a feeling of fullness or stuffiness in your cars? Yes _____ No _____

• Do you ever experience facial numbness, weakness, or tingling? Yes _____ No _____

• Are you ever dizzy, unsteady, or off-balance? Yes _____ No _____
     Is your dizziness accompanied by: Nausea?   Yes _____ No _____
                                                            Vomiting?   Yes _____ No _____
                                                            Noises in your ears?   Yes _____ No _____

• Have you ever had any ear surgery? Yes _____ No _____ Describe: _____

• Have you ever been exposed to loud noises?   Yes _____ No _____
     Describe: _____ How recently? _____

• Does anyone in your family have a hearing problem? Yes _____ No _____

• Are you currently taking medication?   Yes _____ No _____ Describe: _____

• What is your occupation? _____

Authorization is hereby granted to this institution to release test findings. Please provide names and addresses of persons or agencies to which you would like this report sent:

1. _____ 2. _____ 3. _____

_____ _____ _____

_____ _____ _____

Signature: _____ Date: _____

(continued)

Pediatric Case History

Name: _____ Age: _____ Birthdate: _____

Referred by: _____

• Primary complaint: _____

• Do you think your child has a hearing problem? Yes _____ No _____

• Has your child ever had a hearing test before? Yes _____ No _____

  Describe the results: _____

• Does your child have ear infections? Yes _____ No _____ If so, please answer questions on reverse.

• Has your child ever had ear surgery? Yes _____ No _____ Describe: _____

• Do you believe your child's speech and language is developing normally? Yes _____ No _____

• Do you believe your child's physical ability is developing normally? Yes _____ No _____

• Does your child require special services, such as speech therapy or remedial help? Yes _____ No _____

• Was the pregnancy normal? Yes _____ No _____

  Describe complications: _____

• Was the delivery of this child normal? Yes _____ No _____

  Describe complications: _____

• Has your child had any illnesses or medical conditions? Yes _____ No _____

  Describe: _____

• Is your child taking medication? Yes _____ No _____ Describe: _____

• Does anyone in your family have a hearing problem? Yes _____ No _____

• Is there any additional information that you believe might be helpful? _____
  _____

Authorization is hereby granted to this institution to release test findings. Please provide names and addresses of persons or agencies to which you would like this report sent:

1. _____   2. _____   3. _____

   _____   _____   _____

   _____   _____   _____

Signature: _____ Date: _____

Otitis Media
Patient/Parent Questionnaire

Ear infections or middle ear fluid can result in hearing problems. If your child has had recurrent ear infections or persistent middle ear fluid, your answers to the following questions will help us to determine the necessary treatment for your child.

• At what age did the ear infection or middle ear fluid first occur? _____

• How many ear infections have occurred in the last six months? _____
                                    In the last twelve months? _____

• How long has the current middle ear infection or fluid been present?_____

• Has treatment included the use of antibiotics?   Yes _____   No _____

    If you can, please list the medicines used and the duration of use:
    Medicine: _____   Duration of use: _____
              _____   _____
              _____   _____
              _____   _____
              _____   _____

    Has antibiotic prophylaxis (once-a-day dosage for an extended period) been tried?
    Yes _____   No _____   Name of medicine: _____

• Has your child had tubes inserted?   Yes _____   No _____   How many times?_____

• Has your child had a tonsillectomy or adenoidectomy?   Yes _____   No _____

• How many siblings are at home? _____

• Is your child in day care?   Yes _____   No _____

• Does anyone smoke at home?   Yes _____   No _____

• Does your child: snore or have difficulty breathing at night?   Yes _____   No _____
                     have recurrent sinusitis or colored nasal drainage?   Yes _____   No _____
                     have recurrent tonsillitis or sore throats?   Yes _____   No _____
                     have clumsiness, balance, or coordination problems?   Yes _____   No _____
                     have difficulty breathing through the nose?   Yes _____   No _____
                     have nasal allergies or food allergies?   Yes _____   No _____

the hearing impairment being quantified is temporary in nature or is the residual deficit that remains after reversible changes.

Also included on adult case histories are questions related to general health and to specific problems that can accompany hearing disorder. These questions are important because the audiologist is often the entry point into health care and must be knowledgeable about warning signs that dictate appropriate medical referral. This cannot be understated. As a nonmedical entry point into the health-care system, audiologists must maintain a constant vigil for warning signs of medical problems. Thus, questions are asked about dizziness, numbness, weakness, **tinnitus**, and other signs that might indicate the potential for otologic, neurologic, or other medical problems.

The sensation of ringing or other sound heard in the ears or head is called **tinnitus**.

Another very important aspect of the case history involves questions about communication ability. The goal here is to obtain information about whether the patient perceives that the hearing problem is resulting in a communication disorder and whether the patient has or would consider use of hearing-device amplification. The questions about communication disorder begin to give the audiologist an impression of the extent to which a hearing problem is handicapping in some way and the circumstances under which the patient is experiencing the greatest difficulty. The questions about hearing devices are intended to "break the ice" on the issue and promote discussion of potential options for the first step in the rehabilitative process.

Case histories for children are oriented in a slightly different way. Questions are asked of the parents about the nature and any problems associated with pregnancy and delivery. Case histories for children also include a checklist of known childhood diseases or conditions. These questions about health of the mother and the developing child are aimed at obtaining an understanding of factors that might impact hearing ability. They also provide the clinician with a better understanding of any factors that might influence testing strategies.

Case histories for children must also include inquiries about overall development and, specifically, about speech and language development. Children with hearing impairments of any degree should be considered at risk for speech and language delays or disorders. Screening for speech and language problems during an audiologic evaluation is an important role of the audiologist, and that screening should begin with the case history. Questions relating to parental concerns and developmental milestones can serve as important aspects of the screening process. In addition, such information can provide the clinician with valuable insight about which test materials might be **linguistically** appropriate.

Linguistically pertains to language.

Another important aspect of a case history for children relates to academic achievement. Answers to questions about school placement and progress will help the audiologist to orient the evaluation and consequent recommendations toward academic needs.

One main benefit of the case history process is that the interaction with patients can reveal substantial information about their general health and communication abilities. For example, experienced clinicians will observe the extent to which patients rely on lipreading and will notice any speech and language abnormalities. They will also attend carefully to patients' physical appearance and **motoric abilities**.

Motoric abilities are muscle movement abilities.

Once the reason for referral is known and the case history is reviewed with the patient, the evaluative challenge begins. Prepared with a knowledge of why the patient is being evaluated and what information the patient hopes to gain, the audiologist can orient the evaluative strategy appropriately.

THE AUDIOLOGIST'S CHALLENGES

Regardless of the techniques that are used, the audiologist faces a number of clinical challenges during any audiologic evaluation. One of the first challenges is to determine whether the problem is strictly a communication disorder or whether there is an underlying active and/or treatable disease process that requires the patient to be referred for medical consultation. Treatable disorders of the outer and middle ears are common causes of auditory complaints. Thus, the first question in the evaluative process is whether these structures are functioning properly. Following that question, the evaluative strategy includes the determination of hearing sensitivity and type of hearing loss, measurement of speech understanding, assessment of auditory processing ability, and estimate of hearing handicap.

Evaluating Outer and Middle Ear Function

Structural changes in the outer and middle ears can cause functional changes and result in hearing impairment. Problems associated with the outer ear are usually related to obstruction or

Stenosis = narrowing

Cerumen = earwax

Tympanic membrane = eardrum

Perforation = hole

Sclerotic tissue = hardened tissue

Ossicular chain = bones in the middle ear; malleus, incus, and stapes

stenosis (narrowing) of the ear canal. The most common problem is an excessive accumulation or impaction of **cerumen**. When changes such as this occur, sound can be blocked from striking the **tympanic membrane**, and a loss in the conduction of sound will occur. The function of the tympanic membrane can also be reduced by either **perforation** or **sclerotic tissue** adding mass to the membrane. These changes result in a reduction in appropriate tympanic membrane vibration and a consequent loss in conduction of sound to the **ossicular chain**.

The first step in the process of assessing outer and middle ear function is inspection of the ear canal. This is achieved with *otoscopy*. Otoscopy is simply the examination of the external auditory meatus and the tympanic membrane with an *otoscope*. An otoscope is a device with a light source that permits visualization of the canal and eardrum. Otoscopes range in sophistication from a hand held speculumlike instrument with a light source, as shown in Figure 5–1, to a video otoscope, as shown in Figure 5–2. The ear canal is inspected for any obvious inflammation, growths, foreign objects, or excessive cerumen. If possible, the tympanic membrane is visualized and inspected for inflammation, perforation, or any other obvious abnormalities in structure. If an obvious disease process is noted during inspection, the patient should be referred for medical assessment following the audiologic evaluation.

If excessive or impacted cerumen is noted, the audiologist may choose to remove it or refer the patient to appropriate medical personnel for cerumen management. Cerumen management involves removal of the excessive or impacted wax in one of three ways:

■ mechanical removal,
■ suction, or
■ irrigation.

Mechanical removal is the most common method and involves the use of small curettes or spoons to extract the cerumen. This is usually done using a speculum to open and straighten the ear canal. Suction is sometimes used, especially when the cerumen is very soft. Irrigation is commonly used when the cerumen is impacted and is hard and dry. Irrigation involves directing a stream of water from an oral jet irrigator against the wall of the ear canal until the cerumen is loosened and extracted.

Following otoscopic inspection of the structures of the outer ear, the next step in the evaluation process is to assess the function of

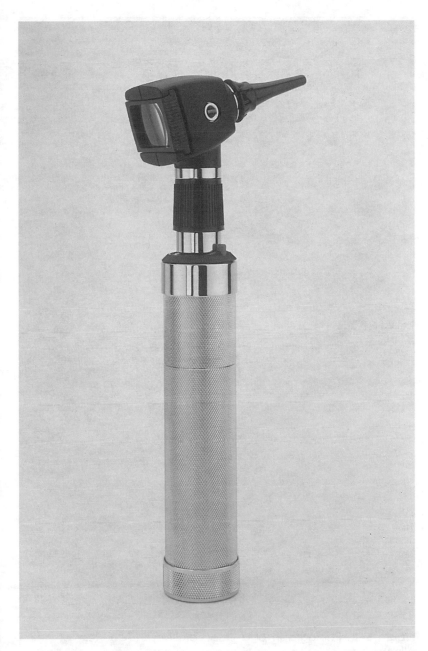

Figure 5-1. Photograph of a hand-held otoscope. (Courtesy of Welch Allyn)

the outer and middle ear mechanisms. Problems in function of the middle ear can be classified into four general categories. Functional deficits can result from

- significant negative pressure in the middle ear cavity,
- an increase in the mass of the middle ear system,

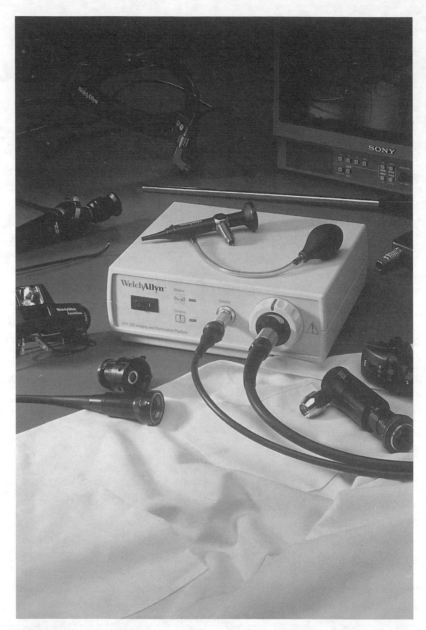

Figure 5–2. Photograph of a video otoscope. (Courtesy of Welch Allyn)

- an increase in the stiffness of the middle ear system, and
- a reduction in the stiffness of the middle ear system.

Negative pressure in the middle ear space occurs when the Eustachian tube is not functioning appropriately due to some form of upper respiratory blockage. Pressure cannot be equalized, and the trapped oxygen is absorbed by the mucosal lining of the middle ear. This results in a reduction in air pressure in comparison to atmospheric pressure and can reduce the transmission of sound through the middle ear.

Increase in the mass of the middle ear system usually occurs as a result of a fluid accumulation behind the tympanic membrane. Following prolonged negative pressure, the mucosal lining of the middle ear begins to excrete fluid that can block the effects of the tympanic membrane and ossicular chain. Mass increases also can occur as a result of abnormal cell growth within the middle ear, which can have an influence similar to the presence of fluid. Any increase in the mass of the system can affect transmission of sound, particularly in the higher frequencies.

Increase in the stiffness of the middle ear system results from some type of fixation of the ossicular chain. Usually this fixation is the result of a **sclerosis** of the bones that results in a fusion of the stapes at the oval window. Increases in stiffness of the ossicular chain can also affect transmission of sound, particularly in the lower frequencies.

Sclerosis is the hardening of tissue.

Reduction in the stiffness can have a similar affect. Abnormal reduction usually results from a break or disarticulation of the ossicular chain, which significantly reduces sound transmission.

It is important to evaluate outer and middle ear function for at least two reasons. First, a reduction in function usually occurs as a result of structural changes that are amenable to medical management. That is, the causes of structural and functional changes in the outer and middle ear usually can be treated with drugs or surgical intervention. Second, the changes in function of the outer and middle ear structures often lead to conductive hearing impairment. Because the ultimate goal of any hearing assessment is the amelioration of hearing impairment, an important early question in the evaluation process is to what extent any impairment is the product of a disease process that can be effectively treated medically. Thus, one of the audiologist's first challenges is to assess outer and middle ear function. If this function is normal, then any hearing impairment is due to changes in the sensory mechanism rather than the conductive mechanism. If this function is abnormal, then it remains to quantify the extent to which changes in function of the conductive mechanism contribute to the overall hearing impairment.

The best means for assessing outer and middle ear function is the use of **immittance audiometry**. Immittance audiometry, as you will learn, is an electroacoustic assessment technique that mea-

Immittance audiometry is a battery of measurements that assesses the flow of energy through the middle ear, including static immittance, typanometry, and acoustic reflex thresholds.

sures the extent to which energy flows freely through the outer and middle ear mechanisms. Its use in the evaluation of middle ear function developed during the late 1960s and early 1970s. It has gained widespread application both for screening middle ear function and for more in-depth assessment. In fact, many clinicians embrace immittance audiometry to the extent that they begin every audiologic assessment with it. They believe that the assessment of outer and middle ear function is among the most important first steps in the hearing evaluation process.

Estimating Hearing Sensitivity

One of the best ways to describe hearing ability is by its sensitivity to sound. Similarly, one of the best ways to describe hearing impairment is by measuring a reduction in sensitivity to sound. Hearing sensitivity is usually defined by an individual's **threshold** of audibility of sound. Measurements are made to determine at what intensity level a tone or a word is just barely audible. That level is considered the threshold of audibility of the signal and is an accepted way of describing the sensitivity of hearing.

Threshold is the level at which a stimulus is just audible.

Substantial progress has been made in understanding hearing and in measuring hearing ability over the past half century. Yet to this day, the best single indicator of hearing impairment, its impact on communication, and the **prognosis** for successful hearing-device use is the **pure-tone audiogram**. The audiogram is a graph, which depicts thresholds of hearing sensitivity, determined behaviorally, as a function of pure-tone frequency. It has become the cornerstone of audiologic assessment and, as a consequence perhaps, the generic indicator of what is perceived to be an individual's hearing ability. Because the audiogram is such a pervasive means for describing hearing sensitivity, it has become the icon for hearing sensitivity itself. It has provided a common language with which to describe an individual's hearing. As a result, when we characterize the hearing ability in an individual, we are likely to think in terms of the pure-tone audiogram.

Prognosis is the prediction of the course or outcome of a disease or treatment.

An **audiogram** is a graph that depicts the amount of hearing loss as a function of frequency.

The audiologist's role in assessment of hearing sensitivity is most often determination of the pure-tone audiogram. In some instances, however, particularly in infants and young children or in individuals who are feigning hearing loss, a reliable pure-tone audiogram cannot be obtained. In these cases, other techniques for estimating hearing sensitivity must be used. Regardless, even in these cases, the challenge remains to try to "predict the audiogram."

The measurement of hearing sensitivity provides a means for describing degree and configuration of hearing loss. If normal listeners have hearing thresholds at one level and the patient being tested has thresholds at a higher level, then the difference is considered the amount of hearing loss compared to normal. By its nature then, a pure-tone audiogram provides a depiction of the amount of hearing loss.

Measurements of sensitivity provide a substantial amount of information about hearing ability. Estimates are made of degree of hearing loss, providing a general statement about the severity of sensitivity impairment. Estimates are also made of degree of loss as a function of frequency, or configuration of hearing loss. The configuration of a hearing loss is a critical factor in speech understanding and in fitting hearing-device amplification.

There are several ways to measure hearing sensitivity. Typically, sensitivity assessment begins with the behavioral determination of a threshold for speech recognition. This speech threshold provides a general estimate of sensitivity of hearing over the **speech frequencies**, generally described as the pure-tone average of thresholds at 500, 1000, and 2000 Hz. Sensitivity assessment proceeds with behavioral pure-tone audiometry for determination of the audiogram. Pure-tone thresholds provide estimates of hearing sensitivity at specific frequencies.

The **speech frequencies** are 500, 1000, and 2000 Hz.

In some cases, behavioral testing cannot be completed. In these instances, estimates can be made via auditory evoked potential measurements. Auditory evoked potentials are responses of the brain to sound. Electrical activity of the nervous system that is evoked by auditory stimuli can be measured at levels very close to behavioral thresholds. Thus, for infants or those who will not or cannot cooperate with behavioral testing, these electrophysiologic estimates of hearing sensitivity provide an acceptable alternative.

Determining Type of Hearing Loss

Another challenge to the audiologist is the determination of the type of hearing loss. If a loss occurs as a result of changes in the outer or middle ear, it is considered a loss in the conduction of sound to the cochlea, or a **conductive hearing loss**. If a loss occurs as a result of changes in the cochlea, it is considered a loss in function at the sensory-neural junction, or a **sensorineural hearing loss**. If a loss occurs as a result of changes in both the outer or

A **conductive hearing loss** is one that occurs as a result of outer or middle ear disorder.

A **sensorineural hearing loss** is one that occurs as a result of cochlear disorder.

A **mixed hearing loss** is one that has both a conductive and sensorineural component.

A **retrocochlear disorder** is one that occurs as a result of VIIIth nerve or auditory brain stem disorder.

middle ear and the cochlea, it will have both a conductive and a sensory component and be considered a **mixed hearing loss**. Finally, if a loss occurs as a result of changes to the VIIIth nerve or auditory brain stem, it is considered a **retrocochlear disorder**.

Determination of the type of hearing loss is an important contribution of the audiologic assessment. A crucial determination is whether a conductive hearing loss is present. Although the function of outer and middle ear structures is readily determined by immittance audiometry, the extent that a disorder in function results in a measurable hearing loss is not. Therefore, one important aspect of the audiologic assessment is measurement of the degree of conductive and sensorineural components of the hearing loss. Knowledge of this is valuable because conductive loss is caused by disorders of the outer or middle ear, most of which are treatable medically. Knowledge of the extent to which a loss is conductive will provide an estimate of the residual sensorineural deficit following medical management. For example, if the loss is entirely conductive in nature, then treatment is likely to return hearing sensitivity to normal. If the loss is partially conductive and partially sensorineural, then a residual sensorineural deficit will remain following treatment. If the loss is entirely sensorineural, then medical treatment is unlikely to be of value.

The transmission of sound through the outer and middle ear to the cochlea is by **air conduction**.

The transmission of sound to the cochlea by vibration of the skull is by **bone conduction**.

To evaluate the type of hearing loss, hearing sensitivity is measured by presenting sounds in two ways. The most common way is to present sound through an earphone to assess hearing sensitivity of the entire auditory mechanism. This is referred to as **air-conduction** testing. The other way to present sound to the ear is by placing a vibrator in contact with the skin, usually behind the ear or on the forehead. Sound is then directed to the vibrator, which transmits signals directly to the cochlea via **bone conduction**. Direct bone-conduction stimulation virtually bypasses the outer and middle ears to assess sensitivity of the auditory mechanism from the cochlea and beyond. The difference between hearing sensitivity as determined by air conduction and the sensitivity as determined by bone conduction represents the contribution of the function of the outer and middle ear. If sound is being conducted properly by these structures, then hearing sensitivity by air conduction is the same as hearing sensitivity by bone conduction. If a hearing loss is present, that loss is attributable to changes in the sensory cells of the cochlea or neural cells of the auditory nervous system and is referred to as a sensorineural hearing loss. If sound is not being conducted properly by the outer and middle ear, then air-conduction thresholds will be poorer than bone-conduction thresholds (i.e., an *air-bone gap* will be present), reflecting a loss in conduction of sound through the outer and middle ears, or a conductive hearing loss.

One other question about type of hearing loss relates to whether the site of disorder is in the cochlear or retrocochlear structures. Retrocochlear disorders result from tumors or other changes in the auditory peripheral and central nervous systems. The underlying disease processes that result in nervous system disorders are often life-threatening. For example, as you learned in Chapter 4, one of the more common retrocochlear disorders results from a tumor growing on the VIIIth cranial nerve, referred to as a **cochleovestibular schwannoma**. A cochleovestibular schwannoma is a benign growth that often emerges from the vestibular branch of the VIIIth nerve. As it grows, it begins to challenge the nerve for space within the internal auditory canal, resulting in pressure on the nerve that can affect its function. As it grows into the brain stem, it begins to compete for space, which results in pressure on other cranial nerves and brain stem structures. If an acoustic tumor is detected early, the prognosis for successful surgical removal and preservation of hearing function is good. Delay in detection can result in substantial permanent neurologic disorder and reduces the prognosis for preservation of hearing.

A **cochleovestibular schwannoma** is a benign tumor of the VIIIth cranial (auditory and vestibular) nerve.

Neurologic disorders of the peripheral and central auditory nervous system may result in hearing loss or other auditory complaints. It is not uncommon for a patient with an acoustic tumor to report a loss of hearing sensitivity, muffled sound, or tinnitus as a first symptom of the effects of the tumor. That patient may seek assistance from a physician or from an audiologist. Thus, the audiologist's responsibility in all cases of patients with auditory complaints is to be alert for factors that may indicate the presence of a retrocochlear disorder. If the audiologic evaluation reveals results that are consistent with retrocochlear site of disorder, the audiologist must make the appropriate referral for medical consultation.

On most of the measures used throughout the audiologic evaluation, there are indicators that can alert the audiologist to the possibility of retrocochlear disorder. Acoustic reflex thresholds, symmetry of hearing sensitivity, configuration of hearing sensitivity, and measures of speech recognition all provide clues as to the nature of the disorder. Any results that arouse suspicion about the integrity of the nervous system should serve as an immediate indicator of the need for medical referral.

Prior to the advent of sophisticated imaging and radiographic techniques, specialized audiologic assessment was an integral part of the differential diagnosis of auditory nervous system disorders. Behavioral measures of differential sensitivity to loudness, loudness growth, and auditory adaptation were designed to assist in the diagnostic process. As imaging and radiographic techniques improved, the ability to visualize ever-smaller lesions of the auditory nervous system was enhanced. These smaller lesions were less likely to have an impact on auditory function. As a result, the sensitivity of the behavioral audiologic techniques diminished.

For a number of years in the late 1970s and early 1980s, auditory evoked potentials were used as a very sensitive technique for assisting in the diagnosis of neurologic disorders. For a time, these measures of neurologic function were thought to be even more sensitive than radiographic techniques in the detection of lesions. However, the advent of magnetic resonance imaging (MRI) techniques, permitting the visualization of even smaller lesions, reduced the sensitivity of these functional measures once again.

Today, auditory evoked potentials, particularly the auditory brain stem response, remains a valuable indicator of VIIIth nerve and auditory brain stem function. Audiologists are often consulted to carry out evoked-potential testing as a first screen in the process of neurologic diagnosis. The procedure has lost some of its stature in the diagnostic process to the more sensitive MRI procedures. Nevertheless, many neurologists and otologists continue to seek an assessment of **neural function** by evoked potentials to supplement the assessment of **structure** provided by the MRI procedures.

> Evoked potentials assess **neural function**; MRI assesses neural **structure**.

Measuring Speech Recognition

Once a patient's hearing thresholds have been estimated, it is important to determine **suprathreshold** function, or function of the auditory system at intensity levels above threshold. Threshold assessment provides only an indicator of the sensitivity of hearing, or the ability to hear faint sounds. Suprathreshold measures provide an indicator of how the auditory system deals with sound at higher intensity levels.

> An intensity level that is above threshold is termed **suprathreshold**.

The most common suprathreshold measure in an audiologic evaluation is that of **speech recognition**. Measures of speech recognition provide an estimate of how well an individual uses

> The ability to perceive and identify speech is called **speech recognition**.

residual hearing to understand speech signals. That is, if speech is of sufficient intensity, can it be recognized appropriately?

Measurement of speech recognition is important for at least two reasons. The most important reason is that it provides an estimate of how well a person will hear speech at suprathreshold levels, thereby providing one of the first estimates of how much a person with a hearing loss might benefit from a hearing device. In general, if an individual has a hearing sensitivity loss and good speech-recognition ability at suprathreshold levels, the prognosis for successful hearing-device use is good. If an individual has poor speech-recognition ability at suprathreshold levels, then making sound louder with a hearing device is unlikely to provide as much benefit.

Measurement of speech recognition is also important as a screen for retrocochlear disorder. In most cases of hearing loss of cochlear origin, speech recognition ability is predictable from the degree and configuration of the audiogram. That is, given a hearing sensitivity loss of a known degree and configuration, the ability to recognize speech is roughly equivalent among individuals and nearly equivalent between ears within an individual. Expectations of speech-recognition ability, then, lie within a certain predictable range for a given hearing loss of cochlear origin. In most cases of hearing loss of retrocochlear origin, however, speech-recognition ability is poorer than would be expected from the audiogram. Thus, if performance on speech-recognition measures falls below that which would be expected from a given degree and configuration of hearing loss, suspicion must be aroused that the hearing loss is due to retrocochlear rather than cochlear disorder.

Speech-recognition ability is usually measured with **monosyllabic word tests**. Several tests have been developed over the years. Most use single-syllable words in lists of 25 or 50. Lists are usually developed to resemble, to some degree, the **phonetic** content of speech in a particular language. Word lists are presented to patients at suprathreshold levels, and the patients are instructed to repeat the words. Speech recognition is expressed as a percentage of correct identification of words presented.

Monosyllabic word tests are tests that consist of one-syllable words that typically are phonetically balanced; that is, they contain speech sounds that occur with the same frequency as those of conversational speech. **Phonetic** pertains to an individual speech sound.

Measuring Auditory Processing

Another suprathreshold assessment is the evaluation of **auditory processing** ability. Auditory processing ability is usually defined

Auditory processing is how the auditory system utilizes acoustic information.

as the process by which the central auditory nervous system transfers information from the VIIIth nerve to the auditory cortex. The central auditory nervous system is a highly complex system that analyzes and processes neural information from both ears and transmits that processed information to other locations within the nervous system.

Much of our knowledge of the way in which the brain processes sound has been gained from studying systems that are abnormal due to neurologic disorders. The central auditory nervous system plays an important role in comparing sound at the two ears for the purpose of sound localization. The central auditory nervous system also plays a major role in extracting a signal of interest from a background of noise. While signals at the cochlea are analyzed exquisitely in the frequency, amplitude, and temporal domains, it is in the central auditory nervous system where those fundamental analyses are eventually perceived as speech or some other meaningful nonspeech sound.

If we understand the role of audiologic evaluation as the assessment of hearing, then we can begin to understand the importance of evaluating more than just the sensitivity of the ears to faint sounds and the ability of the ear to detect single-syllable words presented in quiet. Although both measures provide important information to the audiologic assessment, they stop short of offering a complete picture of an individual's auditory ability. Certainly, as we think of the complexity of auditory perception, the ability to follow a conversation in a noisy room, the effortless ability to localize sound, or even the ability to recognize someone from the sound of footsteps, we begin to understand that the rudimentary assessments of hearing sensitivity and speech recognition do not adequately characterize what it takes to hear. Neither do they adequately describe the possible disorders that a person might have.

Over the past two decades, techniques that were once used to assist in the diagnosis of neurologic disease have been adapted for use in the assessment of communication impairment that occurs as a result of central auditory processing disorder. Speech audiometric measures that are sensitized in certain ways are now commonly used to evaluate auditory processing ability. A typical battery of tests might include:

Competing speech signal = background noise

- the assessment of speech recognition across a range of signal intensities;
- the assessment of speech recognition in the presence of **competing speech signals**; and

■ the measurement of **dichotic listening**, which is the ability to process two different signals presented simultaneously to the two ears.

Listening to different signals presented to each ear simultaneously is called **dichotic listening**.

Results of such an assessment provide an estimate of central auditory processing ability and a more complete profile of a patient's auditory abilities and impairments. Such information is often useful in providing guidance regarding appropriate amplification strategies or other rehabilitation approaches.

Measuring Hearing Disability and Handicap

Assessment of hearing sensitivity, measurement of speech understanding, and estimates of auditory processing abilities are all measures of a patient's hearing ability or hearing impairment. The question that remains to be asked is whether a hearing sensitivity loss, reduction in speech understanding, or auditory processing disorder is having an impact on communication ability. Asked another way, is a hearing impairment causing a hearing disability and/or hearing handicap?

A hearing **impairment** can be thought of as the actual dysfunction in hearing that is described by the various measures of hearing status. Hearing **disability** can be thought of as the functional limitations imposed by the hearing impairment. Hearing **handicap** can be thought of as the obstacles placed on psychosocial function imposed by the disability. Audiologists know that the mere presence of impairment does not necessarily result in disability or handicap. Although there is a relationship between degree of impairment and disability or handicap, it is not necessarily a close one in individual patients. For example, a mild hearing sensitivity loss of slow onset may not result in a disability for an 80-year-old with limited communication demands. The same mild sensitivity loss, if it was of sudden onset in a person whose livelihood was tied to verbal communication, could impose a substantial disability and handicap. Thus, the presence of a mild impairment can impose a significant handicap to one person, whereas the presence of a substantial impairment may only be mildly handicapping to another.

Impairment refers to abnormal or reduced function.
Disability refers to a functional limitation imposed by an impairment.
Handicap refers to the obstacles to psychosocial function resulting from a disability.

Because of the disparity among impairment, disability, and handicap, it is important to assess the degree of disability and handicap that result from the impairment. Such an assessment often leads to a clear set of goals for the rehabilitation process. If the goal of audiologic assessment is to define hearing impairment for the purpose of providing appropriate strategies for amelioration of the resultant handicap, then there is no better way to complete the assessment process than with an evaluation of the nature and extent of the consequences of the impairment.

The most efficacious way of measuring disability and handicap is by self-assessment scales. Several scales have been developed that are designed to assess both the extent of hearing disability and the social and emotional consequences of hearing impairment. That is, the scales were designed to determine the extent to which an auditory disorder is causing a hearing problem and the extent to which the hearing problem is affecting quality of life. Generally, these scales consist of a series of questions designed to provide a profile of the nature and extent of disability and handicap. The patient is typically asked to complete the questionnaire prior to the audiologic evaluation. These scales have also been used following hearing aid fitting in an effort to assess the impact of hearing aids on the disability or handicap. Audiologists also use these scales with spouses or other significant individuals in the patient's life as a way of assessing the impact of the impairment on family and other social interactions. An example of a self-assessment scale is shown in Figure 5–3.

Screening Hearing Function

One other challenge that an audiologist faces involves the screening of hearing sensitivity. Hearing screening is designed to assess the hearing sensitivity of large numbers of individuals rapidly. The challenge of the audiologist in the screening process is usually different than the challenges faced in the conventional audiologic assessment. Typical screening measures of sensitivity are simplified to an extent that the actual procedures can be carried out by technical personnel. The audiologist's role includes education and training of technical staff, continual monitoring of screening results, and follow-up audiologic evaluation of screening failures.

Screening programs are usually aimed at populations of individuals who are at risk for having hearing impairment or individuals whose undetected hearing impairment could have a substantive negative effect on communication ability. There are three major groups that undergo hearing screening:

- newborns,
- children entering school, and

Question:	Response
1. Does a hearing problem cause you to feel embarrassed when meeting new people?	yes sometimes no
2. Does a hearing problem cause you to feel frustrated when talking to members of your family?	yes sometimes no
3. Do you have difficulty hearing when someone speaks in a whisper?	yes sometimes no
4. Do you feel handicapped by a hearing problem?	yes sometimes no
5. Does a hearing problem cause you difficulty when visiting friends, relatives, or neighbors?	yes sometimes no
6. Does a hearing problem cause you to attend religious services less often than you would like?	yes sometimes no
7. Does a hearing problem cause you to have arguments with family members?	yes sometimes no
8. Does a hearing problem cause you difficulty when listening to TV or radio?	yes sometimes no
9. Do you feel that any difficulty with your hearing limits or hampers your personal or social life?	yes sometimes no
10. Does a hearing problem cause you difficulty when in a restaurant with relatives or friends?	yes sometimes no

yes = 4 points; sometimes = 2 points; no = 0 points

Scores range from 0 to 40, with higher scores indicating greater perceived handicap

Figure 5–3. An example of a self-assessment scale, the Hearing Handicap Inventory for the Elderly, administered to determine the impact of hearing loss. (From The Hearing Handicap Inventory for Adults: A New Tool, by I. Ventry and B. Weinstein, 1982, *Ear and Hearing, 3,* 128–134. Reprinted with permission.)

■ adults in occupations that expose them to potentially dangerous levels of noise.

The goal of newborn hearing screening is to identify any child with a substantial sensorineural hearing impairment and to initiate treatment by 6 months of age. To achieve this goal, efforts have focused on screening the hearing sensitivity of newborns before they leave the hospital. Newborn hearing screening became fairly common in the 1970s and 1980s for infants who were determined to be at risk for potential hearing impairment. Risk factors, or indicators, presented in Table 5–1, have been developed that are intended to place the infant in a category that requires hearing screening and follow-up. Although these programs were effective in identifying infants with hearing impairment, research findings suggest that as many as half of all infants with significant sensorineural hearing loss do not have any of the risk-factor indicators. As of the early 1990s, the average age of identification of children with significant hearing impairment remained at an alarming 2.5 to 3 years in many areas of the United States. Because of the failure of the system to identify half of the children with hearing loss and because of the extent of delay in identifying those children who were not detected early, universal newborn hearing screening programs were implemented. Universal newborn screening has as its goal the hearing screening of all children, at birth, before discharge from the hospital. Infant hearing screening is usually carried out by techni-

Table 5–1. The Joint Committee on Infant Hearing has identified the following factors, or indicators, that place an infant into a category of being at-risk for significant sensorineural hearing loss, thereby requiring hearing screening and follow-up.

Risk Factors
Family history of childhood hearing loss
Congenital infections (TORCH)*
Craniofacial anomalies
Birth weight <1500 grams
Hyperbilirubinemia requiring exchange
Bacterial meningitis
Asphyxia
Ototoxic medication
Mechanical ventilation > 10 days
Syndromes that include hearing loss

*TORCH: acronym describing congenital perinatal infections, including *tox*oplasmosis, *o*ther infections (especially syphilis), *r*ubella, *c*ytomegalovirus infection, and *h*erpes simplex

cians, volunteers, and nursing personnel under the direction of hospital-based audiologists.

Not all children who have significant hearing impairment are born with it. Some develop it early in childhood and will be missed by the early screening process. As a result, for many years efforts have been made to screen the hearing of children as they enter school. School screening programs are aimed at identifying children who develop hearing loss later in childhood or whose hearing impairment is mild enough to have escaped early detection. School screening programs are usually carried out by nursing or other school personnel under the direction of an educational audiologist.

Screening programs have also been designed for adults who are at risk for developing hearing impairment, usually due to noise exposure. Two such groups are:

- individuals who are entering the military or
- employees who are starting jobs in work settings that will expose them to potentially damaging levels of noise.

These individuals are usually subjected to pre-enlistment or pre-employment determination of **baseline audiograms**. In addition, they are reevaluated periodically in an effort to detect any changes that may be attributable to noise exposure in the workplace. Much of the screening of adults is accomplished via automated pure-tone audiometry. The audiologist's role is usually to coordinate the program, ensure the validity of the automated screening, and follow up on those who fail the screening and those whose hearing has changed on reevaluation.

> An initial audiogram obtained for comparison with later audiograms to quantify any change in hearing sensitivity is called a **baseline audiogram**.

The screening of newborns requires the use of techniques that can be carried out without active participation of the patient. Two techniques have proven to be most useful. The **auditory brain stem response (ABR)** is an electrophysiologic technique that is used successfully to screen the hearing of infants. It involves attaching electrodes to the infant's scalp and recording electrical responses of the brain to sound. It is a reliable measure that is readily recorded in newborns. Another technique is the measurement of **otoacoustic emissions (OAEs)**. OAEs are echoes that occur in response to sound being delivered to the ear. A sensitive microphone, placed into the ear canal, is used to monitor the presence of the echo following stimulation. OAEs are reliably recorded in infants who have normal cochlear function. There are various advantages and disadvantages to these two techniques.

> An **ABR** or **auditory brain stem response** is an electrophysiological response to sound, consisting of five to seven identifiable peaks that represent neural function of auditory pathways.
>
> **Otoacoustic emissions (OAEs)** are measurable echoes emitted by the normal cochlea related to the function of the outer hair cells.

Most successful programs have developed strategies to incorporate both techniques in the screening of all newborns.

Screening the hearing of children entering school is accomplished using behavioral pure-tone audiometry techniques. Typically, the intensity level of the audiometer is fixed at 20–30 dB HL, and hearing is screened across the audiometric frequency range. Children who fail the screening are referred to the audiologist for a complete audiologic evaluation. Some programs also screen school-age children for middle ear disorder. Since young children are at risk for developing middle ear disease, some of which can go undetected, efforts have been made to evaluate middle ear status. Immittance audiometry screening is used in these cases.

Screening of adults is usually accomplished by automated pure-tone audiometry. Automated screening makes use of microcomputer-based instruments that are programmed to establish hearing sensitivity thresholds across the audiometric frequency range. These automated instruments have proven to be effective when applied to adult populations with large numbers of individuals who have normal hearing sensitivity.

SUMMARY

- The main purpose of a hearing evaluation is to define the nature and extent of hearing impairment.
- The hearing evaluation serves as a first step in the rehabilitation of hearing handicap that results from the impairment.
- Although the fundamental goal of an audiologic assessment is similar for most patients, the specific focus of the evaluation can vary considerably, depending on the nature of the patient and problem.
- The answer to the question *Why is the patient being evaluated?* is an important step in the assessment process because it guides the audiologist to an appropriate evaluative strategy. The nature of the referral source is often a good indicator of why the patient is being evaluated.
- An important starting point of any audiologic evaluation is the case history. An effective case history guides the experienced audiologist in a number of ways.
- Regardless of the techniques that are used, the audiologist faces a number of clinical challenges during any audiologic evaluation.

- One of the first challenges is to determine whether the problem is strictly a communication disorder or whether there is an underlying disease process that requires medical consultation.
- The audiologic evaluation strategy includes determination of hearing sensitivity and type of hearing loss, measurement of speech understanding, assessment of auditory processing ability, and estimate of hearing handicap.
- The best single indicator of hearing impairment, its impact on communication, and the prognosis for successful hearing-device use is the pure-tone audiogram.
- Suprathreshold measures provide an indicator of how the auditory system deals with sound at higher intensity levels. The most common suprathreshold measure in an audiologic evaluation is that of speech recognition.
- Another suprathreshold assessment is the evaluation of auditory processing ability, or the process by which the central auditory nervous system transfers information from the VIIIth nerve to the auditory cortex.
- Because of the disparity among impairment, disability, and handicap, it is important to assess the degree of disability and handicap that result from the impairment. The most efficacious way of measuring disability and handicap is by self-assessment scales.
- One other challenge that an audiologist faces involves the screening of hearing sensitivity of newborns, children entering school, and adults in occupations that expose them to potentially dangerous levels of noise.

SUGGESTED READINGS

Bess, F. H., & Hall, J. W. (Eds.). (1992). *Screening children for auditory function.* Nashville: Bill Wilkerson Center Press.

Gelfand, S. A. (1997). *Essentials of audiology.* New York: Thieme.

Katz, J. (Ed.). (1994). *Handbook of clinical audiology* (4th ed.). Baltimore: Williams & Wilkins.

Wilson, P. L., & Roeser, R. J. (1997). Cerumen management: professional issues and techniques. *Journal of the American Academy of Audiology, 8,* 421–430.

6

The Audiologist's Assessment Tools: Behavioral Measures

THE AUDIOMETER

An audiometer is an electronic instrument used by an audiologist to quantify hearing. An audiometer produces pure tones of various frequencies, attenuates them to various intensity levels, and delivers them to transducers. It also produces **broad-band** and **narrow-band noise**. In addition, the audiometer serves to attenuate and direct speech signals from other sources, such as a microphone, tape player, or compact disc player.

Broad-band noise is sound with a wide bandwidth, containing a continuous spectrum of frequencies with equal energy per cycle throughout the band.

Narrow-band noise is bandpass-filtered noise that is centered at one of the audiometric frequencies.

There are several types of audiometers, and they are classified primarily by their functions. For example, a clinical audiometer includes nearly all of the functions that an audiologist might want to use for behavioral audiometric assessment. In contrast, a screening audiometer might generate only pure-tone signals delivered to earphones.

There are three main components to any audiometer: an **oscillator**, an **attenuator**, and an **interrupter switch**.

Regardless of audiometer type, there are three main components to any audiometer, as shown schematically in Figure 6–1. The primary components are

- an **oscillator**,
- an **attenuator**, and
- an **interrupter switch**.

The *oscillator* generates pure tones, usually at discrete frequencies at the octave and mid-octave frequencies of 125, 250, 500, 750,

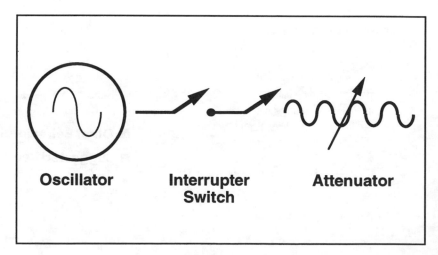

| Oscillator | Interrupter Switch | Attenuator |

Figure 6–1. Schematic representation of the three main components of any audiometer.

1000, 1500, 2000, 3000, 4000, 6000, and 8000 Hz. Some audiometers do not include all of these frequencies; other audiometers extend to higher frequencies. The oscillator is controlled by some form of frequency-selector switch.

The *attenuator* controls the intensity level of the signal, usually in 5 dB steps from −10 dB HL to a maximum output level that varies by frequency. Typical maximum output levels for earphones are: 75 dB at 125 Hz; 90 dB at 250, 6000, and 8000 Hz; and 110 dB from 500 through 4000 Hz. Typical maximum output levels for bone-conduction vibrators are 50 dB at 500 and 750 Hz and 60 dB from 1000 to 4000 Hz. Some audiometers permit dB step sizes smaller than 5 dB. The attenuator is controlled by some form of intensity-selector dial or push button.

The *interrupter switch* controls the duration of the signal that is presented to the patient. The interrupter switch is typically set to the off position for pure-tone signals and is turned on when the presentation button is pressed. The interrupter switch is typically set to the on position for speech signals.

A photograph of an audiometer is shown in Figure 6–2. The appearance of an audiometer and the layout of its dials and buttons vary substantially across manufacturers. Features that are commonly found on most clinical audiometers include:

■ signal selector to choose the type of signal to be presented;
■ signal router to direct the signal to the right ear, left ear, both ears, bone vibrator, loudspeaker, etc.;
■ microphone to present speech;
■ VU meter to monitor the output of the oscillator, microphone, tape player, etc.;
■ external input for tape player or other sound sources;
■ auxiliary output for loudspeakers or other transducers; and
■ patient response indicator to monitor when the patient pushes a patient response button.

Another important component of the audiometer system is the **output transducer**. Transducers are the devices that convert the electrical energy from the audiometer into acoustical or vibratory energy. Transducers used for audiometric purposes are earphones, loudspeakers, or bone-conduction vibrators. Earphones are of two varieties, insert and supra-aural. An insert earphone is a small earphone coupled to the ear canal by means of an ear

A **transducer** is a device that converts one form of energy to another, such as an earphone or bone vibrator.

An older term for supra-aural earphones is circumaural earphones.

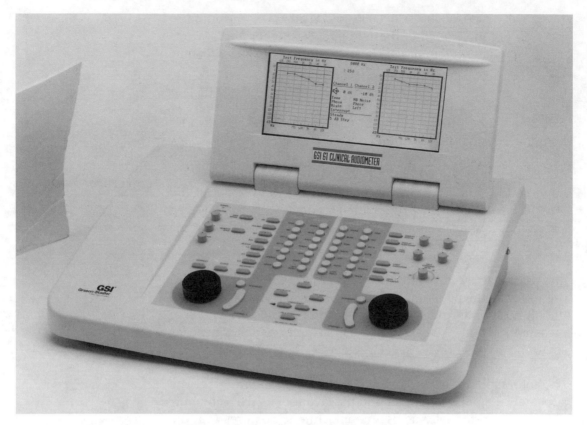

Figure 6-2. Photograph of an audiometer. (Courtesy of Grason-Stadler, Inc.)

insert, which is a device made of foamlike or other soft material used to provide the acoustic coupling between an earphone and the ear canal. A photograph is shown in Figure 6–3. A supra-aural earphone is an earphone mounted in a standard cushion that is placed over the ear. A photograph is shown in Figure 6–4. There are various clinical advantages to using insert earphones over supra-aural earphones. These are delineated in the following Clinical Note. A bone-conduction transducer is a vibrator that is secured to the forehead or mastoid and used to stimulate the cochlea by vibrating the bones of the skull. A photograph is shown in Figure 6–5.

The type of audiometer described and shown here is considered a *manual* audiometer because control over the signal presentation is in the hands of the tester. *Automatic* audiometers also exist. Signal presentation in automatic audiometers is typically under computer control. These devices are often used for screening purposes.

Which Earphones to Use?

Supra-aural, or circumaural, earphones were the standard transducer for many years. In the 1980s, insert earphones arrived on the scene and, in many clinics, became the earphone of choice. Why use one type over the other? There are several important advantages to using insert earphones over supra-aural earphones. They are:

■ **No more collapsing canals**—placement of supra-aural earphones can cause the ear canals to collapse or close. This is especially true in older patients whose ear canal cartilage is more pliable. Collapsed canals generally cause high-frequency conductive hearing loss on the audiogram, a condition that is not experienced in real life without earphones. The alert audiologist will catch this, but it can cause significant consternation during testing. Insert earphones have eliminated this audiometric challenge.

■ **Reduced need for masking**—supra-aural earphones deliver sound to the ear canal, but they also deliver vibration to the skull through the earphone cushion. The more contact the cushion has with the head, the more readily the vibration is transferred. This causes crossover to the other ear, a condition that creates the need to mask or keep the nontest ear busy during audiometric testing. Sound that is delivered to one ear is attenuated or reduced by the head as it crosses over to the other ear. This is called interaural attenuation (IA), or attenuation between the ears. The amount of IA is greater for insert earphones than for supra-aural earphones. This is good news—it means that crossover is less likely, thereby reducing the need to mask.

■ **Enhanced stability of sound delivered to the ear**—earphone placement always affects the intensity of sound delivered to the ear. The size of this effect is smaller with insert earphones than with supra-aural earphones.

Okay, so if insert earphones are so great, why doesn't everyone use them? Good question. There are a few conditions that contraindicate insert earphone use, such as atresia, a stenotic ear canal, or a badly draining ear. For these patients, it is a good idea to keep a set of supra-aural earphones around. Other than that, there are few good reasons to choose supra-aural over insert earphones.

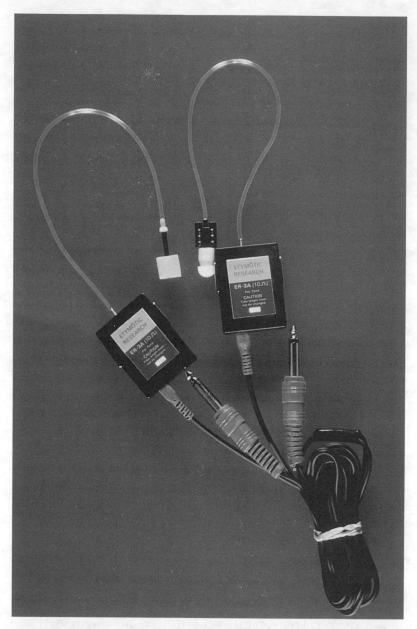

Figure 6–3. Photograph of insert earphones. (Courtesy of Etymotic Research)

PURE-TONE AUDIOMETRY

The Pure-Tone Audiogram

The aim of pure-tone audiometry is to establish hearing threshold sensitivity across the range of audible frequencies important

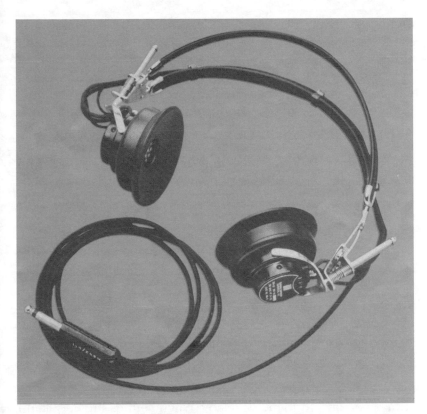

Figure 6-4. Photograph of supra-aural earphones. (Courtesy of Telephonics)

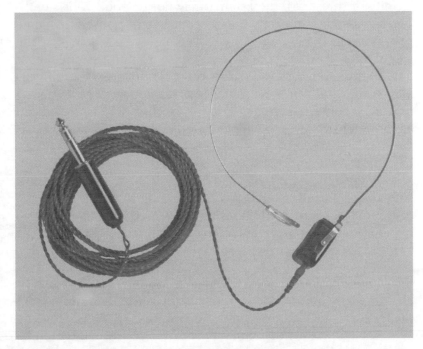

Figure 6-5. Photograph of a bone-conduction transducer.

An **audiogram** depicts the amount of hearing loss across a frequency range of 250 to 8000 Hz.

for human communication. Threshold sensitivity is usually measured for a series of discrete sinusoids or pure tones. The object of pure-tone audiometry is to determine the lowest intensity of such a sinusoid that the listener can "just barely hear." When thresholds have been measured at a number of different sinusoidal frequencies, the results are illustrated graphically, in a frequency-versus-intensity plot, to show how threshold sensitivity changes across the frequency range. This graph is called an **audiogram**. In clinical pure-tone audiometry, thresholds are usually measured at sinusoidal frequencies over the range from 250 Hz at the low end to 8000 Hz at the high end. Within this range, thresholds are determined at octave intervals in the range below 1000 Hz and at mid-octave intervals in the range above 1000 Hz. Thus, the *audiometric frequencies* for conventional pure-tone audiometry are 250, 500, 1000, 1500, 2000, 3000, 4000, 6000, and 8000 Hz.

The concept of threshold as the "just-audible" sound intensity is somewhat more complicated than it seems at first glance. The problem is that, when a sound is very faint, the listener may not hear it every time it is presented. When sounds are fairly loud, they can be presented over and over, and the listener will almost always respond to them. Similarly, when sounds are very faint, they can be presented over and over, and the listener will almost never respond to them. But when the sound intensity is in the vicinity of threshold, the listener may not respond consistently. The same sound intensity might produce a response after some presentations but not after others. Therefore, the search is for the sound intensity that produces a response from the listener about 50% of the time. This is the classical notion of a sensory threshold. Within the range of sound intensities over which the listener's response falls from 100% to 0%, threshold is designated as the intensity level at which response accuracy is about 50%.

A **decibel** is a unit of sound intensity.
Intensity is perceived as loudness.
Frequency is perceived as pitch.

In clinical audiometry, intensity is expressed on a **decibel** (dB) scale relative to "average normal hearing." The zero point on this scale is the **sound intensity** corresponding to the mode of the distribution of threshold intensities measured on a large sample of people with normal hearing. This decibel scale of sound intensities is called the *hearing level* scale, and is abbreviated as the HL scale. An audiogram is a plot of the listener's threshold levels at the various test frequencies, where **frequency** is expressed in Hertz, or Hz, units, and the threshold intensity is expressed on the HL dB scale. Figure 6–6 shows an example of such a plot. The zero line, running horizontally across the top of the graph, is sound intensity corresponding to average normal hearing at each

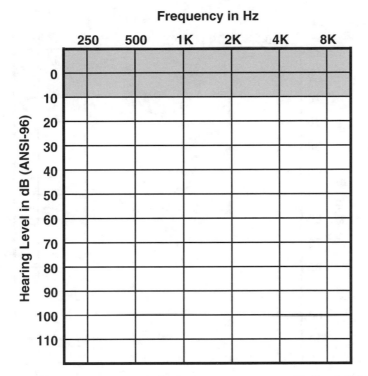

Figure 6–6. An audiogram, with frequency expressed in Hz plotted as a function of intensity expressed in dB HL.

of the test frequencies. Figure 6–7 shows that, for this listener, the threshold at 1000 Hz is 45 dB HL. This means that when 1000 Hz sinusoidal signals were presented to the listener, and the intensity was systematically altered, the threshold, or intensity at which the sound was heard about 50% of the time was at an intensity level 45 dB higher than would be required for a person with average normal hearing.

There are two modes by which pure-tone test signals are presented to the auditory system: through the air via earphones or directly to the bones of the skull via a small vibrator. When test signals are presented by earphones, via the air route, the manner of determining the audiogram is referred to as air-conduction pure-tone audiometry. Through the use of earphones or similar devices, sinusoidal or pure-tone test signals are presented either to the right ear or to the left ear. An audiogram is generated separately for each ear. When test signals are presented via the bone route through a bone vibrator, the manner of determining the audiogram is referred to as bone-conduction pure-tone audiometry.

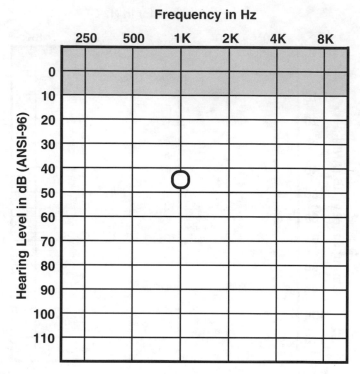

Figure 6–7. An audiogram with a single threshold of 45 dB HL plotted at 1000 Hz.

The complete pure-tone audiogram, then, consists of four different plots, the air-conduction and bone-conduction curves for the right ear and the air-conduction and bone-conduction curves for the left ear. Figure 6–8 illustrates how air- and bone-conduction thresholds are plotted on the audiogram form. The Clinical Note on the next pages shows two different standards that are used to plot audiograms.

The two ears are not completely isolated from one another. Signals presented to one ear can be transmitted, via bone conduction, to the other ear. Therefore, special precautions must be taken when testing one ear to be certain that the other ear is not participating in the response. This is particularly the case with unilateral hearing losses in which one ear has a greater hearing loss than the other. In such a case, the better ear may hear loud sounds presented to the poorer ear. The most common method of prevention is to **mask** the nontest ear with an interfering sound so that it cannot hear the test signal being presented to the test ear. In the case of air-conduction testing, this is done whenever large ear asymmetry exists. In the case of bone-

To **mask** is to introduce sound to one ear while testing the other in an effort to eliminate any influence of crossover of sound from the test ear to the nontest ear.

A Choice of Audiometric Symbols

Although there are standards for audiometric symbols, there are probably as many variations in their use as there are clinics using audiograms. One would think that the standards makers would get the message about what clinicians think of their symbols!

Two different versions of audiometric symbols and audiograms are shown in Figure CN 6–1. One is a standard according to the ASHA. The other is a version of a system that is often used clinically. There are numerous differences between these approaches, including the following:

Separate Graphs for Each Ear? The ASHA system plots both ears on one graph, using separate symbols for each ear for the same type of testing. The clinical system plots each ear separately, using only one symbol for each type of testing. People who ascribe to the single plot believe that it helps them compare ears. Those who ascribe to separating the ears do not think it matters and find the audiogram less cluttered.

Include Masking Levels? The ASHA system includes masking levels so that a record can be kept of the masking level that was used in the nontest ear. This may be useful for teaching purposes or, I suppose, if someone is questioning the validity of the masked thresholds. The clinical system does not record masking levels, under the assumption that audiologists know how to mask effectively and if they are able to successfully mask at a given frequency, then the threshold is masked. In addition, some clinicians use a plateau method, resulting in several effective masking levels from which to choose.

No Response Symbols? The ASHA system records a symbol when the patient does not respond at the limits of the audiometric equipment. This is to signify that testing was actually completed at that level. The clinical system simply does not record a response if none was obtained. The idea here is to reduce clutter on the audiogram and to limit the risk that someone will interpret a no-response symbol as a response symbol. The assumption here, of course is that the clinician is thorough.

A Communication Disorder? Compare the two audiogram systems for results obtained from the same patient, shown in Figure CN 6–2. The clarity of the clinical system is the reason that many clinicians choose to use some variation of it. It is also the reason that the system was used for this textbook. *(continued)*

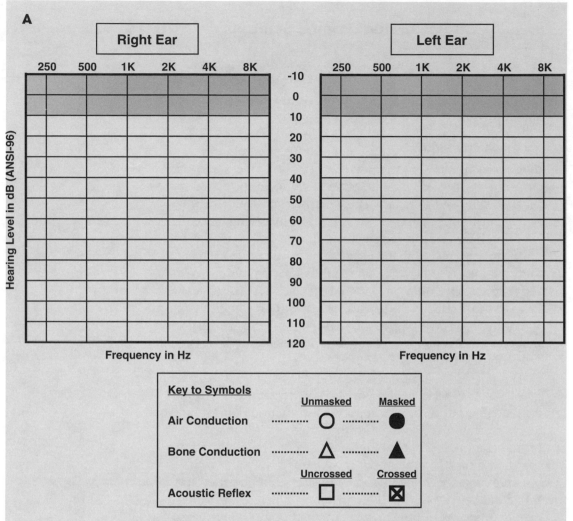

Figure CN 6-1. Clinical version (A) and ASHA standard version (B) of the audiogram and audiometric symbols.

B

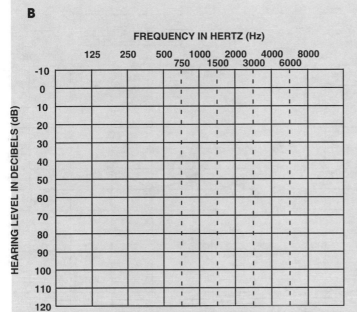

FREQUENCY IN HERTZ (Hz)

EFFECTIVE MASKING LEVELS
TO THE NON-TEST EAR

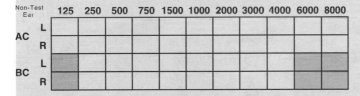

Response

Modality	Ear		
	Left	Unspecified	Right
A C Unmasked	✕		◯
Masked	☐		△
BC - mastoid Unmasked	❭	∧	❬
Masked	❑		❑
BC - forehead Unmasked		∨	
Masked	Γ		⅂
Sound Field	✕	S	∅
Acoustic Reflex Contralateral	⋎		⋏
Ipsilateral	⊢		⊣

No Response

Modality	Ear		
	Left	Unspecified	Right
A C Unmasked	✕		◯
Masked	☐		△
BC - mastoid Unmasked	❭	◆	❬
Masked	❑		❑
BC - forehead Unmasked		∨	
Masked	Γ		⅂
Sound Field	✕	S	∅
Acoustic Reflex Contralateral	⋎		⋏
Ipsilateral	⊢		⊣

(continued)

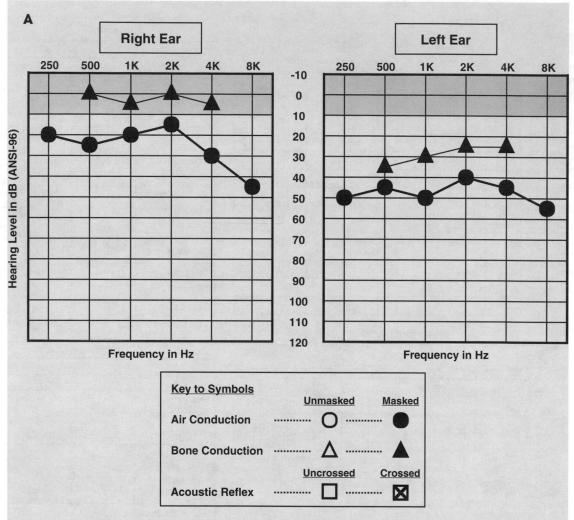

Figure CN 6-2. Audiometric results plotted on the clinical audiogram (A) and on the ASHA standard audiogram (B).

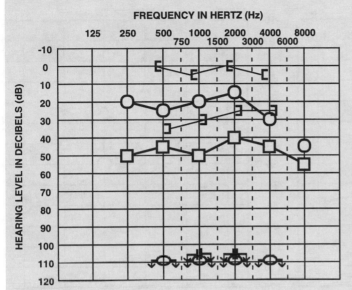

FREQUENCY IN HERTZ (Hz)

Response

Modality	Ear		
	Left	Unspecified	Right
AC			
Unmasked	✕		◯
Masked	☐		△
BC - mastoid			
Unmasked	❭	∧	❬
Masked	]		[
BC - forehead			
Unmasked		∨	
Masked	Γ		⌐
Sound Field	✖	$	∅
Acoustic Reflex			
Contralateral	⟩		⟨
Ipsilateral	⊢		⊣

No Response

Modality	Ear		
	Left	Unspecified	Right
AC			
Unmasked	✕		◯
Masked	☐		△
BC - mastoid			
Unmasked	❭	◈	❬
Masked	]		[
BC - forehead			
Unmasked		∨	
Masked	[		]
Sound Field	✖	$	∅
Acoustic Reflex			
Contralateral	⟩		⟨
Ipsilateral	⊢		⊣

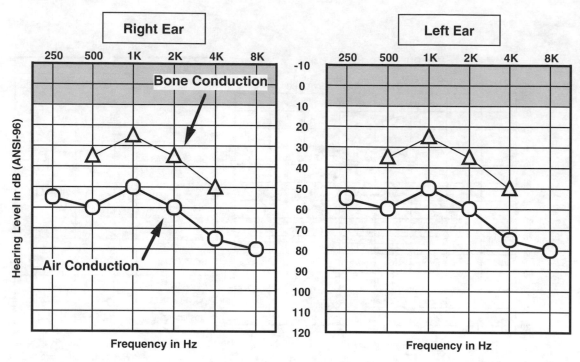

Figure 6-8. Right and left ear audiograms with air conduction and bone conduction thresholds.

conduction testing, however, masking is more often required because of the minimal isolation between ears via bone conduction.

The pure-tone audiogram tells us a number of important things about a person's hearing loss. First, it provides a metric for degree of loss, whether it is:

- minimal (10–25 dB),
- mild (25–40 dB),
- moderate (40–55 dB),
- moderately severe (55–70 dB),
- severe (70–90 dB), or
- profound (more than 90 dB).

Figure 6–9 shows these ranges.

Second, the audiogram describes the shape of loss or the audiometric contour: a hearing loss may be the same at all frequencies and have a flat configuration; the loss may also increase as the curve moves from the low-frequency region to the high-frequency region and have a downward sloping contour; or

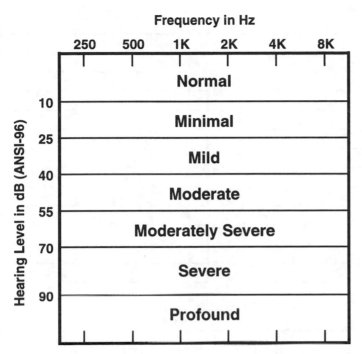

Figure 6–9. Degrees of hearing loss plotted on an audiogram.

the degree of loss may decrease as the curve moves from the low- to the high-frequency region and have a rising contour (Figure 6–10).

Third, the audiogram provides a measure of **interaural symmetry**, or the extent to which hearing sensitivity is the same in both ears or better in one than the other (Figure 6–11).

Interaural means between the ears.

Fourth, the combination of air- and bone-conduction audiometry allows the differentiation of hearing loss into one of three types (Figure 6–12):

■ conductive,
■ sensorineural, or
■ mixed.

These are the three major categories of **peripheral hearing loss**. *Conductive* losses result from problems in the external ear canal or, more typically, from disorders of the middle-ear vibratory system. *Sensorineural* losses result from disorders in the cochlea or auditory nerve. The audiometric signature of a conductive hearing loss is reduced sensitivity via the air-conduction route, but relatively normal sensitivity via the bone conduction route.

A **peripheral hearing loss** can be conductive, sensorineural, or mixed.

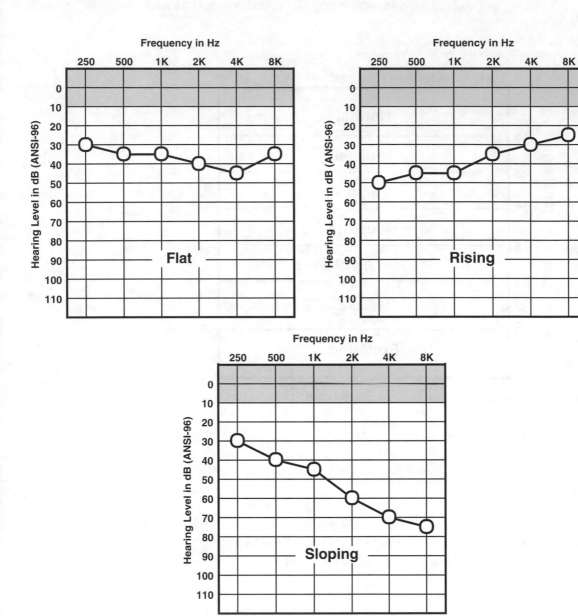

Figure 6-10. Three audiometric configurations: flat, rising, and sloping.

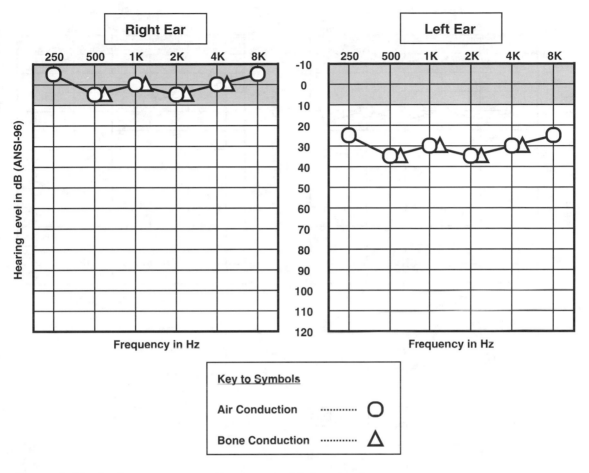

Figure 6-11. Audiogram representing asymmetric hearing loss.

Remember that the air-conduction loss reflects disorders along the entire conductive and sensorineural systems from middle ear to cochlea to auditory nerve. The bone conduction loss, however, reflects only a disorder in the cochlea and auditory nerve. The bone-conducted signal goes directly to the cochlea, in effect by-passing the external and middle-ear portions of the auditory system. Strictly speaking, this is not quite true. Changes in middle-ear dynamics do affect bone-conduction sensitivity in predictable ways, but as a first approximation, this is a useful way of thinking about the difference between conductive and sen-sorineural audiograms. Comparisons of the air-conduction and bone-conduction threshold curves provide us with the broad category of type of loss. In a pure conductive loss, there is reduced sensitivity by air conduction but relatively normal sensitivity by bone conduction. In a pure sensorineural loss, however, both

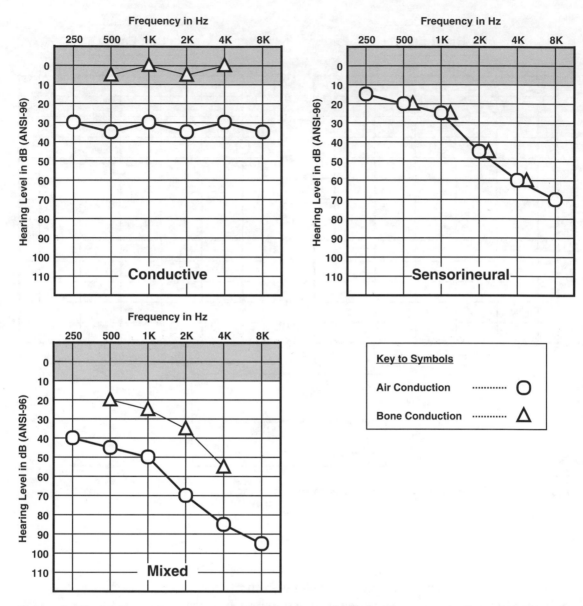

Figure 6-12. Audiograms representing three types of hearing loss: conductive, sensorineural, and mixed.

air-conduction and bone-conduction sensitivity are reduced equally. If there is a loss by both air and bone conduction, but more loss by air than by bone, then the loss is categorized as *mixed.* In a mixed loss, there is both a conductive and a sensorineural component.

Establishing the Pure-Tone Audiogram

Establishing a pure-tone audiogram is the cornerstone of a hearing evaluation. Simple in concept and strategy, it can also be the most difficult of all measures in the audiologic battery. The paradox is complete. On one hand, pure-tone audiometry is so structured and rule-driven that it can be automated easily for computer-based testing. On the other hand, pure-tone audiometry is so challenging that it takes years to master its nuances.

The establishment of pure-tone thresholds is based on a psychophysical paradigm that is a modified method of limits. Although the precise strategy may vary among audiologists, the following strategies and conventions generally apply:

1. Test the better ear first. Based on the patient's report, the better ear should be chosen to begin testing. Knowledge of the better-ear thresholds becomes important later for masking purposes. If hearing is reported to be the same in both ears, begin with the right ear.
2. Begin threshold search at 1000 Hz. This is a relatively easy signal to perceive, and it is often a frequency at which better hearing occurs. You must begin somewhere, and clinical experience suggests that this is a good place to start.
3. Continuous or pulsed tones should be presented for about 1 second. Pulsed tones are often easier for the listener to perceive and can be achieved manually or, on most audiometers, automatically.
4. Begin presenting signals at an intensity level at which the patient can clearly hear. This gives the patient experience listening to the signal of interest. If you anticipate from the case history and from conversing with the patient that hearing is going to be normal or near normal, then begin by testing at 40 dB HL. If you anticipate that the patient has a mild hearing impairment, then begin at a higher intensity level, say 60 dB, and so on.
5. If the patient does not respond, increase the intensity level by 20 dB until a response occurs. Once the patient responds to the signal, threshold search begins.

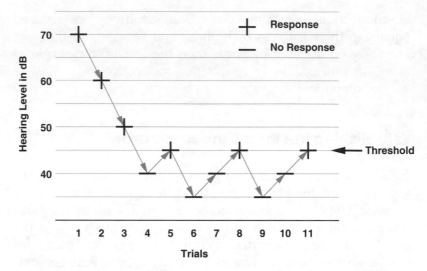

Figure 6–13. Schematic representation of a threshold search, showing the "down -10, up -5" strategy for bracketing hearing threshold level.

6. Threshold search follows the "down 10, up 5" rule. This rule states that if the patient hears the tone, intensity is decreased by 10 dB, and if the patient does not hear the tone, intensity is increased by 5 dB. This threshold search is illustrated in Figure 6–13.

7. Threshold is considered to be the lowest level at which the patient perceives the tone about 50% of the time (either 2 out of 4 or 3 out of 6 presentations).

8. Once threshold has been established at 1000 Hz, proceed to test 2000, 3000, 4000, 6000, 8000, 1000 (again), 500, and 250 Hz. Repeat testing at 1000 Hz in the first ear tested to ensure that the response is not slightly better now that the patient has learned the task.

9. Test the other ear in the same manner.

Air Conduction

Hearing thresholds by air conduction are established to describe hearing sensitivity for the entire auditory system. Air-conduction testing provides an assessment of the functional integrity of the outer, middle, and inner ears. The term *air conduction* is used because signals are presented through the air via earphones.

As you learned earlier, there are two major types of air-conduction transducers, supra-aural earphones and insert earphones. Examples are shown in Figures 6–3 and 6–4. Supra-aural earphones are mounted in cushions that are placed over the outer ear. This type of earphone was the standard for many years. It had as its advantages ease of placement over the ears and ease of **calibration**.

Calibration is the process of adjusting the output of an instrument to a known standard.

The newer type of earphone is called an insert earphone. An insert earphone consists of a loudspeaker mounted in a small box that sends the acoustic signal through a tube to a cuff that is inserted into the ear canal. Insert earphones are becoming a new standard for clinical use. As you learned in the Clinical Note on page 197, insert earphones have several advantages related to sound isolation and interaural attenuation.

If a patient has normal outer and middle ear function, then air-conduction thresholds will tell the entire story about hearing sensitivity of the cochlea. If a patient has a disorder of outer or middle ear function, then air conduction thresholds reflect the additive effects of (1) any sensorineural loss due to inner-ear disorder and (2) any conductive loss imposed by outer- or middle-ear disorder. Bone-conduction testing must be completed to separate the contribution of the two disorders to the overall extent of the loss.

Bone Conduction

Bone-conduction thresholds are established in a manner similar to air-conduction thresholds, but with a different transducer. In this case, a bone vibrator (shown previously in Figure 6–5) is used to generate vibrations of the skull and stimulate the cochlea directly. Theoretically, thresholds by bone conduction reflect function of the cochlea, regardless of the status of the outer or middle ears (Clinical Note on page 216 explains the exceptions). Therefore, if a person has normal middle ear function on one day and middle-ear disorder on the next, hearing by bone conduction will be unchanged, while hearing by air conduction will be adversely affected.

The bone-conduction transducer has changed little over the years, and the only real decisions that have to be made are related to vibrator placement and masking issues. Some clinicians choose to place the vibrator on the mastoid-bone prominence behind the pinna, so called mastoid placement. Others choose to place it on the forehead. There are advantages to each as described in the Clinical Note on page 217.

Contributors to Bone Conduction Hearing

When a sound is delivered to the skull through a bone vibrator, the cochlea is stimulated in several ways. The primary stimulation of the cochlea occurs when the temporal bone vibrates, causing displacement of the cochlear partition. A secondary stimulation occurs as a result of the middle-ear component, due to a lag between the vibrating mastoid process and the vibrating ossicular chain. This is referred to as inertial bone-conduction. That is, the ossicles are moving relative to the head, thereby stimulating the cochlea. A third, and minor, component of bone conducted hearing is sometimes referred to as osseotympanic bone conduction. Here, the vibration of the external ear canal wall is radiated into the ear canal and tranduced by the tympanic membrane.

The result of all of this is that most of the hearing measured by bone conduction is due to direct stimulation of the cochlea—most, but not all. Therefore, in certain circumstances, a disorder of the middle ear can reduce the inertial and osseotympanic components of bone conduction, resulting in an apparent sensorineural component to the hearing loss. We often see this in patients with otosclerosis. They show a hearing loss by bone conduction around 2000 Hz, the so-called Carhart's notch. Once surgery is performed to free the ossicular chain, the "sensorineural" component to the loss disappears. Actually, what appears to occur is that the inertial component to bone-conducted hearing that was reduced by stapes fixation is restored.

Masking

Crossover results when sound presented to one ear through an earphone crosses the head via bone conduction and is perceived by the other ear.

Air-conduction and bone-conduction pure-tone audiometry are often confounded by **crossover** or *contralateralization* of the signal. A signal that is presented to one ear, if it is of sufficient magnitude, can be perceived by the other ear. This is known as crossover of the signal. Suppose, for example, that a patient has normal hearing in the right ear and a profound hearing loss in the left ear. When tones presented to the left ear reach a certain level, they will cross over the head and be heard by the right ear. As a result, although you may be trying to test the left ear, you will actually be testing the right ear because the signal is crossing the head.

Where to Place the Bone Vibrator?

Just like there are Democrats and Republicans, there are audiologists who "do bone" from the forehead and those who "do bone" from the mastoid. Does it matter?

Remember that, regardless of where a bone vibrator is placed on the skull, both cochleas are likely to be stimulated to the same degree. Actually, there is a little interaural attenuation of high-frequency signals when the bone is placed on the mastoid, but it is negligible for lower frequencies. So, how do you choose?

Those who ascribe to mastoid placement cite the following advantages. First, because there is a little interaural attenuation in the high frequencies, you get a little more isolation of the cochlea on the side with the bone vibrator. This may help to reduce the need for masking or to make it easier in some situations. Second, you get slightly better thresholds from mastoid placement, an important factor when a hearing loss is near the level of the maximum output of the bone vibrator. You may be able to measure that threshold with mastoid placement but not with forehead placement.

Most of those who ascribe to forehead placement believe that you should always mask when testing by bone conduction. They say that counting on some level of interaural attenuation is a waste of time and that you should simply always mask. This being the case, forehead placement is simply convenient. When immittance audiometry shows a middle ear disorder, the patient can be placed into the test booth, insert earphones placed into the ears, and a bone vibrator placed on the forehead. Testing of the right ear by bone conduction then simply requires the introduction of masking into the left ear and vice versa. Forehead audiologists cannot understand why mastoid audiologists would want to go back and forth into the test room to fumble with the bone vibrator and masking earphone to switch mastoids.

In terms of thoroughness and care in bone conduction testing, the forehead audiologists probably have the right idea. They create norms for bone-conduction testing by always testing with earphones occluding the ear canals and masking in the nontest ear. In that way, no corrections need to be made for occluding the ears or for introducing masking. This can be done with mastoid testing, but it is slightly more inconvenient. The seasoned audiologist will be prepared to use either mastoid or forehead placement, depending on the nature of the clinical question.

Table 6-1. Lowest values of interaural attenuation for three types of transducers.

Frequency (Hz)	Supra-aural (TDH-49)	Insert (ER-3A)	Bone Vibrator
250	40	75	
500	40	75	0
1000	40	60	0
2000	45	55	0
4000	50	65	0
8000	50	65	

When crossover has occurred, you need to isolate the ear that you are trying to test by *masking* the other (nontest) ear. Masking is a procedure wherein noise is placed in one ear to keep it occupied while the other ear is being tested. In the current example, the right, or normal hearing, ear would need to be masked by introducing sufficient noise to keep it occupied while the left ear was being tested. With appropriate masking noise in the right ear, the left ear can be isolated for determination of thresholds.

Interaural attenuation (IA) is the reduction in sound energy of a signal as it is transmitted by bone conduction from one side of the head to the opposite ear.

One of the most important concepts related to masking is that of **interaural attenuation**. The term interaural attenuation was coined to describe the amount of reduction in intensity (attenuation) that occurs as a signal crosses over the head from one ear to the other (interaural or between ears). Using our example, let us say that the right ear threshold is 10 dB and the left ear threshold is 100 dB at 1000 Hz. As you try to establish threshold in the left ear, the patient responds at a level of, say, 70 dB, because the tone crosses the head and is heard by the right ear. The amount of interaural attenuation in this case is 60 dB (70 dB threshold in the unmasked left ear minus 10 dB threshold in the right ear). That is, the signal level being presented to the left ear was reduced or attenuated by 60 dB as it crossed the head.

The amount of interaural attenuation depends on the type of transducer used. Table 6–1 shows the amount of interaural attenuation for three different types of transducers: supra-aural earphones, insert earphones, and bone-conduction vibrators. Insert earphones have the highest amount of interaural attenuation and, thus, the lowest risk of crossover. This is related to the amount of vibration that is delivered by the transducer to the skin surface. An insert earphone produces sound vibration in a loudspeaker that is separated from the insert portion by a relatively long tube. Very little of the insert is in contact with the skin, and the amount of vibration transferred from it to the skull is minimal. Supra-aural earphones are in contact with more of the surface of the skin, thereby reducing the amount of inter-aural attenuation and increasing the risk of crossover. A bone-conduction transducer vibrates the skin and skull directly, resulting in the lowest amount of interaural attenuation and the highest risk of crossover.

The need to mask the nontest ear is related to the amount of interaural attenuation. If the difference in thresholds between ears exceeds the amount of interaural attenuation, then there is a possibility that the nontest rather than the test ear is responding. Minimum levels of interaural attenuation are usually set to provide guidance as to when crossover may be occurring. These levels are set as a function of transducer type as follows:

Supra-aural earphones:	40 dB
Insert earphones:	50 dB
Bone-conduction vibrator:	0 dB

Thus, if you are using supra-aural earphones, crossover may occur when the threshold from one ear exceeds the threshold from the other ear by 40 dB or more. If you are using insert earphones, crossover may occur if inter-ear asymmetry exceeds 50 dB. If you are using a bone-conduction vibrator, crossover may occur at any time, since the signal is not necessarily attenuated as it crosses the head. These minimum interaural attenuation levels dictate when masking should be used.

Air-Conduction Masking. Masking should be used during air-conduction audiometry whenever the air-conducted threshold of the ear under test exceeds the bone-conduction threshold of the nontest ear by more than the minimum interaural attenuation levels. For example, say you have established air-conduction thresholds in the right ear to be 0 dB throughout the frequency range. Because bone-conduction thresholds cannot be poorer than air-conduction thresholds, then bone-conduction thresholds for that ear are somewhere between 0 and −10 dB. If you are using insert earphones and are testing the left ear, you know that thresholds are valid for the left ear if they are within 50 dB of the right-ear bone-conduction thresholds. You know this because 50 dB is the minimum interaural attenuation for insert earphones. Therefore, if a threshold in the left ear is 50 dB or better, you can safely assume that no masking is needed and that the response is truly a threshold from the left ear. If, however, the threshold exceeds 50 dB, then it could be a response from the right ear due to crossover, and masking is necessary.

The rule for air-conduction masking is relatively simple: *if the thresholds from the test ear exceed the bone-conduction thresholds of the nontest ear by the amount of minimum interaural attenuation, then masking must be used.* An important caveat is that, even though you are testing by air conduction, the critical difference is between the air-conduction thresholds of the test ear and the bone-conduction thresholds of the nontest ear. Remember that the signal crossing over is from vibrations transferred from the transducer to the skull. These vibrations are perceived by the opposite cochlea directly, not by the opposite outer ear. Therefore, if the nontest ear has an air-conduction threshold of 30 dB and a bone-conduction threshold of 0 dB, then masking should be used if the test ear has a threshold of 50 dB, not 80 dB.

It is typical in pure-tone audiometry to establish air-conduction thresholds in the better ear first, followed by air-conducted thresholds in the poorer ear. In many instances this procedure works well. Problems arise when the better ear has a conductive hearing loss, and the air-conduction thresholds are not reflective of the bone-conduction thresholds for that ear. Once bone-conduction thresholds are ultimately established, air-conduction thresholds may need to be re-established if the thresholds from one ear turn out to have exceeded the bone-conduction thresholds from the other ear by more than minimum interaural attenuation.

Bone-Conduction Masking. Masking should be used during bone-conduction audiometry under most circumstances, because the amount of interaural attenuation is negligible. For example, if you place the bone vibrator on the right mastoid, it may stimulate both cochleas identically because there is no attenuation of the signal as it crosses the head. In reality, there is some amount of interaural attenuation of the bone-conducted signal. However, the amount is small enough that it is safest to assume that there is no attenuation and simply always mask during bone-conduction testing. Some clinicians choose to surrender to this notion and test with the bone vibrator placed on the forehead, always masking the non-test ear. You have already discovered the relative merits of bone-vibrator placement in the Clinical Note on page 217.

The rule for bone-conduction masking is very simple: *always use masking in the nontest ear during bone conduction testing.* It is safest

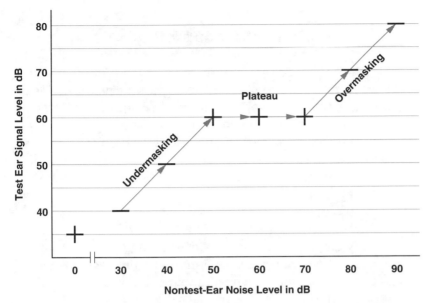

Figure 6–14. Schematic representation of the plateau method of masking. The patient responds to a pure-tone signal presented at 30 dB with no masking in the nontest ear. When 30 dB of masking is introduced, the patient no longer responds, indicating that the initial response was heard in the nontest ear. During the undermasking phase, the patient responds as the pure-tone level is increased but discontinues responding when masking is increased by the same amount. Threshold for the test ear is at the level of the plateau, or 60 dB. At the plateau, the patient continues to respond as masking level is increased in the nontest ear. During overmasking, the patient discontinues responding as masking level is increased.

to assume that no interaural attenuation occurs and that the risk of testing the nontest ear is omnipresent.

Masking Strategies. Once the determination of a need for masking has been made, several techniques can be used for effective masking. One that has stood the test of time is called the **plateau method**, depicted in Figure 6–14. The plateau method can be used for air-conduction and bone-conduction threshold testing. Details of the method are described in the Clinical Note on pages 222–223.

Briefly, threshold for a given pure tone is established in the test ear, narrow-band noise is presented to the nontest ear, and threshold is re-established in the test ear. If the nontest ear is responding, the presence of masking noise in that ear will shift the threshold in the test ear, and the patient will stop responding. The level of the pure tone is then increased and presented. If the

The **plateau method** Is a method of masking the nontest ear in which masking is introduced progressively over a range of intensity levels until a plateau is reached, indicating the level of masked threshold of the test ear.

The Plateau Method

Students who become audiologists will eventually learn how to mask. This will be no easy task at first. The idea seems simple—keep one ear busy while you test the other. But there is a significant challenge in doing that. You must ensure that you have enough masking to keep the nontest ear busy, but you must also ensure that you do not have too much masking in the nontest ear or you will begin to mask the ear you are trying to test.

Throughout your career as a student, you will encounter a number of clinical supervisors, all of whom have a slightly different approach to determining what is effective masking. They will give you formulas and provide you with shortcuts that will be mind-numbing at first. Trust them—they mean well.

There is one masking strategy that you can always count on. It is called the plateau method. A graphic representation of the plateau method is shown in Figure 6–14. The technique is fairly straightforward. First, you establish threshold in the test ear. Then you increase masking noise in the nontest ear. At first, you will likely be undermasking; that is, you will not be presenting masking noise sufficient to occupy the nontest ear. As you increase the masking in the nontest ear, the threshold in the test ear will change accordingly because you are actually testing the nontest ear. When you reach the plateau of the function, you will actually be testing the test ear, and the nontest ear will be effectively masked. This is the threshold for the test ear. Trust me. As you increase the masking beyond a certain level, the masking noise begins to cross over the head, interfering with the test ear, and threshold for the test ear begins to change again as you increase the masking noise. This is called overmasking.

It is just that simple. Learn the plateau method and you will conquer masking. The figure on the facing page is a plateau form that you can sneak into the clinic and use to ensure that you are masking effectively. There are even audiologists who use this approach routinely. They plot a plateau when masking bone conduction and save the plateau form in the patient file as verification that effective masking was achieved.

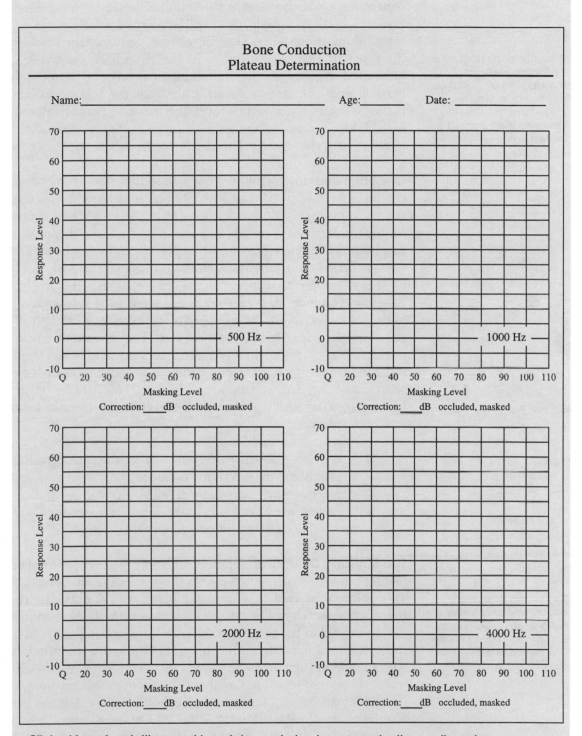

Bone Conduction
Plateau Determination

Name:_____ Age:_____ Date:_____

500 Hz

Response Level

Masking Level

Correction:____dB occluded, masked

1000 Hz

Response Level

Masking Level

Correction:____dB occluded, masked

2000 Hz

Response Level

Masking Level

Correction:____dB occluded, masked

4000 Hz

Response Level

Masking Level

Correction:____dB occluded, masked

Clinical form for plotting masking plateaus during bone-conduction audiometry.

patient responds, the masking level is increased and so on. Eventually a level of *effective masking* will be reached where increasing the masking noise will no longer result in a shift of threshold in the test ear. This is referred to as the *plateau* of the masking function and signifies that the nontest ear has been effectively masked and that responses are truly from the test ear. When masking is raised above this level, the masking noise itself may exceed the interaural attenuation value and actually cross over to interfere with the test ear. This is referred to as **overmasking**.

Overmasking results when the intensity level of masking in the nontest ear is sufficient to cross over to the test ear, thereby elevating the threshold in the test ear.

One other masking technique that is used for establishing bone-conduction thresholds is the sensorineural acuity level (SAL) test. For conventional bone-conduction testing, pure tones are presented through the bone vibrator and masking noise through an earphone. The bone vibrator is often placed on the forehead, and noise is presented to the nontest ear to mask it. The SAL test is done in the opposite manner. Threshold is established in the test ear by air conduction. Bone-conducted noise is then introduced to the bone vibrator on the forehead at a maximum level, and air-conduction thresholds are re-established. The amount of threshold shift that occurs is then compared to a normative level, and the conductive component is calculated. A more thorough description of the SAL can be found in the Clinical Note on the facing page. The SAL test is a very useful clinical technique for at least three reasons:

- it is often a much easier task for young children than conventional masked bone conduction,
- it may be more accurate for small air-bone gaps, and
- it serves as a valuable cross-check for conventional masked bone-conduction audiometry.

The Masking Dilemma. A point can be reached where masked testing cannot be completed due to the size of the air-bone gap. This is often referred to as a *masking dilemma. A* **masking dilemma** occurs when the difference between the bone-conduction threshold in the test ear and the air-conduction threshold in the nontest ear approaches the amount of interaural attenuation. An example of such an audiogram is shown in Figure 6–15. Unmasked bone-conduction thresholds for the right ear are around 0 dB. Unmasked air-conduction thresholds for the left ear are around 60 dB. If we wish to mask the left ear and establish either air-conduction or bone-conduction thresholds in the right ear, we are in trouble from the start, because we need to introduce masking to the left ear at 70 dB, a level that could cross over the head and mask the ear that we are trying to test.

A **masking dilemma** occurs when both ears have large air-bone gaps, and masking can only be introduced at a level that results in overmasking.

The SAL Test

There is another way to estimate the size of an air-bone gap. It is an old test called the sensorineural acuity level (SAL) test. The SAL test is a very handy strategy to have around when conventional bone conduction fails you. There are at least three clinical challenges for which the SAL test can be particularly useful:

- testing young children;
- measuring small air-bone gaps; and
- solving masking dilemmas.

Some young children cannot handle the masking task used in conventional bone-conduction testing. That is, listening to masking in one ear and pure tones in the other can be confusing for children. The SAL is a different perceptual task and can often be obtained in children when masked bone conduction cannot. In addition, SAL seems to be as good or better at resolving small air-bone gaps, and it is occasionally useful in solving masking dilemmas.

What is the SAL test? How does one do it? The SAL test is a technique used to determine the amount of conductive component to a hearing loss. Unlike conventional bone-conduction testing in which pure tones are presented via the bone vibrator and masking noise via an earphone, in the SAL test, masking noise is delivered via the bone vibrator, and pure-tones are presented via the earphone.

Here is how it works. Threshold is established in the ear of interest via air conduction at a specific frequency. Narrow band noise centered at that frequency is introduced at its maximum level via the bone vibrator, and the threshold is re-established via air conduction. If the threshold does not shift, the loss is sensorineural. If the threshold shifts, the loss is conductive. The amount of shift can be compared to a normal shift, and an air bone gap can be estimated. Got it?

Try this: The figure on the next page shows the results from a patient with a sensorineural hearing loss and a patient with a conductive hearing loss. In the case of the sensorineural hearing loss, the masking noise introduced via the bone vibrator has no influence on threshold, because the cochlear hearing loss precludes perception of the noise, and no shift in air-conducted hearing occurs. In contrast,

(continued)

Sensorineural Acuity Level	Conduc-tive	Sensori-neural
AC threshold in quiet	a 25	25
AC threshold in max BC noise	b 60	25
SAL norm	c 35	35
Conductive component (b-c)	d 25	0
SAL threshold (a-d)	0	25

SAL results from a patient with a sensorineural hearing loss and a patient with a conductive hearing loss.

because the patient with the conductive hearing loss has a normal cochlea, the bone-conducted noise masks the cochlea, and the threshold via air conduction shifts accordingly.

There are two things left to do before you get started on the SAL. The first is to determine the maximum bone-conduction level for each narrow-band-noise signal. This is simple. Place the bone vibrator on your forehead and increase the intensity to a level just below that which causes a tactile sensation. If you can feel the bone vibrator vibrating, you are at too high a level. Note the highest level that can be achieved for each frequency. Now you need to determine the SAL norm. Grab 10 of your young, normal-hearing friends. Determine the air-conduction threshold at 1000 Hz. Then determine the threshold again with a 1000 Hz narrow-band noise presented at its maximum level via the bone vibrator placed on the forehead. The difference between the threshold in quiet and the threshold in noise is the SAL norm. Repeat this for all test frequencies. Determine the average SAL norm at each frequency across all 10 of your friends. You are now ready to become a master of bone conduction.

Just in case this is not altogether clear, The figure on the facing page is a computation form that you can use for determining the SAL. Notice that you can also obtain a speech SAL, a particularly useful tool for testing children.

Sensorineural Acuity Level (SAL)
Computation Form

Name:_____ Age:_____ Date: _____

Right Ear	500 Hz	1000 Hz	2000 Hz	4000 Hz	ST
AC Threshold in Quiet **a**					
Max BC Level	45	55	60	60	50
AC Threshold in BC Noise **b**					
SAL Norm **c**	30	35	45	40	30
Conductive Component (b - c) **d**					
SAL Threshold (a - d)					

Left Ear	500 Hz	1000 Hz	2000 Hz	4000 Hz	ST
AC Threshold in Quiet **a**					
Max BC Level	45	55	60	60	50
AC Threshold in BC Noise **b**					
SAL Norm **c**	30	35	45	40	30
Conductive Component (b - c) **d**					
SAL Threshold (a - d)					

Occlusion-effect correction for conductive losses:
Add to 10 dB to conductive component (d) at 500 Hz; 5 at 1000 Hz

Clinical form for computing the SAL.

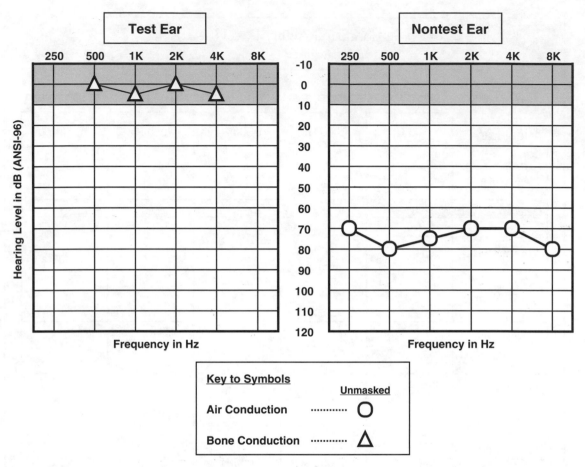

Figure 6-15. An audiogram representing the masking dilemma, in which overmasking occurs as soon as masking noise is introduced into the nontest ear.

Summary

- An audiometer is an electronic instrument used by an audiologist to quantify hearing.
- An audiometer produces pure tones of various frequencies and other signals, attenuates them to various intensity levels, and delivers them to transducers.
- An important component of the audiometer system is the output transducer, which converts electrical energy from the audiometer into acoustical or vibratory energy. Transducers used for audiometric purposes are earphones, loudspeakers, and bone-conduction vibrators.
- The aim of pure-tone audiometry is to establish hearing threshold sensitivity across the range of audible frequencies important for human communication.

- Establishing a pure-tone audiogram is the cornerstone of a hearing evaluation.
- The establishment of pure-tone thresholds is based on a psychophysical paradigm that is a modified method of limits.
- Hearing thresholds by air conduction are established to describe hearing sensitivity for the entire auditory system.
- Hearing thresholds by bone conduction reflect function of the cochlea, regardless of the status of the outer or middle ears.
- Air-conduction and bone-conduction pure-tone audiometry are often confounded by *crossover* or *contralateralization* of the signal.
- When crossover has occurred, the test ear needs to be isolated by *masking* the other (nontest) ear.

SPEECH AUDIOMETRY

Speech audiometry is a key component of audiologic assessment. Because it uses the kinds of auditory signals present in everyday communication, speech audiometry can tell us, in a more realistic manner than with pure tones, how an auditory disorder might impact the communicative problems of daily living. Also, the influence of speech processing can be detected at virtually every level of the auditory system. Speech measures can thus be used diagnostically to examine processing ability and the manner in which it is affected by disorders of the middle ear, cochlea, auditory nerve, brain stem pathways, and auditory centers in the cortex. In addition, there is a predictable relation between a person's hearing for pure tones and hearing for speech. Thus, speech audiometric testing can serve as a cross-check on the validity of the pure-tone audiogram.

The goal of **speech audiometry** is to quantify a patient's ability to understand everyday communication.

In many ways, speech audiometry can be thought of as our best friend in the clinic. Young children usually respond more easily to the presentation of speech materials than to pure tones. As a result, estimates of thresholds for speech recognition are often sought first in children to provide the audiologist guidance in establishing pure-tone thresholds. In adults, suprathreshold speech understanding may be a sensitive indicator of retrocochlear disorder, even in the presence of normal hearing sensitivity. A thorough assessment of speech understanding in such patients may assist in the diagnosis of neurologic disease. In elderly individuals, speech audiometry is a vital component in our understanding of the patient's communication function. The degree of hearing impairment described by pure-tone thresholds often underestimates the amount of communication disorder that a patient has, and suprathreshold speech audiometry can provide a better metric for understanding the degree of hearing impairment resulting from the disorder.

Uses of Speech Audiometry

Speech audiometric measures are used routinely in an audiologic evaluation and contribute in a number of important ways, including:

- measurement of threshold for speech
- cross-check of pure-tone sensitivity
- quantification of suprathreshold speech recognition ability
- assistance in differential diagnosis
- assessment of central auditory processing ability
- estimation of communicative function

Speech Thresholds

A *speech threshold* is the lowest level at which speech can be detected or recognized. The threshold of detection is referred to as the *speech awareness threshold* (SAT) or, less commonly, the *speech detection threshold* (SDT). The threshold of recognition is often referred to as a **spondee threshold (ST)** or a **speech-recognition threshold (SRT)**. The ST is a measure of the threshold of sensitivity for hearing and identifying speech signals. Even in isolation, the ST provides significant information. It estimates hearing sensitivity in the frequency region of the audiogram where the major components of speech fall, thereby providing a useful estimate of degree of hearing loss for speech.

ST or **SRT** is the threshold level for speech recognition, expressed as the lowest intensity level at which 50% of spondaic words can be identified.

Pure-Tone Cross-Check

Often the audiologist will establish an ST first to provide guidance as to the level at which pure-tone thresholds are likely to fall. The ST should agree closely with the pure-tone thresholds averaged across 500, 1000, and 2000 Hz (**pure-tone average** or PTA). That is, if both the pure-tone intensity levels and the speech intensity levels are expressed on the dB HL scale, the degree of hearing loss for speech should agree with the degree of hearing loss for pure tones in the 500 through 2000 Hz region. In

The **pure-tone average** is the average of thresholds obtained at 500, 1000, and 2000 Hz, and should closely agree with the ST or SRT.

practice, speech signals seem to be easier to process and sometimes result in lower initial estimates of threshold than testing with pure tones. In such a case, the audiologist will be alerted to the fact that the pure-tone thresholds may actually be suprathreshold and that the patient will need to be reinstructed. The extreme case of this is the patient who is feigning a hearing loss, often called malingering. In the case of malingering, the ST may be substantially better than the PTA.

Speech Recognition

Pure-tone audiometry and speech awareness thresholds characterize the lowest level at which a person can detect sound, but they provide little insight into how a patient hears above threshold, at suprathreshold levels. Speech recognition testing is designed to provide an estimate of suprathreshold ability to recognize speech. In its most fundamental form, speech recognition testing involves the presentation of single syllable words at a fixed intensity level above threshold. This is often referred to as speech discrimination testing or word-recognition testing. The patient is asked to repeat the words that are presented, and a percentage-correct score is calculated.

Results of word-recognition testing are generally predictable from the degree and configuration of the pure-tone audiogram. It is in this predictability that the value of the test lies. If word recognition scores equal or exceed those that might be expected from the audiogram, then suprathreshold speech recognition ability is thought to be normal for the degree of hearing loss. If word recognition scores are poorer than would be expected, then suprathreshold ability is abnormal for the degree of hearing loss. Abnormal speech recognition is often the result of cochlear distortion or retrocochlear disorder. Thus, word-recognition testing can be useful in providing estimates of communication function and in assisting in the diagnosis of neurologic disorder.

Differential Diagnosis

Speech audiometric measures can be useful in differentiating whether a hearing disorder is due to changes in the outer or middle ear, cochlea, or auditory peripheral or central nervous systems. Again, in the cases of cochlear disorder, word-recognition ability is usually predictable from the degree and slope of the audiogram. Although there are some exceptions, such as hearing loss due to **endolymphatic hydrops**, word recognition ability and performance on other forms of speech audiometric measures are

Endolymphatic hydrops is the cause of Ménière's disease.

highly correlated with degree of hearing impairment in certain frequency regions. When performance is poorer than expected, the likely culprit is a disorder of the VIIIth nerve or central auditory nervous system structures. Thus, unusually poor performance on speech audiometric tests lends a measure of suspicion about the site of the disorder causing the hearing impairment.

Central Auditory Processing

Speech audiometric measures also permit us to evaluate the ability of the central auditory nervous system to process acoustic signals. As neural impulses travel from the cochlea through the VIIIth nerve to the auditory brain stem and cortex, the number and complexity of neural pathways expands progressively. The system, in its vastness of pathways, includes a certain level of redundancy or excess capacity of processing ability. Such redundancy serves many useful purposes, but it also makes the function of the central auditory nervous system somewhat impervious to our efforts to examine it. For example, a patient can have a rather substantial lesion of the auditory brain stem or auditory cortex and still have normal hearing and normal word-recognition ability. As a result, we have to sensitize the speech audiometric measures in some way before we can peer into the brain and understand its function and disorder.

With the use of advanced speech audiometric measures, we are able to measure central auditory nervous system function, often referred to as central auditory processing ability. Such measures are often useful diagnostically in helping to identify the presence of neurologic disorder. They are also helpful in that they provide insight into a patient's auditory abilities beyond the level of cochlear processing. We are often faced with the question of how a patient will hear after a peripheral sensitivity loss has been corrected with hearing aids. Estimates of central auditory processing ability are useful in predicting suprathreshold hearing ability.

Estimating Communicative Function

Speech thresholds tell us about a patient's hearing sensitivity and, thus, what intensity level speech will need to reach to be made audible. Word-recognition scores tell us how well speech can be recognized once it is made audible. Advanced speech audiometric measures tell us how well the central auditory nervous system processes auditory information at suprathreshold levels. Taken together, these speech audiometric measures provide us with a profile of a patient's communication function. If we know only the pure-tone thresholds, we can only guess as to the patient's functional impairment. If, on the other hand, we have estimates of the ability to understand speech, then we have substantive insight into the true ability to hear.

Speech Audiometry Materials

The goal of speech audiometry is to permit the measurement of patients' ability to understand everyday communication. The question of whether patients can understand speech seems like an easy one, but several factors intervene to complicate the issue.

You might think that the easiest way to assess a person's speech understanding ability would be to determine whether the person can understand running speech or **continuous discourse**. The problem with such an assessment lies in the redundancy of information contained in continuous speech. There is simply so much information in running speech that a patient with nearly any degree of disorder of the auditory system can extract enough of it to understand what is being spoken. On the other hand, you might think that the easiest way to assess speech understanding is by determining whether a patient can hear the difference between two **phonemes** such as /p/ and /g/. The problem with this type of assessment is that there is so little redundancy in the speech target, that a patient with even a mild disorder of the auditory system may be unable to discriminate between the sounds.

Continuous discourse is running speech, such as a talker reading a story, used primarily as background competition.

A **phoneme** is the smallest distinctive class of sounds in a language.

In reality, different types of speech materials are useful for different types of speech audiometric measures. The materials of speech audiometry include nonsense syllables, single-syllable or monosyllabic words, two-syllable words, **sentential approximations**, sentences, and sentences with key words at the end.

Sentential approximations are contrived nonsense sentences, designed to be syntactically appropriate but meaningless.

Types of Materials

The materials used in speech audiometry vary from nonsense syllables to complete sentences. Each type of material has unique attributes, and most are used in unique ways in the speech audiometric assessment.

Nonsense syllables, such as *pa, ta, ka, ga,* have been used as a means of assessing a patient's ability to discriminate between phonemes of spoken language. Ability to discriminate small differences relies on an intact peripheral auditory system, somewhat limiting the applicability of such measures clinically, where most individuals have disordered auditory systems.

Single-syllable or monosyllabic words, such as *cat, tie, lick,* have been used extensively in the assessment of word recognition ability. In fact, the most popular materials for the measurement of suprathreshold speech understanding have been monosyllabic words, grouped in lists that were designed to be phonetically balanced across the speech sounds of the English language. These 50-word lists were compiled during World War II as test materials for comparing the speech transmission characteristics of aircraft radio receivers and transmitters. The words were selected from various sources and arranged into 50-word lists so that all of the sounds of English were represented in their relative frequency of occurrence in the language within each list. Hence the lists were considered to be **phonetically balanced** and became known as PB lists.

Phonetically balanced word lists contain speech sounds that occur with the same frequency as those of conversational speech.

Two-syllable or **spondaic words**, such as *northwest, cowboy,* and *hotdog,* are also used routinely in speech audiometric assessment. Spondees are words that can be spoken with equal emphasis on both syllables and have the advantage that, with only small individual adjustments, they can be made *homogeneous with respect to audibility.* That is, they are all just heard at about the same speech intensity level.

Spondaic words are two-syllable words spoken with equal emphasis on each syllable.

Sentences and variations of sentence materials are also used as speech audiometric measures. A novel procedure employing sentences with variable context is the Speech-Perception-In-Noise (SPIN) test. In this case, the test item is a single word that is the last of a sentence. There are two types of sentences, those having high predictability in which word identification is aided by context (e.g. "They played a game of cat and *mouse*") and those having low predictability in which context is not as helpful (e.g. "I'm glad you heard about the *bend*"). Sentences are presented to the listener against a background of competing **multitalker babble**. Another sentence-based procedure is the Synthetic Sentence Identification (SSI) test. Artificially created, seven-word sentential approximations (e.g., "Agree with him only to find out") are presented to the listener against a competing background of single-talker continuous discourse.

Multitalker babble is a recording of numerous people talking at once and is used as background competition.

Redundancy in Hearing

There is a great deal of redundancy associated with our ability to hear and process speech communication. Intrinsically, the cen-

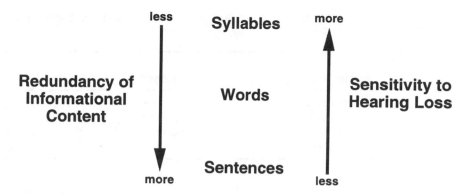

Figure 6–16. Relationship of redundancy of informational content and sensitivity to the effects of hearing loss on three types of speech-recognition materials.

tral auditory nervous system has a rich system of anatomic, physiologic, and biochemical overlap. Among other functions, such **intrinsic redundancy** permits multisensory processing and simultaneous processing of different auditory signals. Another aspect of intrinsic redundancy is that the nervous system can be altered substantially by neurologic disorder and still maintain its ability to process information.

Extrinsically, speech signals contain a wealth of information due to **phonetic, phonemic, syntactic**, and **semantic** content and rules. Such **extrinsic redundancy** allows us to hear only part of a speech segment and still understand what is being said. We are capable of perceiving consonants from the coarticulatory effects of vowels even when we do not hear the acoustic segments of the consonants. We are also capable of perceiving an entire sentence from hearing only a few words that are imbedded into a semantic context. Extrinsic redundancy increases as the content of the speech signal increases. Thus, nonsense syllable are least redundant; continuous discourse is most redundant. The immunity of speech perception to the effects of hearing sensitivity loss varies directly with the amount of redundancy of the signal. The relationship is shown in Figure 6–16. The more redundancy inherent in the signal, the more immune that signal is to the effects of hearing loss. Stated another way, perception of speech that has less redundancy is more likely to be affected by the presence of hearing loss than is perception of speech with greater redundancy.

The issue of redundancy plays a role in the selection of speech materials. If you are trying to assess the effects of a cochlear

Intrinsic redundancy is the abundance of information present in the central auditory system due to the excess capacity inherent in its richly innervated pathways.

Phonetic pertains to an individual speech sound.

Phonemic pertains to the smallest distinctive class of sounds in a language, representing the set of variations of a speech sound that are considered the same sound and represented by the same symbol.

Syntactic refers to the arrangement of words in a sentence.

Semantic refers to the meaning of words.

Extrinsic redundancy is the abundance of information present in the speech signal.

Table 6-2. The relationship of intrinsic (I) and extrinsic (E) redundancy to speech recognition ability.

Intrinsic		Extrinsic		Speech Recognition
normal	+	normal	=	normal
normal	+	reduced	=	normal
reduced	+	normal	=	normal
reduced	+	reduced	=	abnormal

hearing impairment on speech perception, then signals that have reduced redundancy should be used. Nonsense syllables or monosyllable words are sensitive to peripheral hearing impairment and are useful in quantifying its effect. Sentential approximations and sentences, on the other hand, are not. Redundancy in these materials is simply too great to be affected by most degrees of hearing impairment.

If you are trying to assess the effects of a disorder of the central auditory nervous system on speech perception, the situation becomes more difficult. Speech signals of all levels of redundancy provide too much information to a central auditory nervous system that, itself, has a great deal of redundancy. Even if the intrinsic redundancy is reduced by neurologic disorder, the extrinsic redundancy of speech may be sufficient to permit normal processing. The solution to assessing central auditory nervous system disorders is to reduce the extrinsic redundancy of the speech information enough to reveal the reduced intrinsic redundancy caused by neurologic disorder. This concept is shown in Table 6–2. Normal intrinsic redundancy and normal extrinsic redundancy result in normal processing. Reducing the extrinsic redundancy, within limits, will have little effect on a system with normal intrinsic redundancy. Similarly, a neurologic disorder that reduces intrinsic redundancy will have little impact on perception of speech with normal extrinsic redundancy. However, if a system with reduced intrinsic redundancy is presented with speech materials that have reduced extrinsic redundancy, then the abnormal processing caused by the neurologic disorder will be revealed.

To reduce extrinsic redundancy, speech signals must be sensitized in some way. Table 6–3 shows some methods for reducing redundancy of test signals. In the frequency domain, speech can be sensitized by removing high frequencies (passing the lows and cutting out the highs or low-pass filtering), thus limiting the pho-

Table 6–3. Methods for reducing extrinsic redundancy

Domain	Technique
frequency	low-pass filtering
time	time compression
intensity	high-level testing
competition	speech in noise
binaural	dichotic measures

netic content of the speech targets. Speech can also be sensitized in the time domain by time-compression, a technique that removes segments of speech and compresses the remaining segments to increase speech rate. In the intensity domain, speech can be presented at sufficiently high levels at which disordered systems cannot seem to process effectively. Another very effective way to reduce redundancy of a signal is to present it in a background of competition. Yet another way to challenge the central auditory system is to present different but similar signals to both ears simultaneously in what is referred to as a *dichotic* measure.

One confounding variable in the measurement of central auditory nervous system processing is the presence of cochlear hearing impairment. In such cases, signals that have enhanced redundancy need to be used so that hearing sensitivity loss does not interfere with interpretation of the measures. That is, you want to use materials that are not affected by peripheral hearing impairment so that you can assess processing at higher levels of the system. Nonsense-syllable perception would be altered by the peripheral hearing impairment, and any effects of central nervous system disorder would not be revealed. Use of sentences would likely overcome the peripheral hearing impairment, but their redundancy would be too great to challenge nervous-system processing, even if it is disordered. The solution is to use highly redundant speech signals to overcome the hearing sensitivity loss and then to sensitize those materials enough to challenge central auditory processing ability.

Other Considerations in Speech Materials

Another factor in deciding which speech materials to use is whether the measure is open-set or closed-set in nature. **Open-set** speech materials are those in which the choice of a response is limited only to the constraints of a language. For example,

Open-set means the choice can be from among all available targets in the language.

PB-word lists are considered open set because the correct answer can be any single-syllable word from the English language. **Closed-set** speech materials are those that limit the possible choices. For example, picture-pointing tasks have been developed, mostly for pediatric testing, wherein the patient has a limited number of foils from which to choose the correct answer.

Closed-set means the choice is from a limited set; multiple choice.

Some speech materials have been designed specifically to evaluate children's speech perception. Children's materials must be carefully designed to account for language abilities of children and to make the task interesting. Specific target words or sentences must be of a vocabulary level that is appropriate, defined, and confined so that any reduction in performance can be attributable to hearing disorder and not to some form of language disorder. The task must also hold a child's interest for a time sufficient to complete testing. Closed-set picture-pointing tasks have been developed that effectively address both of these issues.

Clinical Applications of Speech Audiometry

For clinical purposes, speech audiometric measures fall into one of four categories:

- speech recognition threshold
- speech awareness threshold
- word recognition score
- sensitized speech measures

In a typical clinical situation, a speech threshold (awareness or recognition) will be determined early as a cross-check for the validity of pure-tone thresholds. Following completion of pure-tone audiometry, word-recognition scores will be obtained as estimates of suprathreshold speech understanding in quiet. Finally, either as part of a comprehensive audiological evaluation or as part of an advanced speech audiometric battery, sensitized speech measures will be obtained to assess processing at the level of the central auditory nervous system.

Speech Thresholds

The first threshold measure obtained during an audiological evaluation is usually the spondee or speech-recognition threshold, also known as the speech reception threshold. The ST is the lowest level at which speech can be identified. The main purpose of

How to Establish an ST

Spondaic thresholds, or speech recognition thresholds, can be obtained in a number of valid and reliable ways. Some ways simply take longer than others. Here is a rapid technique that works well, particularly with adults:

1. Familiarize the patient with the spondees—you will find your measure to be much more stable this way, and it will be worth your time.
2. Instruct the patient to repeat the words, even when they are very faint, and even when guessing is necessary.
3. Present one spondee at the lowest attenuator setting (or 30 dB below a ST established during a previous hearing evaluation). Ascend in 10 dB steps, presenting one word at each level, until the patient responds correctly.
4. Descend 15 dB.
5. Present up to five spondees until:
   a. the patient misses three spondees, after which you should ascend 5 dB and try again; or
   b. the client first repeats two spondees correctly—this level is the ST.

Adapted from A Fast Valid Method to Measure Speech Recognition Threshold, by D. Downs and P. Dickinson Minard, 1996, *The Hearing Journal*, *49*, (8), 39–44. Adapted with permission.

obtaining an ST is to provide an anchor against which to compare pure-tone thresholds.

The preferred materials for the measurement of a speech threshold are spondaic words. In theory, almost any materials could be used, but the spondees have the advantage of being homogeneous with respect to audibility, or just audible at about the same speech intensity level. This helps greatly in establishing a threshold for speech. By presenting a series of spondaic words and systematically varying the intensity, one can determine the lowest level at which the individual can identify about 50% of the test items. One procedure for determining the ST is described in the Clinical Note above.

An important clinical value of this ST is that it should agree closely with the pure-tone thresholds averaged across 500, 1000, and 2000 Hz. If both the pure-tone intensity levels and the speech intensity levels are expressed on a hearing threshold level (HL) decibel scale, then the degree of hearing loss for speech should agree with the degree of hearing loss for pure tones in the 500 through 2000 Hz region. In clinical practice, the ST and the PTA should be in fairly close agreement, differing by no more than ±6 dB. If, for example, the ST is 45 dB, the PTA should be at some level between 39 and 51 dB. If there is a larger discrepancy between the two numbers, then one or the other is probably an invalid measure.

Speech Awareness Threshold

Speech awareness threshold (SAT) is the lowest level at which the presence of a speech signal can just be detected.

A **speech awareness threshold**, sometimes referred to as speech detection threshold, is the lowest level at which a patient can just detect the presence of a speech signal. Determination of SAT is usually not a routine part of the audiometric evaluation and is used only when an ST cannot be established. The SAT is established by presenting speech, often spondaic words, and determining the lowest level at which the individual can just detect the presence (not the understanding) of words about 50% of the time.

An SAT is determined in place of an ST in patients who do not have the language competency to identify spondaic words, especially in young children who have not yet developed the vocabulary to identify words or pictures representing words. It may also be necessary to establish SATs rather than STs in patients who do not speak a language for which spondees have been recorded or in patients who have lost language function due to a cerebrovascular accident or other neurologic insult.

The important clinical value of the SAT is that it should agree closely with the best pure-tone threshold within the audiometric frequency range. For example, if the best pure-tone threshold is at 0 dB at 250 Hz, then the SAT should be around 0 dB. Or, if the best pure-tone threshold is 25 dB at 1000 Hz, then the SAT should be approximately 25 dB. Because speech is composed of a broad spectrum of frequencies, speech awareness thresholds will reflect hearing at the frequencies with the best sensitivity.

Word Recognition

The most common way that we describe suprathreshold hearing ability is with word-recognition measures. Word-recognition testing, also referred to as speech discrimination, word discrimination, and PB-word testing, is an assessment of a patient's ability to identify and repeat single-syllable words presented at some suprathreshold level.

The words used for word-recognition testing are contained in lists of 50 items that are phonetically balanced with respect to the relative frequency of occurrence of phonemes in the language. Raymond Carhart, one of the early pioneers of audiologic evaluation, adapted these so-called PB lists to audiologic testing. He reasoned that if you first established the threshold for speech, the ST, then presented a PB list at a level 25 dB above the ST, the percent correct word repetition for a PB list would tell you something about how well the individual could understand speech in that ear. This measure, the PB score at a constant suprathreshold level, came to be called the *discrimination score,* on the assumption that it was proportional to the individual's ability to "discriminate" among the individual sounds of speech. This basic speech audiometric paradigm, a percent-correct score at a defined **sensational level** above the ST, formed the framework for audiologic and aural rehabilitation procedures that remain in use today. Subsequent modifications of the original PB lists include the W-22 lists, developed at the Central Institute for the Deaf (CID), and the NU-6 lists, developed at Northwestern University. Other modifications involve the use of half lists of 25 words each or the use of lists that are rank-ordered in terms of difficulty, both of which are designed to enhance the efficiency of word-recognition measures. Use of monitored live-voice testing is another way to enhance efficiency, but not without a substantial loss in quality of test results, as described in the Clinical Note on the next page.

Sensation level (SL) is the intensity level of a sound in dB above an individual's threshold.

Interpretation of word-recognition measures is based on the predictable relation of maximum word-recognition scores to degree of hearing loss. If the maximum score falls within a given range for a given degree of hearing loss, then the results are considered to be within expectation for a cochlea hearing loss. If the score is poorer than expected, then word-recognition ability is considered to be abnormal for the degree of hearing loss and consistent with retrocochlear disorder. Table 6–4 can be used to determine whether a score exceeds expectations based on degree of hearing loss, in this case the PTA or pure-tone average of thresholds at 500, 1000, and 2000 Hz. The number represents the lowest maximum score that 95% of individuals with hearing loss will obtain on this particular measure, the 25-item NU-6 word lists. Any score below this number for a given hearing loss is considered to be abnormal.

Monitored Live Voice is a Bad Idea

Word-recognition scores are a simple measure of a patient's ability to recognize single-syllable words presented in quiet. They do not say much about a patient's ability to function in the real world, and they are quite predictable from the audiogram. Because word-recognition testing is an expected part of the clinical routine, and because the results are seldom surprising, the testing is often carried out as expediently as possible.

One simple way to expedite testing is to present words via monitored live voice. Here the audiologist presents the words into a microphone, waits for the patient's response, and presents the next word. For most individuals, this can be completed fairly rapidly. The other option for testing word recognition is to use taped speech stimuli. Here, words are prerecorded onto standardized tapes and CDs, and words are presented at a fixed time interval. In most cases, this is slower than testing by monitored live voice.

The advantages of using recorded speech are important and numerous. Yet monitored live voice testing persists in clinical practice, again, based on the expediency of its use. In reality, the audiologist who chooses to assess word recognition in this manner would do better to just skip it and save even more time than to do it so poorly that the results are uninterpretable anyway.

Word-recognition testing is carried out as a matter of routine for the times when results are not predictable or significant changes in functioning have occurred. In both of these cases, the underlying cause of the results may signal health concerns that alert the audiologist to make appropriate medical referrals.

The first question, then, is whether results are predictable from the degree of hearing loss. For example, is a score of 68% normal for a person with a moderate hearing loss? This can be assessed by comparing the score to published data for patients with known cochlear hearing loss. If the score falls within the expected range, then it is consistent with the degree of hearing loss. If not, then there is reason for concern that the underlying cause of the disorder is retrocochlear in nature. These published data are, of course, based on standard recordings of word-recognition targets. If you used monitored live voice, you simply do not know if 68% is normal or not. Why would you carry out a test if you cannot interpret the outcome?

A similar problem results when you begin looking for changes in performance. On many occasions as an audiologist, you will encounter patients who are being monitored for one reason or another. The question is often whether the patient is getting worse. If you encounter a significant decline on recorded speech measures, you can be fairly confident that a real change has occurred. If the same decline is noted on monitored-live voice testing, you have no basis for making a decision. Again, why are you bothering to do this if your results have so little meaning?

The provision of health care is not a matter of expediency. Given a choice, and you do have one, why not do word-recognition testing well?

Table 6-4. Values used to determine whether a maximum word-recognition score on the 25-item NU-6 word lists meets expectations based on degree of hearing loss, expressed as the pure-tone average (PTA) of 500, 1000, and 2000 Hz.

PTA (in dB HL)	Maximum Word- Recognition Scores
0	100
5	96
10	96
15	92
20	88
25	80
30	76
35	68
40	64
45	56
50	48
55	44
60	36
65	32
70	28

Source: Adapted from Confidence Limits for Maximum Word-recognition Scores, by J. R. Dubno, F. Lee, A. J. Klein, L. J. Matthews, and C. F. Lam, 1995, *Journal of Speech and Hearing Research, 38,* 490–502.

Another more recent modification of Carhart's original paradigm has been the exploration of speech understanding across the patient's entire dynamic range of hearing rather than at just a single suprathreshold level. The goal here is to determine a maximum score regardless of test level. The issues surrounding presentation levels are described in the Clinical Note on the following page.

Performance-intensity function (PI function) is a graph of percentage-correct speech recognition scores plotted as a function of presentation level of the target signals.

To obtain a maximum score, lists of words or sentences are presented at 3 to 5 different intensity levels, extending from just above the speech threshold to the upper level of comfortable listening. In this way, a **performance versus intensity** or **PI function** is generated for each ear. The shape of this function often has important diagnostic significance. Figure 6–17 shows examples of PI functions. In most cases, the PI function rises systematically as speech intensity is increased, to an asymptotic level representing the best speech understanding that can be achieved in the test ear. In some cases, however, there is a para-doxical **rollover** effect, in which the function declines substan-tially as speech intensity increases beyond the level producing the maximal performance score. In other words, as speech inten-sity increases, performance rises to a maximum level, then de-clines or "rolls over" sharply as intensity continues to increase. This rollover effect is commonly observed when the site of the hearing loss is retrocochlear, in the auditory nerve or the auditory pathways in the brain stem.

Rollover is a decrease in speech recognition ability with increasing intensity level.

The use of PI functions is a way of sensitizing speech by challeng-ing the auditory system at high intensity levels. Because of its ease of administration, many audiologists use it routinely as a screening measure for retrocochlear disorders. The most effica-cious clinical strategy is to present a PB list simply at the highest intensity level (usually 80 dB HL). If the patient scores above 80%, then rollover of the function will be minimal, and testing can be terminated. If the patient scores below 80%, then rollover could occur, and the function is completed by testing at lower intensity levels.

Sensitized Speech Measures

Some problems in speech understanding appear to be based not on the distortions introduced by peripheral hearing loss, but on deficits resulting from disorders in the auditory pathways within the central nervous system. Revealing these disorders relies on the use of sensitized speech materials that reduce the extrinsic redundancy of the signal. Although redundancy can be reduced by low-pass filtering or time compression, these methods have not proven to be clinically useful because of their susceptibility to the effects of cochlear hearing loss. Perhaps the most successfully

Word-Recognition Testing: What Level?

Early in the development of word-recognition testing as a clinical tool, the choice of an intensity level to carry out testing was based on the performance of normal-hearing listeners. Data from groups of subjects with normal hearing showed that, by 25–40 dB above the speech recognition threshold, most subjects achieve 100% recognition of single-syllable words on the clinical word lists. As a result, the early clinical standard was to test patients at 40 dB sensation level (SL). SL was referenced to either the pure-tone average or the speech-recognition threshold.

Over the years, this notion of testing at 40 dB SL began to be questioned as clinicians realized that the audibility of speech signals varied with both degree *and* configuration of hearing loss. If a person had a flat hearing loss in both ears, then the parts of speech that would be audible to the listener would be equal for both ears at 40 dB SL. If however, one ear had a flat loss and the other had a sloping hearing loss, then the ear with the sloping loss would be at a disadvantage in terms of the speech signals that were audible to that ear. Lo and behold, the word-recognition score would be lower in that ear, for it is certainly more difficult to perceive speech that is not audible. Thus, differences between ears could be accounted for on the basis of the audiometric configuration, and little was learned from the exercise of measuring word recognition. Worse still, when differences did occur, their importance was difficult to judge because of the audibility question.

Current clinical practice has largely abandoned the notion of equating the ears by using SL, or even equating the ears by using comfort levels. Instead, these strategies have been replaced with the practice of testing and comparing ears at equal SPL and in searching for the maximum word-recognition scores at high intensity levels.

The notion is a simple one. If we obtain the best or maximum score for both ears, then intensity level is likely removed from the equation. Maximum scores can then be compared between ears and to normative data to see if they are acceptable for the degree of hearing loss.

There is one other important issue regarding level. Some patients with retrocochlear disorder actually have poorer word-recognition scores as intensity increases. If you

(continued)

were to plot their performance, as in Figure 6–17, you would see a function that "rolls over" at high intensity levels. This rollover is consistent with retrocochlear disorder and serves as a useful clinical screening device.

Combining these ideas then, one common clinical strategy for word-recognition testing is to present words at the highest reasonable level, which is 80 dB HL for most patients. If the patient obtains a score of better than 80%, then there is no chance of measuring significant rollover, and testing is completed. If the score is poorer than 80%, the level should be reduced by 10 dB and testing repeated until a function is defined and the maximum score determined.

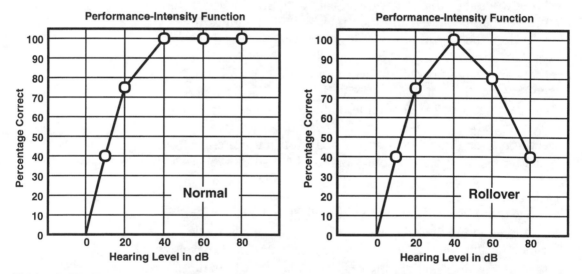

Figure 6–17. Examples of two performance-intensity functions, one normal and one with rollover.

used sensitized speech measures are those in which competition is presented either in the same ear or the opposite ear as a means of stressing the auditory system.

Two examples of speech-in-competition measures are the SPIN test and the SSI test. The SPIN, or Speech-Perception-In-Noise test, has as its target a single word that is the last in a sentence. In half of the sentences, the word is predictable from the context of the sentence. These signals are presented in a background of multitalker competition. The SSI, or Synthetic Sentence Identification test, also uses sentence materials presented in competition. The SSI uses sentential approximations that are presented in a closed-set format. The patient is asked to identify the sentence from a list of 10. Sentences are presented in the presence of single-talker competition. Testing typically is carried out with the signal and the competition at the same intensity level, a **message-to-competition** (MCR) of 0 dB.

The ratio in dB of the presentation level of a speech target to that of background competition is called the **message-to-competition ratio** (MCR).

Another effective approach for assessing central auditory processing ability is the use of dichotic tests. In the dichotic paradigm, two different speech targets are presented simultaneously to the two ears. The patient's task is usually either to repeat back both targets in either order or to report only the word heard in the precued ear. In this latter case, the right ear is precued on half the trials and the left on the other half. Two scores are determined, one for targets correctly identified from the right ear, the other for targets correctly identified from the left ear. The patterns of results can reveal auditory processing deficits, especially those due to disorders of the temporal lobe and corpus callosum. Dichotic tests have been constructed using nonsense syllables, monosyllabic words, **staggered spondaic words** (SSW), and synthetic sentences (Dichotic Sentence Identification or DSI).

Staggered spondaic words are used in tests of dichotic listening, in which two spondaic words are presented so that the second syllable delivered to one ear is heard simultaneously with the first syllable delivered to the other ear.

Speech Recognition and Site of Lesion

Speech audiometric measures can be useful in predicting where the site of lesion might be for a given hearing loss. A summary is presented in Table 6–5.

If a hearing loss is conductive due to middle ear disorder, the effect on speech recognition will be negligible, except to elevate

Table 6–5. Probable speech-recognition results for various disorder sites.

Site of Disorder	Speech-Recognition	Ipsilateral/Contralateral
Middle ear	normal	ipsi
Cochlea	predictable	ipsi
VIIIth nerve	poor	ipsi
Brain stem	reduced	ipsi/contra
Temporal lobe	reduced	contra

the ST by the degree of hearing loss in the ear with the disorder. Suprathreshold speech recognition will not be affected.

If a hearing loss is sensorineural due to cochlear disorder, the ST will be elevated in that ear to a degree predictable by the pure-tone average. Suprathreshold word recognition scores will be predictable from the degree of hearing sensitivity loss. Sensitized speech measures will be normal or predictable from degree of loss. Dichotic measures will be normal. One exception is in the case of endolymphatic hydrops or Ménière's disease, in which the cochlear disorder causes such distortion that word recognition scores are poorer than predicted from degree of hearing loss.

If a hearing loss is sensorineural due to an VIIIth nerve lesion, the ST will be elevated in that ear to a degree predictable by the pure-tone average. Suprathreshold word recognition ability is likely to be substantially affected. Maximum scores are likely to be poorer than predicted from the degree of hearing loss, and rollover of the performance-intensity function is likely to occur. Speech-in-competition measures are also likely to be depressed. Abnormal results will occur in the same, or ipsilateral, ear in which the lesion occurs. Dichotic measures will be normal.

If a hearing disorder occurs as a result of a brain stem lesion, the ST will be predictable from the pure-tone average. Suprathreshold word recognition ability is likely to be affected substantially. Word recognition scores in quiet may be normal, or they may be depressed or show rollover. Speech-in-competition measures are likely to be depressed in the ear ipsilateral to the lesion. Dichotic measures will likely be normal.

If a hearing disorder occurs as the result of a temporal lobe lesion, hearing sensitivity is unlikely to be affected, and the ST and word recognition scores are likely to be normal. Speech-in-competition measures may or may not be abnormal in the ear contralateral to the lesion. Dichotic measures are the most likely of all to show a deficit due to the temporal-lobe lesion.

Predicting Speech Recognition

As you learned earlier, word-recognition ability is predictable from the audiogram in most patients. This has been known for many years. Essentially, speech recognition can be predicted based on the amount of speech signal that is audible to a patient. The original calculations for making this prediction resulted in what was referred to as an **articulation index**, a number between 0 and 1.0 that described the proportion of the average speech signal that would be audible to a patient based on his or her audiogram.

Articulation index (AI) is also known as audibility index and speech intelligibility index.

Over the years, the concept and clinical techniques have evolved into the measurement that is now referred to as the audibility index, reflecting its intended purpose of expressing the amount of speech signal that is audible to a patient. From the *audibility index* (AI), an estimate can be made of recognition scores for syllables, words, and sentences. A simple clinical technique for calculating the AI and for predicting these scores is described in the Clinical Note on pages 250–252.

The strategy of using the AI to describe communication impairment is a useful one, particularly in terms of describing improvement with hearing aid amplification. In many ways, the idea of audibility of speech information is a more useful way of describing the impact of a hearing loss than the percentage correct score on single-syllable word-recognition measures.

Summary

- Speech audiometry can be thought of as our best friend in the clinic.
- Speech audiometric measures are used to measure threshold for speech, cross-check pure-tone sensitivity, quantify suprathreshold speech recognition ability, assist in differential diagnosis, assess central auditory processing ability, and estimate communicative function.
- The goal of speech audiometry is to permit the measurement of patients' ability to understand everyday communication.
- Different types of speech materials are useful for different types of speech audiometric measures. The materials used in speech audiometry vary from nonsense syllables to complete sentences.
- Speech audiometric measures fall into one of four categories: speech recognition threshold, speech awareness threshold, word recognition score, and sensitized speech measures.
- The first threshold measure obtained during an audiological evaluation is usually the spondee or speech-recognition threshold.

Count the Dots

The *audibility index* (AI) is a measure of the proportion of speech cues that are audible. It was originally called the *articulation index* and is sometimes referred to as the *speech intelligibility index.* The audibility index is usually expressed as the proportion, between 0 and 1.0, of the average speech signal that is audible to a given listener. Calculations for determination of the AI are based on dividing the speech signal into frequency bands, with various weightings attributed to each band based on their likely contribution to the ability to hear speech. For example, consonant sounds are predominantly higher frequency sounds, and because their audibility is so important to understanding speech, the higher frequencies are weighted more heavily in the AI calculation.

This concept of audibility of average speech has not had much impact clinically, where word-recognition testing has prevailed as a means of estimating the ability to recognize speech. One of the problems with the AI is that it is not well understood, and it has been rather cumbersome to calculate.

In 1988, Chas Pavlovic described a simplified way to calculate audibility. The method has been variously adapted and is now known clinically as the "count the dots" procedure. An illustration of a count-the-dots audiogram form is shown in the top figure on the facing page. Here the weighting of frequency components by intensity is shown as the number of dots in the range on the audiogram.

Calculating the AI from this audiogram is very simple. The bottom figure on the facing page shows a patient's audiogram superimposed on the count-the-dots audiogram. Those components of average speech that are below (or at higher intensity levels than) the audiogram are audible to the patient, and those that are above the audiogram are not. To calculate the AI, simply count the dots that are audible to the patient. In this case, the AI is 0.60. This essentially means that 60% of average speech is audible to the patient.

The AI has at least three useful clinical applications. First, it can serve as an excellent counseling tool for explaining to a patient the impact of a hearing loss on the ability to understand speech. Second, the AI has a known relationship to word-recognition ability. Thus word-recognition

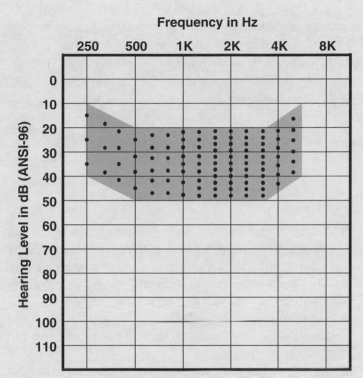

Illustration of a count-the-dots audiogram form.

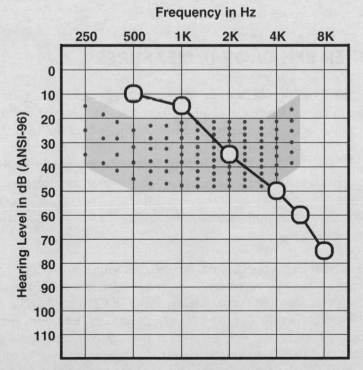

Results of an audiometric evaluation superimposed on the count-the-dots audiogram. *(continued)*

scores can be predicted from the AI or, if measured directly, can be compared to expected scores based on the AI. Third, the count-the-dots procedure can be very useful in hearing aid fitting in serving as a metric of how much average speech is made audible by a given hearing aid.

Pavlovic, C. (1988). Articulation index predictions of speech intelligibility in hearing aid selection. *Asha*, 30(6/7), 63–65.

■ A speech awareness threshold, sometimes referred to as speech detection threshold, is the lowest level at which a patient can just detect the presence of a speech signal.
■ The most common way to describe suprathreshold hearing ability is with word-recognition measures.
■ Sensitized speech audiometric measures are used to quantify deficits resulting from disorders in the central auditory pathways.
■ Speech audiometric measures can be useful in predicting where the site of lesion might be for a given hearing loss.

OTHER BEHAVIORAL MEASURES

A number of other behavioral measures are used for various purposes in the audiologic evaluation. For example, you will learn in Chapter 8 about some behavioral techniques that are useful in identifying and quantifying hearing loss that is *functional*, or exaggerated. Other bone-conduction measures, based on old tuning-fork tests, can be useful in determining the presence of an air-bone gap. In addition, a number of specialized speech audiometric measures are available for various audiometric purposes.

One special class of behavioral measures is important to be aware of from an historic perspective. Prior to the discovery of the objective measures that you will learn about in Chapter 7 and prior to the development of modern imaging and radiographic techniques, a battery of psychophysical measures was used to differentiate cochlear from retrocochlear disorder. This has become known as the *classic test battery,* and it is based primarily on measures of auditory *adaptation* and *recruitment.*

Recall from Chapter 3 that one of the consequences of cochlear hearing loss is *recruitment,* or abnormal loudness growth. That is, loudness grows more rapidly than normal at intensity levels just above threshold in an ear with cochlear site of disorder. Clinically this means that if recruitment is present, then the site of disorder is cochlear rather than retrocochlear. Two measures, loudness balancing and difference limen for intensity, were used to assess recruitment as part of the classic test battery.

One popular measure of recruitment was the *alternate binaural loudness balance* (ABLB) test. The ABLB was designed to be used in patients with unilateral hearing loss. To carry out the ABLB test, the same tone is presented alternately between ears. The intensity level in the impaired ear is fixed at a level above threshold of 20 dB SL. The patient's task is to adjust the level of normal hearing ear until the sounds in the two ears are of equal loudness. The intensity level in the impaired ear is then increased by 10 or 20 dB and the loudness matching is repeated. The ABLB is interpreted by assessing the nature of loudness differences at high intensity levels. If the perception of loudness is at the same intensity level (in HL or SPL) for both ears, then *complete recruitment* occurred in the impaired ear, because the loudness caught up to the normal ear at high levels. This finding is consistent with cochlear site of disorder. In cases of retrocochlear disorder, the opposite, or *decruitment,* might occur. Here the loudness in the impaired ear grows more slowly than in the normal ear.

The measurement of difference limen for intensity was another method used to take advantage of the recruitment phenomenon. The clinical measure was known as the *short increment sensitivity index* (SISI). To carry out the SISI test, a constant tone is presented to the ear at 20 dB SL. Superimposed on that tone is a series of 20 increments of 1 dB. The patient's task is to count the number of increments that are perceived. A patient with cochlear hearing loss can perceive those increments, whereas a patient with retrocochlear site of disorder cannot. One successful modification of the SISI involves the presentation of the signal at a high level, 75 dB HL or 20 dB SL, whichever is higher. A positive SISI, in which 70 to 100% of the increments are identified, is consistent with cochlear hearing loss or normal hearing. A negative SISI, in which only 0 to 30% of the increments are identified, is consistent with retrocochlear site.

You may also recall from Chapter 3 that one of the consequences of retrocochlear hearing loss is abnormal *auditory adaptation.* The normal auditory system tends to adapt to ongoing sound, especially at near-threshold levels, so that, as adaptation occurs, an audible signal becomes inaudible. At higher intensity levels, ongoing sound tends to remain audible without adaptation. However, in an ear with retrocochlear disorder, the audibility may diminish rapidly due to excessive auditory adaptation even at higher intensity levels.

Two popular measures of adaptation from the classic test battery are the tone decay test (TDT) and diagnostic Békésy audiometry.

The *tone decay test* is essentially a measure of the intensity level at which the perception of a tone can be sustained for 60 seconds. In its original form, a tone is presented at 5 dB SL, and the patient is asked to respond for as long as it is audible. If the patient responds for 60 seconds, testing is stopped. If not, the intensity level is increased by 5 dB and the process repeated. Tone decay is quantified in dB as the final test level minus the threshold level. Tone decay is considered positive for retrocochlear disorder if it exceeds 30 dB.

One modification of the tone decay test that is still sometimes useful today is the *suprathreshold adaptation test* (STAT). The STAT is carried out by presenting a tone at 110 dB SPL and determining if patient can hear it for 60 seconds. If not, adaptation occurred, consistent with retrocochlear disorder. The STAT test is useful as a screening measure for retrocochlear disorder in patients with hearing loss severe enough to preclude testing with objective audiometric measures.

Another way to measure auditory adaptation is with *diagnostic Békésy audiometry*. Békésy audiometry is an automated form of hearing sensitivity assessment in which the patient controls the attenuation of the signal. By pushing a button, the patient increases intensity of the signal until it is audible. The patient then releases the button until the signal is inaudible, presses it until it is audible again, releases it, presses it, and so on. These *tracking* responses are displayed on a computer screen or plotter, and threshold is calculated as the midpoint of the excursion between audible and inaudible. While the tracking occurs, the frequency of the signal is slowly swept from low to high, so that an audiogram is measured across the frequency range.

In diagnostic Békésy audiometry, both continuous (C) and interrupted (I) tones are presented. If adaptation occurs, it will affect the continuous tone but not the interrupted tone. Results fall into one of 5 classic types. Békésy Type I, in which the I and C tracings are overlapped, is consistent with cochlear site of disorder, as is Békésy Type II, in which the C tracing is only slightly worse than the I tracing. Békésy Type III, in which the C tracing drops off the graph due to adaptation to the continuous signal, is consistent with retrocochlear site of disorder. So is Békésy Type IV, in which the C tracing is more that 20 dB below the I tracing. In Békésy Type V, the I tracing is poorer than the C tracing, indicating that the patient is probably faking a hearing loss.

All of these measures, ABLB, SISI, TDT, and Békésy audiometry, were useful in the diagnosis of retrocochlear site in the days when tumors or other disorders had to reach a substantial size before they could be diagnosed radiographically. As imaging and radiographic techniques improved, smaller lesions that had less functional impact on the auditory system could be visualized, and the sensitivity of the classic test battery diminished. Today, these measures are relegated mostly to history, although, as noted above, results can occasionally be useful in patients with severe hearing loss.

One behavioral diagnostic measure that has stood the test of time is a measure of lower brain stem function known as the *masking level difference* (MLD). The MLD measures binaural release from masking due to interaural phase relationships. The binaural auditory system is an exquisite detector of differences in timing of sound reaching the two ears. This helps in localizing low frequency sounds, which reach the ears at different points in time. An illustration may help you to understand how sensitive the ears are to these timing, or phase, cues. Suppose that identical low-frequency tones are presented to both of your ears and those tones are adjusted so that the phase is identical. Enough noise is then added to both ears to mask the tones. If the phase of the tone delivered to one earphone is then reversed, the tone will becomes audible again. This is called *binaural release from masking,* and it occurs as a result of processing in the brain stem at the level of the superior olivary complex.

The MLD test is the clinical strategy designed to measure binaural release from masking. To carry out the MLD, a 500 Hz interrupted tone is split and presented in phase to both ears. Narrow band noise is also presented, at a fixed level of 60 dB HL. Using the Békésy tracking procedure, threshold for the in-phase tones is determined in the presence of the noise. Then the phase of one of the tones is reversed, and threshold is tracked again. The MLD is the difference in threshold between the in-phase and the out-of-phase conditions. For a 500 Hz tone, the MLD should be greater than 7 dB and is usually around 12 dB.

Pure-tone audiometry, speech audiometry, and these other procedures constitute the basic *behavioral* measures available to quantify hearing impairment and determine the type and site of auditory disorder. In the next chapter, you will learn about the objective measures that are used for the same purposes.

SUGGESTED READINGS

Dirks, D. D. (1994). Bone-conduction threshold testing. In J. Katz (Ed.), *Handbook of clinical audiology* (4th ed., pp. 132–146). Baltimore: Williams & Wilkins.

Gelfand, S. A. (1997). *Essentials of audiology.* New York: Thieme.

Jerger, J. (1987). Diagnostic audiology: Historical perspectives. *Ear and Hearing, 8,* 7S–12S.

Jerger, J., & Hayes, D. (1977). Diagnostic speech audiometry. *Archives of Otolaryngology, 103,* 216–222.

Jerger, J., & Jordon, C. (1980). Normal audiometric findings. *American Journal of Otology, 1,* 157–159.

Jerger, S. (1987). Validation of the pediatric speech intelligibility test in children with central nervous system lesions. *Audiology, 26,* 298–311.

Keith, R. W. (1996). The audiologic evaluation. In J. L. Northern (Ed.), *Hearing disorders* (3rd ed., pp. 45–56). Needham Heights, MA: Allyn & Bacon.

Silman, S., & Silverman, C. A. (1991). *Auditory diagnosis: Principles and applications.* San Diego: Singular Publishing Group.

Stach, B. A. (1998). Central auditory disorders. In A. K. Lalwani & K. M. Grundfast (Eds.), *Pediatric otology and neurotology.* Philadelphia: J. B. Lippincott Company.

Yantis, P. A. (1994). Puretone air-conduction threshold testing. In J. Katz (Ed.), *Handbook of clinical audiology* (4th ed., pp. 97–108). Baltimore: Williams & Wilkins.

7

The Audiologist's Assessment Tools: Electroacoustic and Electrophysiologic Measures

IMMITTANCE AUDIOMETRY

Immittance audiometry is one of the most powerful tools available for the evaluation of auditory disorder. It serves at least three functions in audiologic assessment:

- it is sensitive in detecting middle ear disorder,
- it can be useful in differentiating cochlear from retro-cochlear disorder, and
- it is helpful in estimating degree of peripheral hearing sensitivity and is often used as a cross check to pure-tone audiometry.

As a result of its comprehensive value, immittance audiometry is a routine component of the audiologic evaluation and is often the first assessment administered in the test battery (Clinical Note on facing page). When immittance audiometry was first introduced into clinical practice during the 1970s, the tendency was to use it to assess middle ear function only if the possibility of middle ear disorder was indicated by the presence of an air-bone gap on the audiogram. That is, the audiologist would assess pure-tone audiometry by air conduction and bone conduction. If an air-bone gap did not exist, the loss was thought to be purely sensorineural. The assumption was made that middle ear function was normal. In contrast, if an air-bone gap existed, indicating a conductive component to the hearing loss, the assumption was made that middle ear disorder was present and should be investigated by immittance audiometry. As the utility of immittance measures became clear, however, this practice changed. The realization was made that the presence of middle ear disorder and the existence of a conductive component to the hearing loss, although related, are independent phenomena. That is, middle ear disorder can be present without a measurable conductive hearing loss. Also, a minor abnormality in middle ear function can result in a significant conductive component.

As a result of the relative independence of the measurement of middle ear function and that of air- and bone-conducted hearing thresholds, immittance audiometry became a routine component of the audiologic assessment. The overall strategy is a simple one: the goal of audiologic testing is to rehabilitate; the first question is whether the problem is related to middle ear disorder that is medically treatable; the best measure of middle ear disorder is immittance audiometry; therefore, the first question is best addressed by immittance audiometry. If middle ear disorder is identified, the next question is whether it is causing a conductive

Why Immittance First?

By the time immittance audiometry became clinically viable, the comparison of air- and bone-conduction thresholds was well entrenched as the method for evaluating indirectly whether outer or middle ear disorder was contributing a conductive component to the hearing loss. The clinical approach was to evaluate the patient and look for an air-bone gap. When an air-bone gap existed, the assumption was that the conductive hearing loss was caused by middle ear disorder. When no air-bone gap existed, the assumption was that there was no middle ear disorder.

The advent of immittance audiometry affected our thinking in two ways. First, it proved to be a sensitive indicator of middle ear function, thereby permitting a direct assessment of middle ear disorder. Second, it taught us to respect the difference between middle ear disorder and conductive hearing loss. We learned that middle ear disorder could exist with or without a significant air-bone gap.

Despite this growing knowledge, clinical practice was sometimes slow to adopt to the changes. The clinical strategy, based solely on the conventional way of doing things, was to measure air-conduction and bone conduction thresholds. If no air-bone gap existed, immittance audiometry was not carried out, under the mistaken assumption that there could not be a middle ear disorder. If an air-bone gap was measured, immittance audiometry was carried out to identify the underlying middle ear disorder responsible for the air-bone gap. That such a practice still exists today is a testament to the resiliency of bad ideas. The irony of this approach is that immittance audiometry is significantly more sensitive to middle ear disorder than the assessment of air-bone gaps.

Current clinical practice argues for carrying out immittance audiometry first, before pure-tone audiometry. If all immittance measures, tympanometry, static immittance, and crossed and uncrossed reflexes, are normal, then whatever hearing loss is determined by pure-tone audiometry is sensorineural in nature. In fact, if an air-bone gap exists, then either air-conduction thresholds or bone-conduction thresholds are not accurate. Many clinicians will not bother testing bone conduction if all immittance measures are normal. This is reasonable practice, since the weakest link in

continued

this chain is bone conduction audiometry. If immittance measures are abnormal, the next clinical question is whether the middle ear disorder is causing a conductive hearing loss, which can then be addressed by air- and bone-conduction audiometry.

Remember this:

■ the goal of audiologic testing is to rehabilitate;
■ the first question is whether the problem is related to middle ear disorder that is medically treatable;
■ the best measure of middle ear disorder is immittance audiometry;
■ therefore, the first question is best addressed by immittance audiometry.

There are other practical reasons for starting an evaluation with immittance audiometry. One has already been mentioned. If immittance measures are normal, there is no need to test by bone-conduction, a large saving in time and effort. The other is more subtle but very important. Immittance audiometry is an excellent indicator of what to expect from pure-tone audiometry. You will begin to understand this the more you do it. Anyone accustomed to carrying out immittance audiometry first will feel rather unprepared to carry out pure-tone audiometry without it.

hearing loss, which is determined by air- and bone-conduction testing. If middle ear function is normal, the next question is whether a sensorineural hearing loss exists, which is determined by air-conduction testing.

Instrumentation

An immittance meter is used for these measurements. A simplified schematic drawing of the components is shown in Figure 7–1, and a photograph of an immittance meter is shown in Figure 7–2.

One major component of an immittance meter is an oscillator that generates a probe tone. The typical frequency of the probe tone is 220 Hz. The probe tone is delivered to a transducer that converts the electronic signal into the acoustic signal, which in

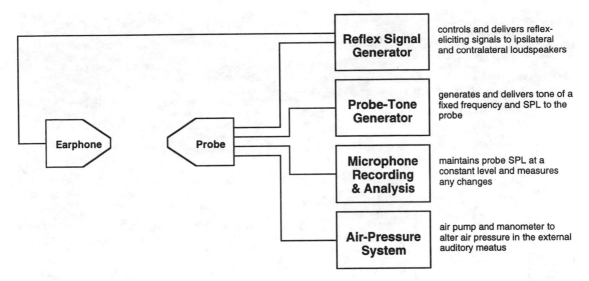

Figure 7-1. Schematic representation of the instrumentation used in immittance measurement.

turn is delivered to a probe that is sealed in the ear canal. The probe also contains a microphone that monitors the level of the probe tone. The immittance instrument is designed to maintain the level of the probe tone in the ear canal at a constant SPL and to record any changes in that SPL on a meter or other recording device.

Another major component of the immittance meter is an air pump that controls the air pressure in the ear canal. Tubing from the probe is attached to the air pump. A manometer measures the air pressure that is being delivered to the ear canal.

An immittance meter also contains a signal generator and trans-ducers for delivering high-intensity signals to the ear for eliciting acoustic reflexes, which you will learn about later in this chapter. The signal generator produces pure tones and broad-band noise. The transducer that is used is either an earphone on the ear opposite to the probe ear or a speaker within the probe itself.

Measurement Technique

Immittance is a physical characteristic of all mechanical vibratory systems. In very general terms, it is a measure of how readily a system can be set into vibration by a driving force. The ease with which energy will flow through the vibrating system is called its **admittance**. The reciprocal concept, the extent to which the

Admittance is the total energy flow through a system.

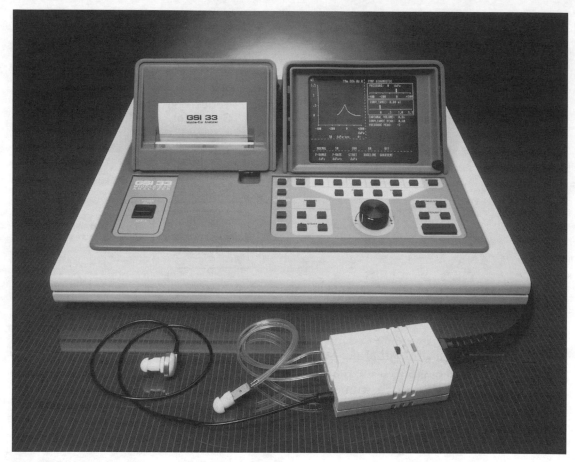

Figure 7-2. Photograph of an immittance meter. (Courtesy of Grason-Stadler, Inc.)

Impedance is the total opposition to energy flow or resistance to the absorption of energy.

system resists the flow of energy through it, is called its **impedance**. If a vibrating system can be forced into motion with little applied force, we say that the admittance is high and the impedance is low. On the other hand, if the system resists being set into motion until the driving force is relatively high, then we say that the admittance of the system is low and the impedance is high. *Immittance* is a term that is meant to encompass both of these concepts.

Immittance audiometry can be thought of as a way of assessing the manner in which energy flows through the outer and middle ears to the cochlea. The middle ear mechanism serves to transform energy from acoustic to hydraulic form. Air-pressure waves from the acoustic signal set the tympanic membrane into vibration, which in turn sets the ossicles into motion. The footplate of the stapes vibrates and sets the fluids of the cochlea into motion.

Immittance measures serve as an indirect way of assessing the appropriateness of energy flow through this system. If the middle ear system is normal, energy will flow in a predictable way. If it is not, then energy will flow either too well (high admittance) or not well enough (high impedance).

Immittance is measured by delivering a pure-tone signal of a constant sound pressure level into the ear canal through a mechanical probe that is seated at the entrance of the ear canal. The signal, which is referred to by convention as the probe tone, is a 220 Hz pure tone that is delivered at 85 dB SPL. The SPL of the probe tone is monitored by an immittance meter, and any change is noted as a change in energy flow through the middle ear system.

Basic Immittance Measures

Three immittance measures are commonly used in the clinical assessment of middle ear function:

- ■ tympanometry,
- ■ static immittance, and
- ■ acoustic reflex thresholds.

Tympanometry

Tympanometry is a way of measuring how acoustic immittance of the middle ear vibratory system changes as air pressure is varied in the external ear canal. Transmission of sound through the middle ear mechanism is maximal when air pressure is equal on both sides of the tympanic membrane. For a normal ear, maximum transmission occurs at, or near, atmospheric pressure. That is, when the air pressure in the external ear canal is the same as the air pressure in the middle ear cavity, the immittance of the normal middle ear vibratory system is at its optimal peak, and energy flow through the system is maximal. Middle ear pressure is assessed by varying pressure in the sealed ear canal until the SPL of the probe tone is at its minimum, reflecting maximum transmission of sound through the middle ear mechanism. But, if the air pressure in the external ear canal is either more than (positive pressure) or less than (negative pressure) the air pressure in the middle ear space, the immittance of the system changes, and energy flow is diminished. In a normal system, as soon as the air pressure changes even slightly below or above the air pressure that produces maximum immittance, the energy flow

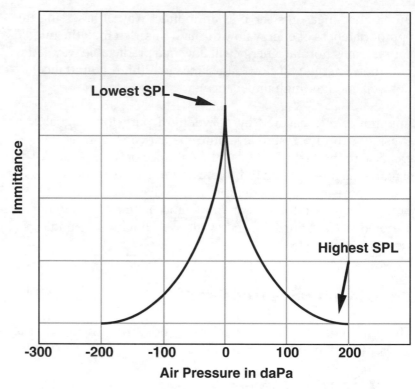

Figure 7–3. A tympanogram, showing that as the pressure is varied above or below the point of maximum transmission, the sound-pressure level (SPL) of the probe tone in the ear canal increases, reflecting a reduction in sound transmission through the middle ear mechanism.

drops quickly and steeply to a minimum value. As the pressure is varied above or below the point of maximum transmission, the SPL of the probe tone in the ear canal increases, reflecting a reduction in sound transmission through the middle ear (Figure 7–3).

The clinical value of tympanometry is that middle ear disorder modifies the shape of the tympanogram in predictable ways. Various patterns of tympanometric shapes are related to various auditory disorders. The conventional classification system designates three tympanogram types, Types, A, B, and C.

Figure 7–4 is an example of the results of tympanometry from a person with normal middle ear function. Air pressure is expressed as negative or positive relative to atmospheric pressure. The unit of measure of air pressure is the **decaPascal, or daPa**. The unit of measure of immittance is the **millimhO, or mmhO**.

decaPascals or daPa = unit of pressure in which 1 daPa equals 10 Pascals

millimhO or mmhO = one-thousandth of a mho, which is a unit of electrical conductance, expressed as the reciprocal of ohm

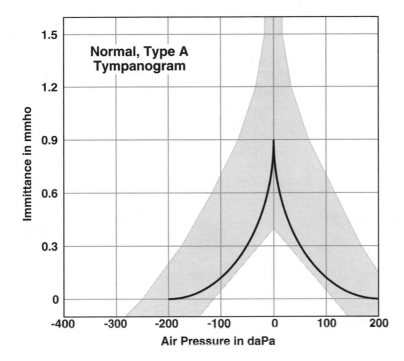

Figure 7–4. A Type A tympanogram, representing normal middle ear function.

This plot of immittance against air pressure is referred to as a tympanogram. In the case of the normal system, the tympanogram has a characteristic shape. There is a sharp peak in immittance in the vicinity of 0 daPa of air pressure and a rapid decline in immittance as air pressure moves away from 0, either in the negative or positive direction. This characteristically normal shape is designated **Type "A."**

Type A = normal

If the middle ear space is filled with fluid, as is an ear with otitis media with effusion, then the tympanogram will lose its sharp peak and become relatively flat or only slightly rounded. This is due to the mass added to the ossicular chain by the fluid. This tympanogram's shape is designated **Type "B"** and is depicted in Figure 7–5. In this case, the SPL in the ear canal remains fairly constant, regardless of the change in air pressure. Because of the increase in mass behind the tympanic membrane, varying the air pressure in the ear canal has little effect on the amount of energy that flows through the middle ear, and the SPL of the probe tone in the ear canal does not change.

Type B = flat

A common cause of middle ear disorder is faulty Eustachian tube function. The Eustachian tube connects the middle ear space to

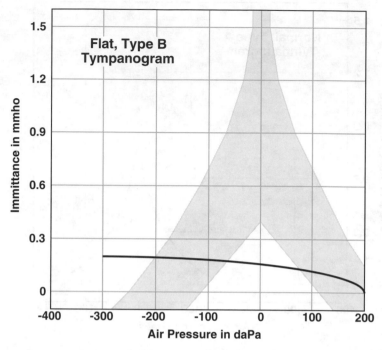

Figure 7-5. A Type B tympanogram, representing middle ear disorder characterized by an increased mass in the middle ear system.

the nasopharynx and is ordinarily closed. The tube opens briefly during swallowing, and fresh air is allowed to reach the middle ear. Sometimes the tube does not open during swallowing. This often occurs as a result of swelling in the nasopharynx that blocks the orifice. When the Eustachian tube does not open, the air that is trapped in the middle ear is absorbed by the mucosal lining. This results in a reduction of air pressure in the middle ear space relative to the pressure in the external ear canal. This pressure differential will retract the tympanic membrane inward. The effect on the tympanogram is to move the sharp peak away from 0 daPa and into the negative air pressure region. The reason for this is simple. Remember that energy flows maximally through the system when the air pressure in the ear canal is equal to the air pressure in the middle ear cavity. In normal ears this occurs at atmospheric pressure. But, if the pressure in the middle ear space is less than atmospheric pressure, because of the absorption of trapped air, then the maximum energy flow will occur when the pressure in the ear canal is negative and matches that in the middle ear space. When this balance has been achieved, energy flow through the middle ear system will be at its maximum and the tympanogram will be at its peak. This tympanogram, normal in shape, but with a peak at substantial negative air pressure, is designated **Type "C."**

Type C = negative pressure

Anything that causes the ossicular chain to become stiffer than normal can result in a reduction in energy flow through the middle ear. The added stiffness simply attenuates the peak of the tympanogram. The shape will remain normal Type "A," but the entire tympanogram will become shallower. Such a tympanogram is designated **Type "A$_s$"** to indicate that the shape is normal, with the peak at or near 0 daPa of air pressure, but with significant reduction in the height at the peak. The subscript "s" denotes *stiffness* or *shallowness*. The disorder most commonly associated with a Type A$_s$ tympanogram is otosclerosis, a disease of the bone surrounding the footplate of the stapes.

Type A$_s$ = normal shape, but height is significantly decreased or shallow

Anything that causes the ossicular chain to lose stiffness can result in too much energy flow through the middle ear. For example, if there is a break or discontinuity in the ossicles connecting the tympanic membrane to the cochlea, the tympanogram will retain its normal shape, but the peak will be much greater than normal. With the heavy load of the cochlear fluid system removed from the chain, the tympanic membrane is much more free to respond to forced vibration. The energy flow through the middle ear is greatly enhanced, resulting in a very deep tympanogram. This shape is designated **"A$_d$"** to indicate that the shape of the tympanogram is normal, with the peak at or near 0 daPa of air pressure, but the height is significantly increased. The subscript "d" denotes *deep* or *discontinuity*.

Type A$_d$ = normal shape, but height is significantly increased or deep

The four abnormal tympanogram types are shown in Figure 7–6. Their diagnostic value lies in the information that they convey about middle ear function, which provides valuable clues about changes in the physical status of the middle ear. The usefulness of tympanometry is enhanced when it is viewed in combination with two other components of the total battery, static immittance and the acoustic reflex.

Static Immittance

In contrast to the dynamic measure of middle ear function represented by the tympanogram, the term **static immittance** refers to the isolated contribution of the middle ear to the overall acoustic immittance of the auditory system. It can be thought of as simply the absolute height of the tympanogram at its peak. The static immittance is measured by comparing the probe-tone SPL or immittance when the air pressure is at 0 daPa, or at the air pres-

Static immittance is the measure of the contribution of the middle ear to acoustic impedance.

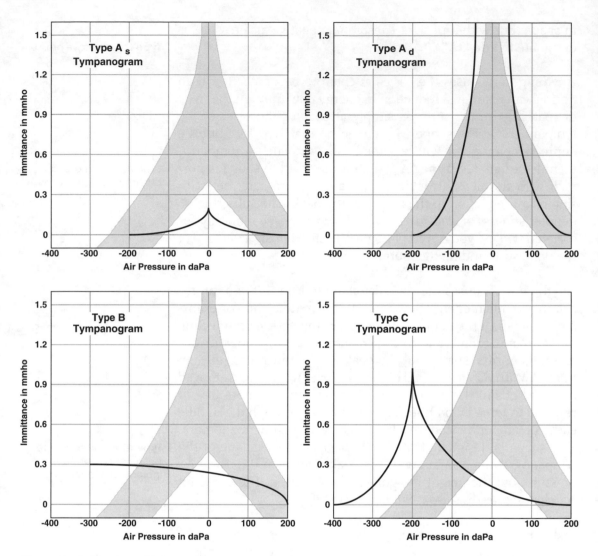

Figure 7-6. The four abnormal tympanogram types.

sure corresponding to the peak, with the immittance when the air pressure is raised to positive 200 daPa. It is convenient to express these immittance measures as equivalent volumes of air in cubic centimeters (cc). The idea is a simple one. When a signal of equivalent intensity is placed into different sized cavities, the SPL of the signal varies. The SPL of the signal in a small cavity is relatively higher and in a large cavity is relatively lower. Therefore, if the probe-tone SPL increases when the air pressure is raised to +200 daPa as less energy flows through the middle ear, it is as if the cavity is smaller. Conversely, if the SPL decreases at 0 daPa as more energy flows through the middle ear, it is as if the cavity is larger. Thus these changes in SPL can be converted to the notion of volume changes and expressed in units of *equivalent volume.* It is important to remember that little actual volume change occurs. Only the SPL of the probe-tone changes due to energy flowing through the middle ear, *as if* the volume changed. When the air pressure is at +200 daPa, this measure is equivalent to the volume of air in the external ear canal. The contribution from the middle ear system is negligible. Volume of air in the external ear canal varies from 0.5 cc to 1.5 cc in children and adults. When the air pressure is at 0 daPa, however, the measured volume is larger because it includes the equivalent volume of the middle ear system. Remember that, as the air pressure is adjusted from +200 to 0, the energy flow through the normal middle ear system is enhanced, resulting in a decrease in probe-tone SPL, as if the volume of the system had increased. The static immittance, then, is the difference between the volume measurement at the two different air pressures. In adults with normal middle ear function, the difference ranges from 0.3 to 1.6 cc.

There are two diagnostic applications of the static immittance. First, values lying below 0.3 cc or above 1.6 cc are strong evidence of middle ear disorder. This information is useful in deciding whether a Type A tympanogram is normal, shallow, or deep. For example, if the tympanogram is Type A and the static immittance is 0.2, then the tympanogram can be considered shallow and indicative of increased stiffness of the middle ear mechanism. Unfortunately, the range of normal static immittance is so large that many of the milder forms of middle ear disorder will fall within the normal boundaries. Thus, the test lacks transitivity in that only one outcome is meaningful. That is, if the static immittance falls outside the normal range, it is safe to predict middle ear disorder. But, values within the normal range do not necessarily exclude the possibility of middle ear disorder.

The second, and perhaps more useful clinical application of the static immittance measure lies in its ability to detect small perforations of the tympanic membrane. Recall that the first volume measurement taken, with the air pressure in the external canal at +200 daPa, is indicating the equivalent volume of air in the external ear canal. If there is any hole in the tympanic membrane through which air can travel, then the measurement will be of both the ear canal and the much larger volume of air in the middle ear space. Therefore, if the initial volume measurement in the static immittance procedure is considerably larger than 1.5 cc, such as 4.5 or 5.0 cc, it means that there is a perforation in the tympanic membrane through which air can pass. This method for detecting perforations can be more sensitive to small perforations than visual inspection of the tympanic membrane.

Acoustic Reflexes

When a sound is of sufficient intensity, it will elicit a reflex of the middle ear musculature. In humans, the reflex consists primarily of the **stapedius muscle**. In other animals, the **tensor tympani muscle** contributes to a greater degree to the overall reflex.

The two muscles of the middle ear are the **stapedius** and the **tensor tympani**.

The stapedius muscle is attached by a tendon from the posterior wall of the middle ear to the head of the stapes. When the muscle contracts, the tendon exerts tension on the stapes, stiffens the ossicular chain, and reduces low-frequency energy transmission through the middle ear. The result of this reduced energy transmission is an increase in probe-tone SPL in the external ear canal. Therefore, when the stapedius muscle contracts in response to high-intensity sounds, a slight change in immittance can be detected by the circuitry of the immittance instrument.

Both middle ear muscles contract in response to sound delivered to either ear. Therefore, **ipsilateral** (uncrossed) and **contralateral** (crossed) reflexes are recorded with sound presented to each ear. For example, when a signal of sufficient magnitude is presented to the right ear, a stapedius reflex will occur in both the right (ipsilateral or uncrossed) and the left (contralateral or crossed) ears. These are called the *right uncrossed* and the *right crossed* reflexes, respectively. When a signal is presented to the left ear and a reflex is measured in that ear, it is referred to as a *left uncrossed* reflex. When a signal is presented to the left ear and a reflex is measured in the right ear, it is referred to as a *left crossed* reflex.

Ipsilateral = uncrossed; **contralateral** = crossed

Threshold Measures. The threshold is the most common measure of the acoustic stapedial reflex and is defined as the lowest intensity level at which a middle ear immittance change can be detected in response to sound. In people having normal hearing and normal middle ear function, reflex thresholds for pure tones will be reached at levels ranging from 70 to 100 dB HL. The average threshold level is approximately 85 dB. These levels are constant across the frequency range from 500 to 4000 Hz. Threshold measures are useful for at least two purposes: (a) differential assessment of auditory disorder and (b) prediction of hearing sensitivity.

Reflex threshold measurement has been valuable in both the assessment of middle ear function and the differentiation of coch-

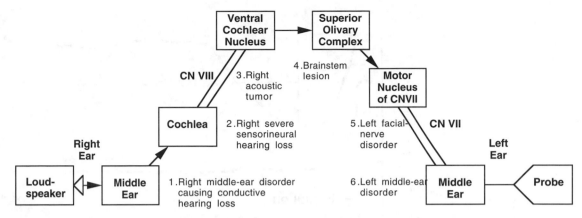

Figure 7-7. Schematic representation of the auditory and nervous-system structures involved in a crossed acoustic reflex, with six possible causes for the absence of a right crossed acoustic reflex.

lear from retrocochlear disorder. In terms of the latter, whereas reflex thresholds occur at reduced sensation levels in ears with cochlear hearing loss, they are typically elevated or absent in ears with VIIIth nerve disorder. Similarly, reflex thresholds are often abnormal in patients with brain stem disorder. Comparison of crossed and uncrossed thresholds has also been found to be helpful in differentiating VIIIth nerve from brain stem disorders.

Although threshold measures are valuable, interpretation of the absence or abnormal elevation of an acoustic reflex threshold can be difficult because the same reflex abnormality can result from a number of pathologic conditions. For example, the absence of a right crossed acoustic reflex can result from:

- ■ a substantial conductive loss on the right ear that keeps sound from being sufficient to cause a reflex,
- ■ a severe sensorineural hearing loss on the right ear that keeps sound from being sufficient to cause a reflex,
- ■ right VIIIth nerve tumor that keeps sound from being sufficient to cause a reflex,
- ■ a lesion of the crossing fibers of the central portion of the reflex arc,
- ■ left facial nerve disorder that restricts neural impulses from reaching the stapedius muscle, or
- ■ left middle ear disorder that keeps the stapedius contraction from having an influence on middle ear function.

A schematic example of these six possibilities is shown in Figure 7–7. It is for this reason that the addition of uncrossed reflex

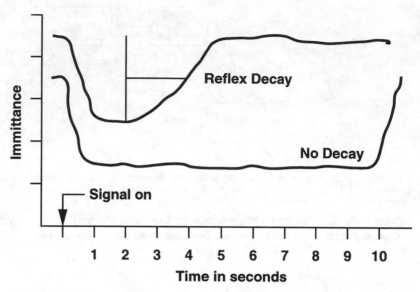

Figure 7-8. Examples of no acoustic reflex decay and abnormal acoustic reflex decay. Abnormal decay occurs when the amplitude of the reflex decreases to at least half of its initial maximum value.

measurement, tympanometry, and static immittance is important in reflex threshold interpretation.

Acoustic reflex thresholds have also been used for the prediction of peripheral auditory sensitivity. Cochlear bandwidth effects on the acoustic reflex have been exploited to predict degree of hearing loss and have been applied successfully in the clinic. Although not altogether precise, use of acoustic reflexes for the general categorization of normal versus abnormal cochlear sensitivity is clinically useful as a powerful crosscheck to behavioral audiometry, especially in children.

Suprathreshold Measures. Suprathreshold analysis of the acoustic reflex includes such measures as **decay, latency**, and **amplitude**. Acoustic reflex decay is often a component of routine immittance measurement used to differentiate cochlear from VIIIth nerve disorder. Although various measurement techniques and criteria for abnormality have been developed, reflex decay testing is typically carried out by presenting a 10-second signal at 10 dB above the reflex threshold. Results are considered abnormal if amplitude of the resultant reflex decreases to less than half of its initial maximum value (Figure 7–8). Reflex decay has been shown to be a sensitive measure of VIIIth nerve, brain stem, and

Decay is the diminution of the physical properties of a stimulus or response.

Latency is the time interval between two events, as a stimulus and a response.

Amplitude is the magnitude of a sound wave, acoustic reflex, or evoked potential.

neuromuscular disorders. One of the problems associated with reflex decay testing, however, is a high false-positive rate in patients with cochlear hearing loss. For example, positive reflex decay has been reported in as many as 27% of patients with cochlear loss due to Ménière's disease. This is considered a false-positive result in that it is positive for retrocochlear disorder when the actual disorder is cochlear in nature.

Other suprathreshold measures include latency and amplitude. Various studies have suggested that these measures may provide additional sensitivity to the immittance battery, especially in the differentiation of retrocochlear disorder. Reflex latency and rise time have been used as diagnostic measures and have been shown to be abnormal in ears with VIIIth nerve disorder, multiple sclerosis, and other brain stem disorders. Similarly, depressed reflex amplitudes have been reported in patients with VIIIth nerve tumors, multiple sclerosis, and other brain stem disorders.

Principles of Interpretation

The key to the successful interpretation of immittance data lies not in the examination of individual results, but in the examination of the pattern of results characterizing the entire audiometric assessment. Within this frame of reference the following observations are relevant.

1. *Certain tympanometric shapes are diagnostically useful.* The Type C tympanogram, for example, clearly indicates reduced air pressure in the middle ear space. Similarly the Type B tympanogram suggests mass loading of the vibratory mechanism. The Type A tympanogram, however, may be ambiguous to interpret.
2. *Static immittance is also subject to ambiguous interpretation.* Certain pathologies of the middle ear act to render the static immittance abnormally low, while others should have the opposite effect. But the distribution of static immittance in normal ears is so broad (95% interval from 0.3 to 1.6 cc) that only very extreme changes in immittance are sufficient to drive the static immittance outside the normal boundaries.
3. *The acoustic reflex is exceedingly sensitive to middle ear disorder.* Only a 5 to 10 dB air-bone gap is usually sufficient to eliminate the reflex when the immittance probe is in the ear with conductive loss. As a corollary, the most common reason for an abnormality of the acoustic reflex is middle ear disorder. Thus,

the possibility of middle ear disorder as an explanation for any reflex abnormality must always be considered.

4. *Crossed reflex threshold testing is usually carried out at frequencies of 500, 1000, 2000, and 4000 Hz.* However, even in normal ears, results are unstable at 4000 Hz. Apparent abnormality of the reflex threshold at this test frequency may not be diagnostically relevant. Uncrossed reflex threshold testing is usually carried out at frequencies of 1000 and 2000 Hz.

5. *Reflex-eliciting stimuli should not exceed 110 dB HL, for any signal, unless there is clear evidence of a substantial air-bone gap in the ear to which sound is being delivered.* Duration of presentation must be carefully controlled and kept short (i.e., less than 1 second). There is a danger that stimulation at these exceedingly high levels will be upsetting to the patient. Several case reports have documented temporary or permanent auditory changes in patients following reflex testing. It is for this reason that very judicious use be made of the reflex decay test, in which stimulation is continuous for 5 to 10 seconds.

Clinical Applications

Middle Ear Disorder

Principles of Clinical Application. Middle ear function is assessed by measurement of static immittance, tympanometry, and acoustic reflexes. Each measure is evaluated in isolation against normative data and then in combination to determine the pattern. The typical immittance pattern associated with middle ear disorder includes:

1. some abnormality of the normal tympanometric shape,
2. some abnormality of the static immittance, and
3. no observable acoustic reflex to either crossed or uncrossed stimulation when the probe is in the affected ear.

In addition, if the middle ear disorder results in a substantial conductive hearing loss, no crossed reflex will be observed when the reflex-eliciting signal is presented to the affected ear. Patterns fall into one of six categories, which are described in Table 7–1. The six patterns include:

1. results consistent with normal middle ear function,
2. results consistent with an increase in the mass of the middle ear mechanism,

Table 7-1. Patterns of immittance-measurement results in various middle-ear disorders.

Middle-Ear Condition	Tympanogram	Static Immittance	Acoustic Reflex
Normal	A	normal	normal
Increased mass	B	low	absent
Increased stiffness	A_s	low	absent
Excessive compliance	A_d	high	absent
Negative pressure	C	normal	abnormal
TM perforation	B	high	absent

3. results consistent with an increase in the stiffness of the middle ear mechanism,
4. results consistent with excessive immittance of the middle ear system,
5. results consistent with significant negative pressure in the middle ear space.
6. results consistent with tympanic-membrane perforation, and

Normal Middle Ear Function. Figure 7–9 shows immittance results on a young adult. Both ears are characterized by Type A tympanograms, normal static immittance, and normal reflex thresholds.

Increased Mass. Figure 7–10 shows immittance results on a young girl. The right ear results are characterized by a Type B tympanogram, excessively low static immittance, and absent right uncrossed and left crossed acoustic reflexes. These results are consistent with increased mass of the right middle ear mechanism. The left ear immittance results are normal. The tympanogram is a Type A, static immittance is within normal limits, and left uncrossed reflexes are present. The absence of right crossed reflexes in the presence of left uncrossed reflexes suggests that the right middle ear disorder has produced a substantial conductive hearing loss on the right ear. The middle ear disorder characterized here was caused by otitis media with effusion.

Increased Stiffness. Figure 7–11 shows immittance results on a middle-aged woman. Both the right and left ears are characterized by Type A tympanograms, relatively low static immittance, and absent acoustic reflexes. These results are consistent with an increase in stiffness of both middle ear mechanisms. This middle ear disorder was caused by otosclerosis.

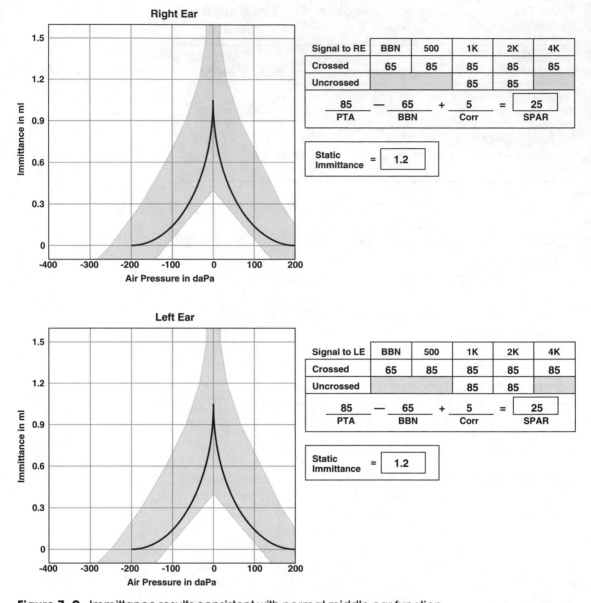

Right Ear

Signal to RE	BBN	500	1K	2K	4K
Crossed	65	85	85	85	85
Uncrossed			85	85	

$$\frac{85}{\text{PTA}} - \frac{65}{\text{BBN}} + \frac{5}{\text{Corr}} = \boxed{\frac{25}{\text{SPAR}}}$$

Static Immittance = 1.2

Left Ear

Signal to LE	BBN	500	1K	2K	4K
Crossed	65	85	85	85	85
Uncrossed			85	85	

$$\frac{85}{\text{PTA}} - \frac{65}{\text{BBN}} + \frac{5}{\text{Corr}} = \boxed{\frac{25}{\text{SPAR}}}$$

Static Immittance = 1.2

Figure 7–9. Immittance results consistent with normal middle ear function.

Excessive Immittance. Figure 7–12 shows immittance results on a 24-year-old man who was evaluated following mild head trauma. The left ear results are characterized by a Type A tympanogram, excessively high static immittance, and absent acoustic reflexes, probe left (left uncrossed and right crossed). The right ear immittance results are normal. The tympanogram is a Type A, static immittance is within normal limits, and right uncrossed reflexes are present. The absence of left crossed reflexes in the

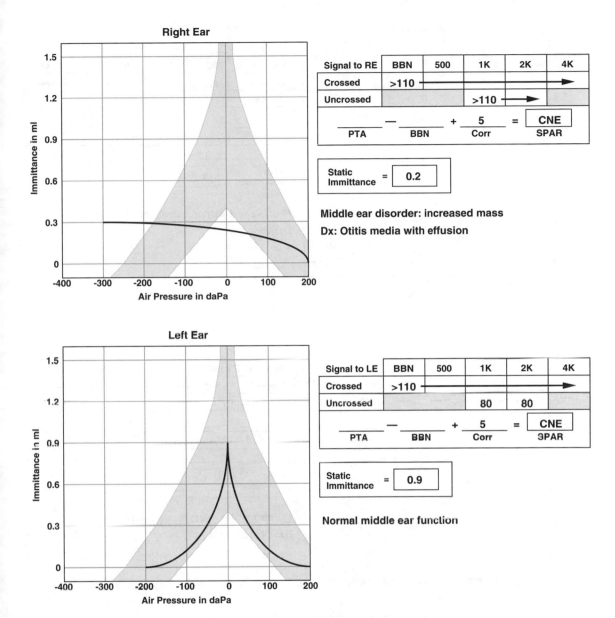

Figure 7-10. Immittance results consistent with right middle ear disorder, characterized by increased mass of the middle ear system caused by otitis media with effusion.

presence of right uncrossed reflexes suggests that the left middle ear disorder is causing a substantial conductive hearing loss on the left ear. This middle ear disorder was caused by ossicular discontinuity.

Tympanic-Membrane Perforation. Figure 7–13 shows immittance results on a young boy. The right ear results are character-

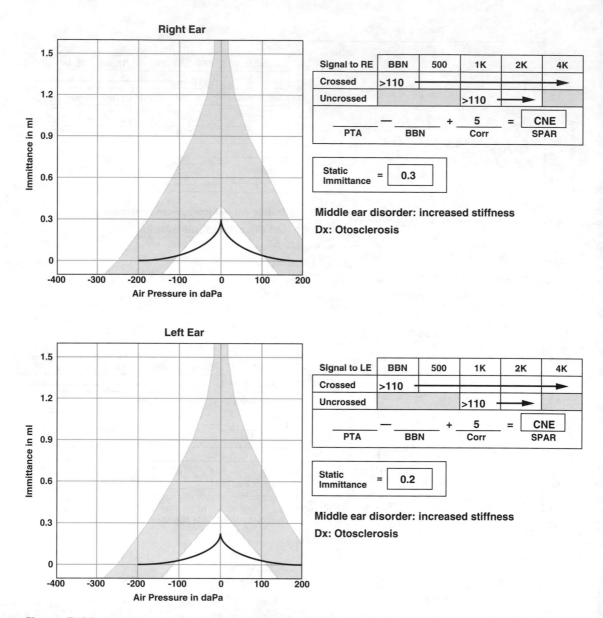

Figure 7-11. Immittance results consistent with bilateral middle ear disorder, characterized by increased stiffness of the middle ear system caused by otosclerosis.

ized by an inability to measure a tympanogram, excessive volume, and unmeasurable acoustic reflexes from the right probe (right uncrossed and left crossed). These results are consistent with a perforated tympanic membrane. The left ear immittance results are normal. The tympanogram is a Type A, static immittance is within normal limits, and left uncrossed reflexes are present. The slight elevation of right crossed reflexes in the presence

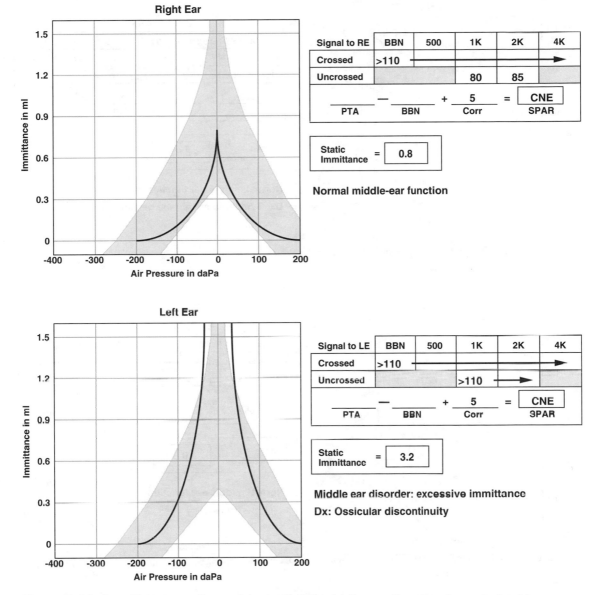

Figure 7-12. Immittance results consistent with left middle ear disorder, characterized by excessive immittance caused by ossicular discontinuity.

of normal left uncrossed reflexes suggests that the right middle ear disorder is causing a mild conductive hearing loss on the right ear.

Negative Middle Ear Pressure. Figure 7–14 shows immittance results on a 2-year-old boy. Results are identical on both ears and are characterized by Type C tympanograms (peak at −200 and

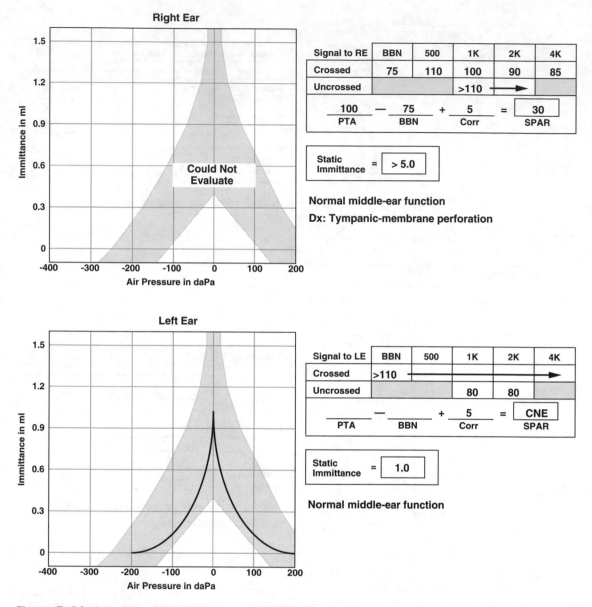

Figure 7-13. Immittance results consistent with right middle ear disorder, characterized by excessive volume caused by tympanic membrane perforation.

−250 daPa in the right and left ear respectively), normal static immittance, and absent acoustic reflexes. These results are consistent with significant negative pressure in the middle ear space.

Cochlear Disorder

The typical immittance pattern associated with cochlear disorder includes:

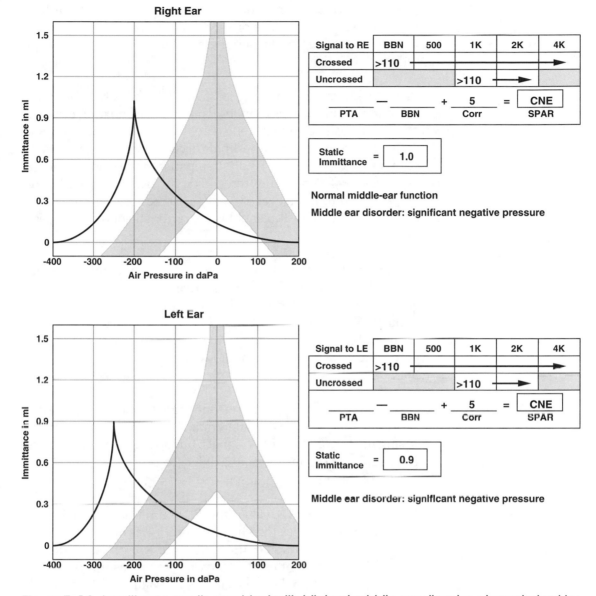

Figure 7-14. Immittance results consistent with bilateral middle ear disorder, characterized by significant negative pressure in the middle ear space.

- normal tympanogram,
- normal static immittance, and
- normal reflex thresholds.

Reflex thresholds will only be normal, however, as long as the sensitivity loss by air conduction does not exceed 50 dB HL. Above this level, the reflex threshold is usually elevated in proportion to the degree of loss. Once a behavioral threshold exceeds 70 dB, the absence of a reflex is equivocal, because it can be due to the degree of peripheral hearing loss as well as to retrocochlear disorder.

In ears with cochlear hearing loss, acoustic reflex thresholds are present at reduced sensation levels. In normal-hearing ears, behavioral threshold to pure tones are, by definition, at or around 0 dB HL. Acoustic reflex thresholds occur at or around 85 dB HL, or at a sensation level of 85 dB. In a patient with a sensorineural hearing loss of 40 dB, reflex thresholds still occur at around 85 dB HL, or at a sensation level of 45 dB. This reduced sensation level of the acoustic reflex threshold is characteristic of cochlear hearing loss.

Several methods have been developed for using acoustic reflex thresholds to predict hearing sensitivity. One method that has gained some popularity is the Sensitivity Prediction by the Acoustic Reflex (SPAR) test. The SPAR test is based on the well-documented difference between acoustic reflex thresholds to pure-tones versus broad-band noise (BBN) and on the change in BBN thresholds, but not pure-tone thresholds, as a result of sensorineural hearing loss. That is, thresholds to BBN signals are lower than thresholds to pure-tone signals. However, sensorineural hearing loss has a differential effect on the two signals, raising the threshold to BBN signals, but not to pure-tone signals. The SPAR test capitalizes on this effect to provide a general prediction of the presence or absence of hearing loss.

SPAR = Reflex PTA − BBN

To compute the **SPAR** value, the BBN threshold is subtracted from the average reflex threshold to pure-tones of 500, 1000, and 2000 Hz. The magnitude of this difference will vary according to the specific equipment used to carry out the measures. A correction factor is then applied to yield a SPAR value of 20 in normal-hearing subjects. If a patient's SPAR value is less than 15, there is a high probability of a sensorineural hearing loss. An example of the SPAR calculation in a normal-hearing individual is shown in Figure 7–15. Note the low value of the BBN threshold in comparison to the thresholds for pure tones. The difference between the average pure-tone thresholds and BBN threshold is large, resulting in a large or normal SPAR. An example of the SPAR calculation in a patient with a high-frequency sensorineural hearing impairment is shown in Figure 7–16. Note the higher BBN threshold and how it affects the SPAR value.

Use of the SPAR or other techniques based on acoustic reflex thresholds is only effective at predicting general degree of hear-

Crossed Reflex Thresholds	BBN	500	1K	2K	4K
	65	85	85	85	85

$$\underset{\text{PTA}}{85} - \underset{\text{BBN}}{65} + \underset{\text{Corr}}{5} = \boxed{\underset{\text{SPAR}}{25}}$$

Figure 7-15. The SPAR calculation in a normal-hearing ear, calculated by subtracting the broadband noise (BBN) threshold from the pure-tone average (PTA) and adding a correction (Corr) factor.

Crossed Reflex Thresholds	BBN	500	1K	2K	4K
	80	80	85	95	100

$$\underset{\text{PTA}}{85} - \underset{\text{BBN}}{80} + \underset{\text{Corr}}{5} = \boxed{\underset{\text{SPAR}}{10}}$$

Figure 7-16. The SPAR calculation in an ear with a high-frequency sensorineural hearing loss.

ing loss. Clinical application of such techniques appears to be most effective when used to predict presence or absence of a sensorineural hearing loss.

Prediction of hearing sensitivity by acoustic reflex thresholds can be very valuable in testing a child on whom behavioral thresholds cannot be obtained. Figure 7–17 shows immittance results of a 2-year-old child who fits this description. Regardless of the nature or intensity of effort, behavioral audiometry could not be completed, and a startle reflex could not be elicited at equipment intensity limits. Tympanograms were Type A, with maximum immittance at 0 daPa. Static immittance was symmetric and within normal limits. Crossed acoustic reflex thresholds were present and normal at 500 and 1000 Hz, elevated at 2000 Hz, and absent at 4000 Hz, bilaterally. The SPAR value was only 4 dB bilaterally, suggesting a significant sensorineural hearing loss. Based on the SPAR and on the configuration of the crossed threshold pattern, these immittance measures predicted a sensorineural hearing

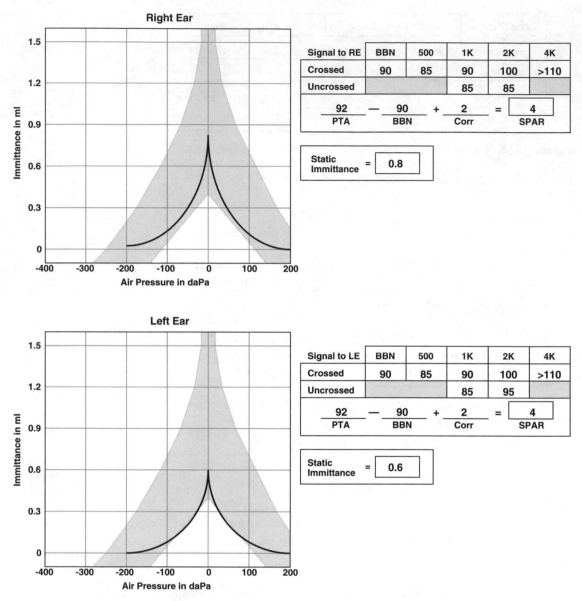

Right Ear

Signal to RE	BBN	500	1K	2K	4K
Crossed	90	85	90	100	>110
Uncrossed			85	85	

$$\frac{92}{\text{PTA}} - \frac{90}{\text{BBN}} + \frac{2}{\text{Corr}} = \boxed{4}\ \text{SPAR}$$

Static Immittance = 0.8

Left Ear

Signal to LE	BBN	500	1K	2K	4K
Crossed	90	85	90	100	>110
Uncrossed			85	95	

$$\frac{92}{\text{PTA}} - \frac{90}{\text{BBN}} + \frac{2}{\text{Corr}} = \boxed{4}\ \text{SPAR}$$

Static Immittance = 0.6

Figure 7–17. Immittance results, with SPARs predicting significant sensorineural hearing loss, on a 2-year-old child from whom behavioral thresholds could not be obtained.

loss, greater in the high-frequency region of the audiogram than in the low.

A second application of reflex measurement for sensitivity prediction is in the case of a patient who is feigning hearing loss. Figure 7–18 shows immittance results on a 34-year-old male patient who was evaluated for a right-ear hearing loss. He reported

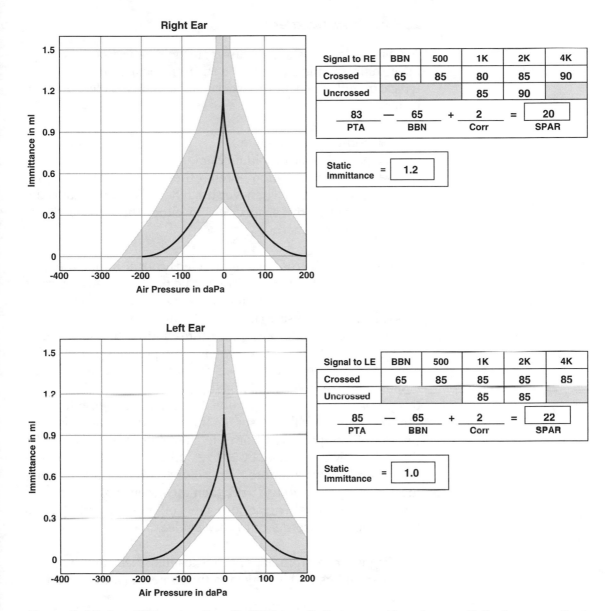

Figure 7-18. Immittance results, with SPARs predicting normal hearing sensitivity, from a patient who was feigning a right-ear hearing loss.

that the loss occurred as the result of an industrial accident, during which he was exposed to high intensity-noise as a result of steam release from a broken pipe at an oil refinery. The tympanogram, static immittance, and acoustic reflex thresholds were all within normal limits. SPARs of 20 and 22 dB and a flat reflex threshold configuration predicted normal hearing sensitivity bilaterally.

Retrocochlear Disorder

Acoustic reflex threshold or suprathreshold patterns can be helpful in differentiating cochlear from retrocochlear disorder. The typical immittance pattern associated with retrocochlear disorder includes:

- normal tympanogram,
- normal static immittance, and
- abnormal elevation of reflex threshold, or absence of reflex response, whenever the reflex-eliciting signal is delivered to the suspect ear in either the crossed or the uncrossed mode.

For example, in the case of a right-sided acoustic tumor, the tympanograms and static immittance would be normal. Abnormality would be observed for the right uncrossed and the right-to-left crossed reflex responses. The key factor differentiating retrocochlear from cochlear elevated reflex thresholds is the audiometric level at the test frequency. As you learned previously, in the case of cochlear loss, reflex thresholds are not elevated at all until the audiometric loss exceeds 50 dB HL, and even above this level the degree of elevation is proportional to the audiometric level. In the case of retrocochlear disorder, however, the elevation is more than would be predicted from the audiometric level. The reflex threshold may be elevated by 20 to 25 dB even though the audiometric level shows no more than a 5 or 10 dB loss. If the audiometric loss exceeds 70 to 75 dB, then the absence of the acoustic reflex is ambiguous. The abnormality could be attributed either to retrocochlear disorder or to cochlear loss.

For diagnostic interpretation, acoustic reflex measures are probably best understood if viewed in the context of a three-part reflex arc:

- the sensory or input portion (afferent),
- the central nervous system portion that transmits neural information (central), and
- the motor or output portion (efferent).

An afferent abnormality occurs as the result of a disordered sensory system on one ear. An example of a pure afferent effect would result from a profound unilateral sensorineural hearing loss on the right ear. Both reflexes with signal presented to the right ear (right uncrossed and right-to-left crossed) would be absent. An efferent abnormality occurs as the result of a disordered motor system or middle ear mechanism on one ear. An example of a pure efferent effect would result from right unilateral facial nerve paralysis. Both reflexes measured by the probe in the right ear (right uncrossed and left-to-right crossed) would be absent. A central pathway abnormality occurs as the result of brain stem disorder and is manifested by the elevation or absence of one or both of the crossed acoustic reflexes in the presence of normal uncrossed reflex thresholds.

Cochlear Hearing Loss. Figure 7–19 shows the immittance results of a patient with a sensorineural hearing loss. The patient was diagnosed as having acute **labyrinthitis** resulting in a unilateral hearing loss and dizziness. Tympanograms, static immittance, and acoustic reflex thresholds are within normal limits. Even though the patient has a substantial sensorineural hearing loss in the left ear, reflex thresholds remain within normal limits. The presence of left uncrossed and left-to-right crossed reflexes argues for a cochlear site of disorder.

Labyrinthitis is the inflammation of the labyrinth, affecting hearing, balance, or both.

Afferent Abnormality. Figure 7–20 shows the immittance results of a patient with an afferent acoustic reflex abnormality resulting from retrocochlear disorder. The patient was diagnosed as having a right acoustic tumor. Tympanograms and static compliance were normal. Acoustic reflexes, with sound presented to the left ear (left uncrossed and left-to-right crossed), were normal. However, reflexes with sound presented to the right ear (right uncrossed and right-to-left crossed) were absent. This pattern of abnormality suggests an afferent disorder which, in the absence of a severe degree of hearing loss, is consistent with retrocochlear disorder.

Efferent Abnormality. Figure 7–21 shows the immittance results of a patient with an efferent acoustic reflex abnormality resulting from facial-nerve disorder. The patient had experienced a sudden left-sided facial paralysis of unknown etiology. She had no history of previous middle ear disorder and no auditory complaints. The tympanogram and static immittance were normal on both ears. Acoustic reflexes were present at normal intensity levels when recorded from the right probe (right uncrossed and left-to-right crossed). However, no reflexes could be measured from the left ear, regardless of which ear was being stimulated (absent left uncrossed and right-to-left crossed). This pattern of abnormality suggests an efferent disorder which, in the absence of any middle ear disorder, is consistent with a neurologic disorder affecting the **VIIth cranial nerve**.

VIIth cranial nerve = facial nerve

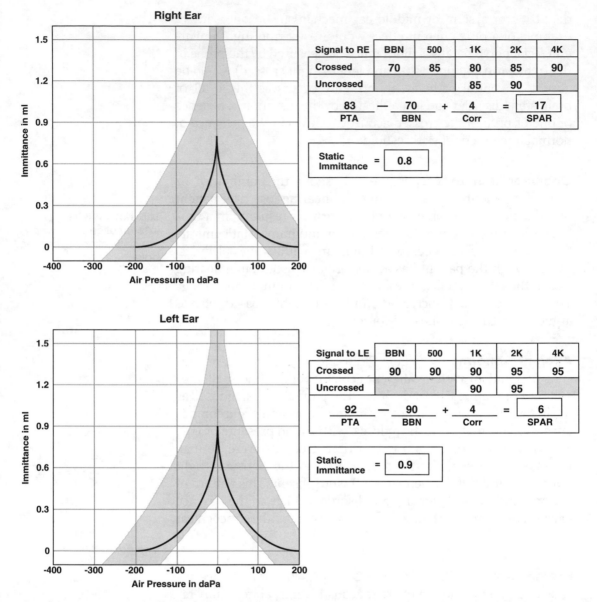

Right Ear

Signal to RE	BBN	500	1K	2K	4K
Crossed	70	85	80	85	90
Uncrossed			85	90	

$$\frac{83}{\text{PTA}} - \frac{70}{\text{BBN}} + \frac{4}{\text{Corr}} = \boxed{\frac{17}{\text{SPAR}}}$$

Static Immittance = 0.8

Left Ear

Signal to LE	BBN	500	1K	2K	4K
Crossed	90	90	90	95	95
Uncrossed			90	95	

$$\frac{92}{\text{PTA}} - \frac{90}{\text{BBN}} + \frac{4}{\text{Corr}} = \boxed{\frac{6}{\text{SPAR}}}$$

Static Immittance = 0.9

Figure 7-19. Immittance results consistent with normal middle ear function and a left sensorineural hearing loss.

Central Pathway Abnormality. Figure 7–22 shows immittance results of a patient with a central pathway abnormality resulting from brain stem disorder. The patient has multiple sclerosis, a disease that causes lesions throughout the brain stem and often results in auditory-system abnormalities. Static immittance and tympanograms were normal bilaterally. Uncrossed reflexes were normal for both ears. In addition, right-to-left crossed reflexes

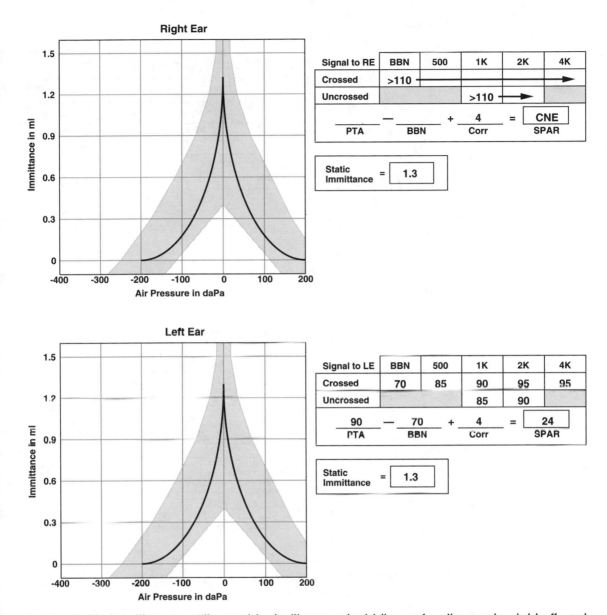

Figure 7-20. Immittance results consistent with normal middle ear function and a right afferent acoustic reflex abnormality resulting from a right acoustic tumor.

were present at normal levels. However, left-to-right crossed reflexes were absent. The presence of a left uncrossed reflex rules out the possibility of either a substantial hearing loss or an acoustic tumor on the left side. The presence of a right uncrossed reflex rules out the possibility of middle ear disorder on the right side. The absence of a left crossed reflex, then, can only be explained as the result of a brain stem disorder.

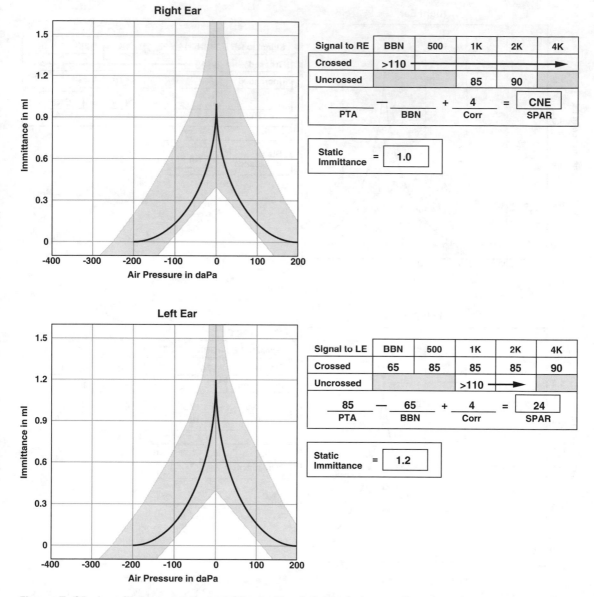

Figure 7–21. Immittance results consistent with a left efferent acoustic reflex abnormality, resulting from a left facial nerve paralysis of unknown cause.

Summary

- Immittance is a physical characteristic of all mechanical vibratory systems. In very general terms, it is a measure of how readily a system can be set into vibration by a driving force.
- Immittance audiometry can be thought of as a way of assessing the manner in which energy flows through the outer and middle ears to the cochlea.

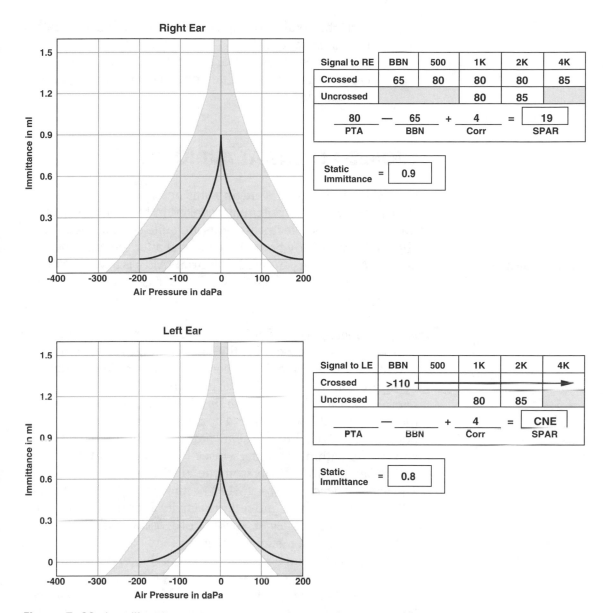

Figure 7–22. Immittance results consistent with a central pathway abnormality, resulting from brain stem disorder secondary to multiple sclerosis.

■ Immittance audiometry is a powerful tool for the evaluation of auditory disorder.

■ Three immittance measures are commonly used in the clinical assessment of middle ear function: tympanometry, static immittance, and acoustic reflex thresholds.

■ The key to successful use of the immittance battery in clinical evaluation is to view the results in combination with the totality of the audiometric examination rather than in isolation.

■ Immittance measures are useful in quantifying middle ear disorders and in differentiating cochlear from retrocochlear disorders.

EVOKED POTENTIAL AUDIOMETRY

By means of computer averaging, it is possible to extract the tiny electrical voltages, or potentials, evoked in the brain by acoustic stimulation. These electrical events are quite complex and can be observed over a fairly broad time interval after the onset of stimulation. An **auditory evoked potential** (AEP) is a waveform that reflects the electrophysiologic function of a certain portion of the central auditory nervous system in response to sound.

Auditory evoked potentials include ECoG, ABR, MLR, and LLR.

For audiologic purposes, it is convenient to group the AEPs into categories based loosely on the latency ranges over which the potentials are observed. The earliest of the evoked potentials, occurring within the first 5 msec following signal presentation, is referred to as an *electrocochleogram* (ECoG) and reflects activity of the cochlea and VIIIth nerve. The most commonly used evoked potential is referred to as the *auditory brain stem response* (ABR) and occurs within the first 10 msec following signal onset. The ABR reflects neural activity from the VIIIth nerve to the midbrain. The *middle latency response* (MLR) occurs within the first 50 msec following signal onset and reflects activity at or near the auditory cortex. The *late latency response* (LLR) occurs within the first 250 msec following signal onset and reflects activity of the primary-auditory and association areas of the cerebral cortex.

Auditory evoked potentials provide an objective means of assessing the integrity of the peripheral and central auditory systems. For this reason, evoked potential audiometry has become a powerful tool in the measurement of hearing of young children and others who cannot or will not cooperate during behavioral testing. It also serves as a valuable diagnostic tool in measuring the function of auditory nervous system structures.

There are four major applications of auditory evoked potential measurement:

■ prediction of hearing sensitivity;
■ neonatal hearing screening;

- diagnostic assessment of central auditory nervous system function; and
- monitoring of auditory nervous system function during surgery.

The use of auditory evoked potentials for prediction of hearing sensitivity and infant hearing screening has had a major impact on our ability to identify hearing impairment in children. The ABR is used in these cases either to screen newborns to identify those in need of additional testing or to predict hearing sensitivity levels in children with suspected hearing impairment.

Diagnostic assessment is usually made with the ABR, MLR, and LLR. The ABR is highly sensitive to disorders of the VIIIth nerve and auditory brain stem and is often used in conjunction with imaging and radiologic measures to assist in the diagnosis of acoustic tumors and brain stem disorders. Surgical monitoring of evoked potentials is usually carried out with ECoG and ABR. These evoked potentials are monitored during VIIIth nerve tumor removal surgery in an effort to preserve hearing.

Measurement Techniques

The brain processes information by sending small electrical impulses from one nerve to another. This electrical activity can be recorded by placing sensing electrodes on the scalp and measuring the ongoing changes in electrical potentials throughout the brain. This technique is called *electroencephalography*, or EEG, and is the basis for recording evoked potentials. The passive monitoring of EEG activity reveals the brain in a constant state of activity; electrical potentials of various frequencies and amplitudes are measured continually. If a sound is introduced to the ear, the brain's response to that sound is just another of a vast number of electrical potentials that occur at that instant in time. Evoked potential measurement techniques are designed to extract those tiny signals from the ongoing electrical activity.

Recording evoked potentials requires sophisticated amplification of the electrical activity, computer signal averaging, proper stimuli to evoke an auditory response, and intricate timing of stimulus delivery and response recording. A schematic representation of the instrumentation is shown in Figure 7–23. Basically, at the same moment in time that a stimulus is presented to an earphone, a computer measures electrical activity from electrodes affixed to the scalp over a fixed period of time. The process is

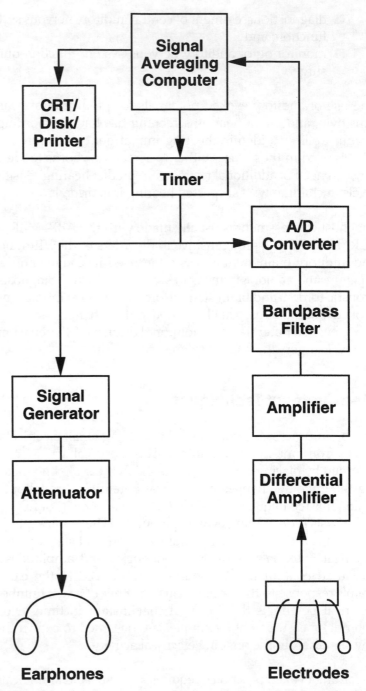

Figure 7-23. Schematic representation of the instrumentation used in recording auditory evoked potentials.

repeated many times, and the computer averages the responses. This results in a series of waveforms that reflect synchronized electrical activity from various structures of the peripheral and central auditory nervous system.

Recording EEG Activity

To record EEG activity, electrodes are affixed to the scalp. These electrodes are usually gold or silver plated and are pasted to the scalp with a gel that facilitates electrical conduction. For measuring auditory evoked potentials, electrodes are placed on the center of the scalp, called the vertex, and on both earlobes or behind the ear on the mastoid area. A ground electrode is usually placed on the forehead. The electrical activity measured at the vertex is compared to that measured at the earlobe.

Electrical potentials related specifically to an auditory signal are quite small in comparison to other electrical activity that is occurring at the same moment in time. The electrodes pick up all electrical activity, and activity related to the auditory stimulation need to be extracted from the other activity. The process involved is designed to enhance the signal in relation to the noise or the **signal-to-noise ratio (S/N)**. The first step in the extraction process occurs at the preamplifier stage. The preamplifier is known as a *differential amplifier,* which is designed to provide **common-mode rejection**. A differential amplifier cancels out activity that is common to both electrodes. For example, 60 Hz noise from lights or electrical fixtures is quite large in amplitude in comparison to the auditory evoked potential. This noise will be seen identically at both the vertex and the earlobe electrodes. The differential amplifier takes the activity measured at the earlobe, inverts it, and subtracts it from the activity measured at the vertex. If the activity is identical or common to both electrodes, it will be eliminated. This process is shown in Figure 7–24. So the first step in the process of extracting the auditory evoked potential is to differentially amplify in a way that eliminates some of the potential background noise. The remaining electrical activity is then amplified significantly, up to 100,000 times its original voltage.

The next step in reducing electrical noise not related to the auditory evoked potential is to filter the EEG activity. Electrical potentials that emanate from the structures of the brain cover a wide range of frequencies. For each of the auditory evoked potentials, we are interested in only a narrow band of frequencies surrounding those that are characteristic of that evoked potential. For example, the auditory brain stem response has five major peaks of

The difference in dB between a sound of interest and background noise is called the **signal-to-noise ratio (S/N)**.

Common mode rejection is a noise-rejection strategy used in electrophysiologic measurement in which noise that is identical at two electrodes is subtracted by a differential amplifier.

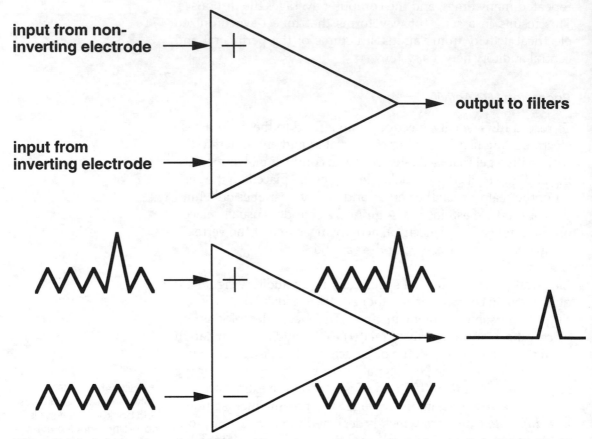

Figure 7-24. Schematic representation of the process of common mode rejection. Activity that is identical or common to both electrodes is eliminated by inverting the input from one electrode and subtracting it from the input to the other.

interest, referred to as waves I through V, which occur about 1 msec apart. Any waveform that repeats every 1 msec has a frequency component of 1000 Hz. Similarly, the largest peaks of the ABR are I, III, and V, which occur at 2 msec intervals. Any waveform that repeats every 2 msec has a frequency component of 500 Hz. As a result, the ABR has two major frequency components, approximately 500 and 1000 Hz. By filtering, electrical activity that occurs above and below these frequencies is reduced in a further effort to focus on the response of interest. Even after differentially amplifying the signal and filtering around the frequencies of interest, the auditory evoked responses remain buried in a background of ongoing electrical activity of the brain. It is only through signal averaging of the response that these potentials can be effectively extracted.

Signal Averaging

Signal averaging is a very effective technique for extracting a signal from a background of noise. The signal that we are pursuing here is a small electrical potential that is buried in a background of ongoing electrical activity of the brain. The purpose of signal averaging is to eliminate the unrelated activity and reveal the auditory evoked potential.

The averaging of samples of EEG activity designed to enhance the response is called **signal averaging**.

Signal averaging is a computer-based technique in which multiple samples of electrical activity are taken over a fixed time base. A key component of the signal averaging process is time-locking of the signal presentation to the recording of the response. That is, a stimulus is delivered to the earphone at the same moment in time that electrical activity is recorded from the electrodes. The sequence is then repeated. For example, when recording an ABR, a click stimulus is presented, and the electrical activity is recorded for 10 msec following stimulus onset. Another click is then presented, and another 10 msec segment of electrical activity is recorded. This process is repeated 1000 to 2000 times.

The segment of time that is designated for electrical-activity recording is sometimes referred to as an *epoch,* after the Greek word meaning a period of time in terms of noteworthy events. Noteworthy is in the eyes of the beholder, and some choose not to use this term but prefer a more common term such as *window* to describe the time segments. The number of time segments that are signal averaged are often referred to as *samples* or *sweeps.*

During each sampling period, the EEG activity is pre-amplified, filtered, and amplified. It is then converted from its analog (A) form to digital (D) form by analog-to-digital (A/D) conversion. Essentially, the A/D converter is activated at the same instant that the stimulus is delivered to the earphone. The A/D converter samples the amplifier and converts the amplitude of the EEG activity at that moment in time to a number. The converter then dwells momentarily and samples again. This continues for the duration of the sample. The process is then repeated for a predetermined number of samples. In the case of the ABR, 1000 to 2000 samples are collected and then averaged. The A/D conversion process is shown schematically in Figure 7–25.

The averaging process is critical to measuring evoked potentials. The concept is a fairly simple one. EEG activity that is not related to the auditory stimulus is being measured at the electrodes along with the EEG activity that is related to the stimulus. This activity

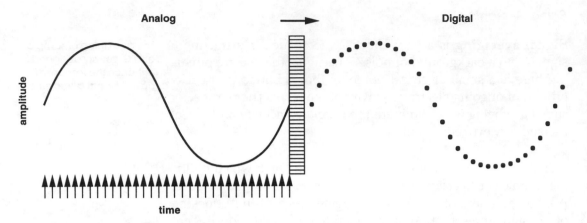

Figure 7–25. Schematic drawing of the conversion of an analog waveform to a digital representation.

Microvolts = μV

is expressed in **microvolts** and will appear as either positive or negative voltage, centering around 0 μV. The unrelated activity is much larger in amplitude, but it is occurring randomly with regard to the stimulus onset. The related activity is much smaller, but it is time-locked to the stimulus. Therefore, over a large number of samples, the randomly occurring activity will be averaged out to near 0 μV. That is, if the activity is random, it is as likely to have a positive voltage as a negative voltage. Averaging enough samples of random activity will result in an average that is nearly zero. Alternatively, if a response is occurring to the presentation of the signal, that response will occur each time and will begin to add to itself with each successive sample. In this way, any true auditory activity that is time-locked to the stimulus will begin to emerge from the background of random EEG.

The result of all of this signal averaging will be a waveform that reflects activity of auditory nervous system structures. The waveform has a series of identifiable positive and negative peaks that serve as landmarks for interpreting the normalcy of a response.

The Family of Auditory Evoked Potentials

For audiologic purposes, it is convenient to group the auditory evoked potentials into four categories, based loosely on the latency ranges over which the potentials are observed. The earliest is the ECoG, and it reflects activity of the most peripheral structures of the auditory system. The remaining three categories are

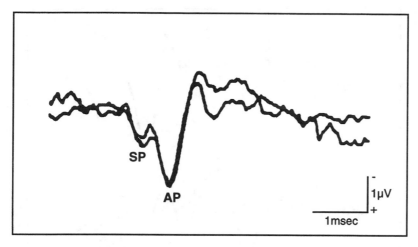

Figure 7–26. A normal electrocochleogram. (AP = action potential; SP = summating potential)

often labeled as *early, middle,* and *late.* These responses measure neural function at successively higher levels in the auditory nervous system.

Electrocochleogram

The ECoG is a response comprised mainly of the **compound action potential (AP)** that occurs at the **distal** portion of the VIIIth nerve (Figure 7–26). A click stimulus is used to elicit this response. The rapid onset of the click provides a stimulus that is sufficient to cause the fibers of the VIIIth nerve to fire in synchrony. This synchronous discharge of nerve fibers results in the AP. There are two other, smaller components of the ECoG. One is referred to as the cochlear microphonic (CM), which is a response from the cochlea that mimics the input stimulus. The other is the summating potential (SP), which is a direct current response that reflects the **envelope** of the input stimulus.

The ECoG is best recorded as a *near-field* response, with an electrode close to the source. Unlike the ABR, MLR, and LLR, which can readily be recorded as far-field responses with remote electrodes, it is more difficult to record the ECoG from surface electrodes. Thus, the best recordings of the ECoG are made from electrodes that are placed, invasively, through the tympanic membrane and onto the promontory of the temporal bone. An alternative arrangement is the use of an electrode in the ear canal placed near the tympanic membrane. Regardless, because of the

A **compound action potential** is the synchronous change in electrical potential of nerve or muscle tissue.

Distal means away from the center of origin.

In acoustics, an **envelope** is the representation of a waveform as a smooth curve joining the peaks of the oscillatory function.

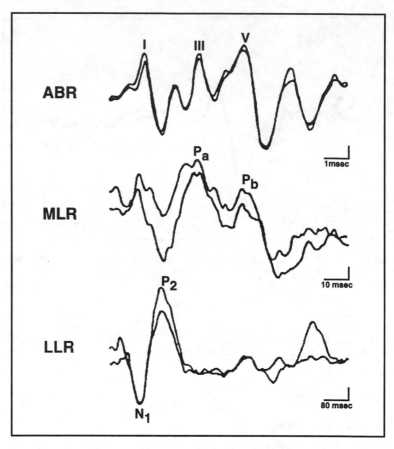

Figure 7-27. Normal auditory brain stem response (ABR), middle latency response (MLR), and late latency response (LLR) waveforms.

relatively invasive nature of this technique, and because the ECoG measures only the most peripheral function of the auditory system, its clinical use remains limited to a small number of specialized diagnostic applications. However, it has proven to be a very useful response for monitoring cochlear function in the operating room where electrode placement is simplified.

Auditory Brain Stem Response

The ABR occurs within the first 10 msec following signal onset and consists of a series of five positive peaks or waves. An ABR waveform is shown in Figure 7–27. The ABR has properties that make it very useful clinically:

1. the response can be recorded from surface electrodes;

2. the waves are robust and can be recorded easily in patients with adequate hearing and normal auditory nervous system function;
3. the response is immune to the influences of patient state, so that it can be recorded in patients who are sleeping, sedated, comatose, etc.;
4. the latencies of the various waves are quite stable within and across people so that they serve as a sensitive measure of brain stem integrity;
5. the time intervals between peaks are prolonged by auditory disorders central to the cochlea, which makes the ABR useful for differentiating cochlear from retrocochlear sites of disorder; and
6. the most robust component, wave V, can be observed at levels very close to behavioral thresholds so that it can be used very effectively to estimate hearing sensitivity in infants, young children, and other difficult-to-test patients.

The ABR is generated by the auditory nerve and by structures in the auditory brain stem. Wave I originates in the distal, or peripheral, portion of the VIIIth nerve near the point at which the nerve fibers leave the cochlea. Wave II originates from the proximal portion of the nerve near the brain stem. Wave III has contribution from this proximal portion of the nerve and from the cochlear nucleus. Waves IV and V have contributions from the cochlear nucleus, superior olivary complex, and lateral lemniscus.

Middle Latency Response

The *middle-latency response* (MLR) is characterized by two successive positive peaks, the first (Pa) at about 25 to 35 msec and the second (Pb) at about 40 to 60 msec following stimulus presentation. The MLR is probably generated by some combination of projections to the primary auditory cortex and the cortical area itself. Although the MLR is the most difficult AEP to record in clinical patients, it is sometimes used diagnostically and as an aid to the identification of central auditory processing disorder.

Late Latency Response

The *late latency response* (LLR) is characterized by a negative peak (N1) at a latency of about 90 msec followed by a positive peak (P2) at about 180 msec following stimulus presentation. This potential is greatly affected by subject state. It is best recorded when the patient is awake and carefully attending to the sounds being presented. There is an important developmental effect on the

LLR during the first 8 to 10 years of age. In older children or adults, however, it is robust and relatively easy to record. In children or adults with relatively normal hearing sensitivity, abnormality or absence of the LLR is associated with central auditory processing disorder.

Taken as a whole, this family of evoked potentials is quite versatile. Both ABR and LLR can be used to estimate auditory sensitivity independently of behavioral response. In addition, ABR can be used to differentiate cochlear from retrocochlear site of disorder. Finally, the array of ABR, MLR, and LLR is an effective tool for exploring central auditory processing disorders.

Clinical Applications

Evoked potentials are used for several purposes in evaluating the auditory system. Because early evoked potentials can be recorded without regard to subject state of consciousness, they have become an invaluable part of pediatric assessment. The ABR is now used routinely to screen the hearing of babies who are at risk for hearing loss and to assess the degree of hearing loss in those who have failed a screening or are otherwise at risk for hearing loss. The same evoked potentials provide a window for viewing the function of the brain's response to sound, which has proven to be useful in the diagnostic assessment of neurologic function. Finally, auditory evoked potentials can be recorded during surgery to provide a functional measure of structural changes that occur during VIIIth nerve tumor removal.

Prediction of Hearing Sensitivity

The audiologist is faced with two challenges that often require the use of auditory evoked potentials to predict hearing sensitivity. The main challenge is trying to measure the hearing sensitivity of infants or young children who cannot or will not cooperate enough to permit assessment by behavioral techniques. The other challenge is assessing hearing sensitivity in older individuals who are feigning some degree of hearing impairment. Regardless, the goal of testing is to obtain an electrophysiologic prediction of both degree and slope of hearing loss.

The process in hearing-sensitivity prediction is simply determining the lowest intensity level at which an auditory evoked potential can be identified. Click or tone-burst stimuli are presented at an intensity level that evokes a response. The level is then low-

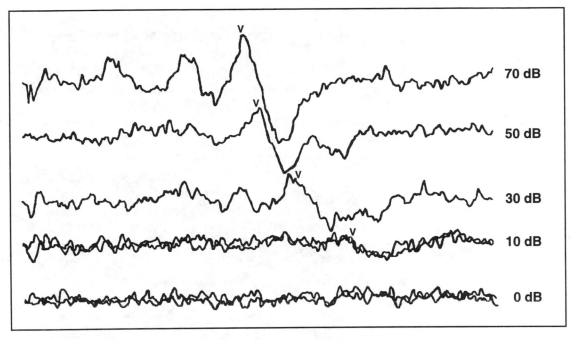

Figure 7-28. The prediction of hearing sensitivity with the ABR, showing the tracking of wave V as click intensity level is reduced.

ered, and the response is tracked until an intensity is reached at which the response is no longer observable (Figure 7–28). This level corresponds closely to behavioral threshold.

Evaluation of infants and young children must be carried out in natural sleep or with mild sedation. Thus, testing is best accomplished with use of the ABR, which is not affected by patient state. A typical strategy is to determine ABR threshold to click stimuli as an estimate of hearing sensitivity in the 1000 to 4000 Hz audiometric frequency range. Once a threshold ABR to clicks has been established, low-frequency tone-bursts may be used to predict the degree of hearing loss in the lower frequency range of the audiogram. The result of ABR threshold testing is an estimate of both degree and slope of hearing loss. The Clinical Note on pages 304–305 describes a clinical technique for rapid estimation of thresholds.

Evaluation of older patients is probably best accomplished by use of the late latency response to tonal stimuli. A typical strategy is to determine LLR thresholds to tonal stimuli across the audiometric frequency range. A response is usually identified at some suprathreshold level and then tracked as the intensity level is

A Rapid Approach to Threshold Prediction

When testing young children, the challenge is simple: get as much information as possible as quickly as possible before the baby wakes up from natural sleep or before the sedation wears off. Many a clinician has been caught with only partial ABR information about one ear when a child awakened. No one wants to repeat the pediatric ABR procedure, especially if sedation is involved. Clinical techniques designed for rapid assessment are important in this population.

One technique that works particularly well is the binaural approach to ABR threshold prediction. The idea here is simple. If you establish an ABR threshold with clicks presented to both ears and the baby wakes up, at least you know the hearing of the better-hearing ear. For example, suppose that a child has no cochlear function in the left ear, but the right ear is normal. The binaural ABR threshold search will yield a prediction of normal hearing because of responses from the good right ear. If the baby wakes up at that point, you at least know how the better-hearing ear is functioning. If you had the misfortune of testing the left ear first, you would still probably be searching for a threshold when the baby awakened, and you would have learned little about the baby's overall hearing ability.

Once you have established the binaural threshold, the next step is to test each ear independently at 10 to 20 dB above the binaural threshold. If the waveforms are present and symmetric, you are finished testing. If responses are obtained in only one ear, then the binaural threshold reflects that ear, and you can spend the rest of your time pursuing threshold in the other ear.

An example of the binaural approach is shown in the figure on the facing page. You can learn a lot about a child's hearing in a short period of time using this approach.

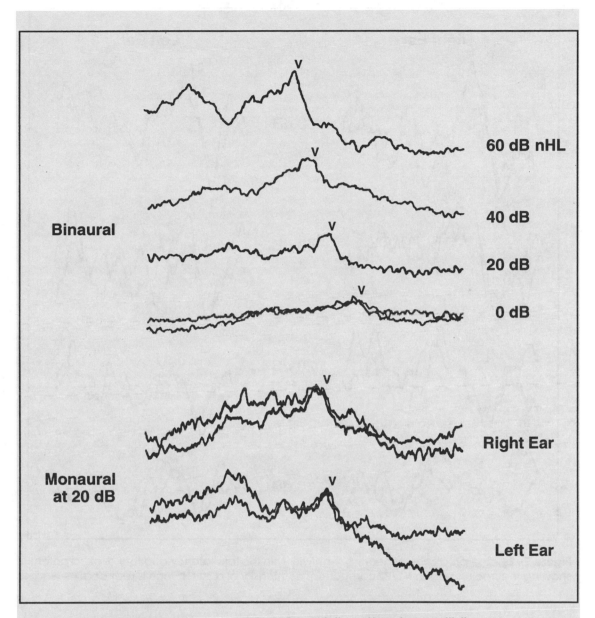

Binaural

60 dB nHL

40 dB

20 dB

0 dB

Monaural at 20 dB

Right Ear

Left Ear

An example of the binaural approach to ABR prediction of hearing sensitivity.

lowered until the response can no longer be identified (Figure 7–29). This level is considered threshold and corresponds well with behavioral thresholds. LLR testing is relatively time consuming, and some clinicians opt for using a combined approach wherein click ABR thresholds are used to predict high-

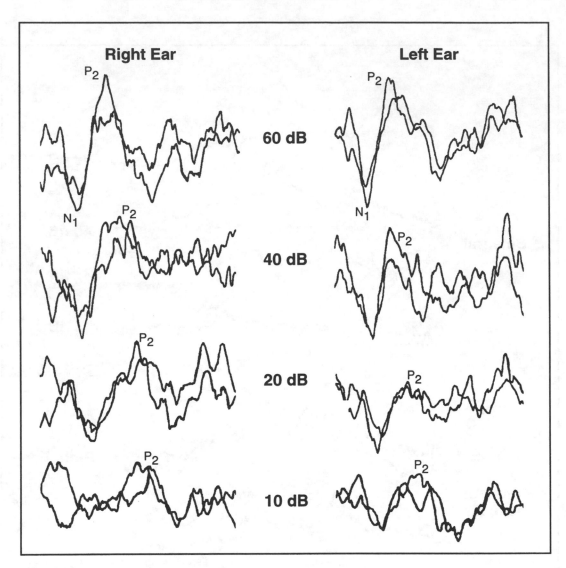

Figure 7–29. The prediction of hearing sensitivity with the late-latency auditory evoked potential, showing the tracking of the N1/P2 component as intensity of a 500 Hz tone is reduced.

frequency hearing and LLR thresholds to predict low-frequency hearing.

Neonatal Hearing Screening

The goal of neonatal hearing screening is to categorize auditory function as either normal or abnormal in order to identify newborns who have significant sensorineural hearing loss. By screening hearing, those with normal cochlear function are eliminated from further consideration, and those with a suspicion of hearing loss are referred for clinical testing.

The ABR is the evoked-potential method of choice for infant hearing screening. Surface electrodes are used to record the ABR and can easily be affixed to the infants' scalp. Because of its immunity to subject state, the ABR can be recorded reliably in sleeping neonates.

A typical screening strategy is to present click stimuli at a fixed intensity level, usually 30 to 40 dB, and determine whether a reliable response can be recorded. If an ABR is present, the child is likely to have normal or nearly normal hearing sensitivity in the 1000 to 4000 Hz frequency region of the audiogram. The underlying assumption here is that such hearing is sufficient for speech and oral language development and that children who pass the screening are at low risk for developing communication disorders due to hearing loss. If an ABR is absent, it is concluded that the child is at risk for significant sensorineural hearing loss and further audiologic assessment is warranted.

Conventional ABR testing of neonates has been largely replaced by *automated* ABR testing. The driving force behind the development of automated testing is that the number of babies who require screening far exceeds the highly skilled personnel available to carry out conventional ABR measures. An automated approach allows less-skilled personnel to provide hearing screening. One commonly used automated screener is designed to present click stimuli at fixed intensity levels, record ABR tracings, and compare the recorded tracings to a template that represents expected results in neonates. The system was designed with several fail-safe mechanisms that halt testing in the presence of excessive environmental or physiologic noise. When all conditions are favorable, the device proceeds with testing until it reaches a decision regarding the presence of an ABR. It then alerts the screener as to whether the infant has passed or needs to be referred for additional testing. This automated system has proven to be a valid and reliable way to screen the hearing of infants.

Infant screening by ABR has been restricted largely to **neonatal intensive care units (NICU)** where the prevalence of auditory disorder is much higher than in the newborn population in general. Although children in the NICU are at increased risk for hearing loss, estimates suggest that risk factors alone identify only about one half of all children with significant sensorineural hearing loss. As a result, efforts have emerged to screen *all* newborns, regard-

The hospital unit designed to take care of newborns needing special care is the **neonatal intensive care unit (NICU)**.

less of setting. Automated ABR strategies are an integral part of the *universal screening* process and are often used in conjunction with otoacoustic-emissions screening for identification purposes.

Two variables unrelated to significant sensorineural hearing loss can interfere with correct identification of these infants. One is the presence of middle ear disorder that is causing conductive hearing loss. If the loss is of a sufficient magnitude, the infant may fail the screening and be referred for additional testing. The other is **neuromaturational delay** or disorder that results in an abnormal ABR. That is, some children's brain stem function has not matured to a point, or is disordered to an extent, that it cannot be measured adequately to provide an estimate of hearing sensitivity. These children will also fail the screening and be referred for additional testing. Although their problems may be important, they are considered false-alarms from the perspective of identifying significant sensorineural hearing loss. As a result of these factors, the false-alarm or false-positive rate can be high in ABR screening of neonates. If these rates are excessive, the value of screening is somewhat diminished.

Neuromaturational delay occurs when a nervous system function has not developed as rapidly as normal.

The opposite problem, failure to identify a child with significant hearing loss, or false negative, is seldom an issue with ABR testing. If it does occur, it is usually in children who have reverse-slope hearing loss, wherein low-frequency hearing is poorer than high-frequency hearing. The click stimulus used in ABR measurement is effective in assessing higher audiometric frequencies. Thus, an infant with normal high-frequency hearing and abnormal low-frequency hearing would likely pass the screening, and the loss would go undetected. Such losses are rare and are considered to have minimal impact on communication development. Thus, the failure to identify these children, although important, is a small cost in comparison to the value of identifying those with significant high-frequency sensorineural hearing loss.

Diagnostic Applications

One of the most important applications of evoked potentials is in the area of diagnosis of disorders of the peripheral and central auditory nervous system. In fact, at one time in the late 1970s and early 1980s, the ABR was probably the most sensitive diagnostic tool available for identifying the presence of VIIIth nerve tumors. However, progress in imaging and radiographic assessment of structural changes has advanced to a point where functional measures such as the ABR have lost some of their sensitivity and, thus, importance. That is, imaging studies have permitted the visualization of ever smaller lesions in the brain. Sometimes the lesions are of a small enough size or are in such a location that they result in little or no measurable functional consequence. Thus, measures of function, such as the ABR, may not detect their presence. Although this trend has been occurring over the past decade, evoked potentials are still used for diagnostic testing, often for screening purposes.

The ABR is a sensitive indicator of functional disorders of the VIIIth nerve and lower auditory brain stem. It is often the first test of choice if such a disorder is suspected. For example, a cochleovestibular schwannoma is a tumor that develops on the VIIIth nerve. A patient with a cochleovestibular schwannoma will often complain of tinnitus, hearing loss, or both, in the ear with the tumor. Based on audiometric data and a physical examination, further testing to rule out this tumor may be pursued. It is likely that the physician who is making the diagnosis will request a magnetic resonance imaging (MRI) scan of the brain, which is currently the gold standard for identifying these space-occupying lesions. However, depending on the level of suspicion of a tumor, ABR testing may be carried out as a screening tool to decide on further imaging studies or as an adjunct to these studies. These basic strategies also apply to other types of disorders that affect the VIIIth nerve or auditory brain stem, such as multiple sclerosis, brain stem neoplasms, and so on.

The ABR component waves, especially waves I, III, and V are easily recordable and are very reliable in terms of their latency. For example, depending on the equipment and recording parameters, we expect to see a wave I at about 2 msec following signal presentation, a wave III at 4 msec, and a wave V at 6 msec. Although these absolute numbers will vary across clinics, the latencies are quite stable across individuals. The I–V interpeak interval in most adults is approximately 4 msec, and the standard deviation of this interval is about 0.2 msec. Thus, 95% of the adult population have I–V interpeak intervals of 4.4 or less. If the I–V interval exceeds this amount, it can be considered abnormal.

These latency measures are amazingly consistent across the population. In newborns, they are prolonged compared to adult values, but in a reasonably predictable way. Once a child reaches 18 months, we expect normal adult latency values that continue throughout life. Because of the consistency of latencies within an individual over time and across individuals in the population, we can rely confidently on assessment of latency as an indicator of integrity of the VIIIth nerve and auditory brain stem. The decision about whether an ABR is normal is usually based on the following considerations:

- interaural difference in I–V interpeak interval;
- I–V interpeak interval;
- interaural difference in wave V latency;
- absolute latency of wave V;
- interaural differences in V/I amplitude ratio;
- V/I amplitude ratio;
- selective loss of late waves; and
- grossly degraded **waveform morphology**.

Morphology is the qualitative description of an auditory evoked potential, related to the replicability of the response and the ease with which component peaks can be identified.

Again, the ABR is used to assess integrity of the VIIIth nerve and auditory brain stem in patients who are suspected of having acoustic tumor or other neurologic disorders. In interpreting ABRs, we exploit the consistency of the response across individuals and ask whether our measured latencies compare well between ears and with the population in general. With this strategy, the ABR has become a useful adjunct in diagnosis of neurological disease.

The MLR and LLR are less useful than the ABR in identifying discrete lesions. Sometimes the influence of an acoustic tumor that affects the ABR will also affect the MLR. Also, sometimes a cerebral vascular accident or other type of discrete insult to the brain will result in an abnormality in the MLR. However, these measures have tended to be more useful as indicators of generalized disorders of auditory processing ability than in the diagnosis of a specific disease process. For example, MLRs and LLRs have been found to be abnormal in patients with multiple sclerosis and Parkinson's disease. Although neither response has proven to be particularly useful in helping to diagnose these disorders, the fact that MLR and LLR abnormalities occur has proven to be valuable in describing the resultant auditory disorders. That is, patients with neurologic disorders often have auditory complaints that cannot be measured on an audiogram or with simple speech audiometric measures. The MLR and LLR are sometimes helpful in quantifying such auditory complaints.

Surgical Monitoring

Auditory evoked potentials are also useful in monitoring the function of the cochlea and VIIIth nerve during surgical removal of a tumor on or near the nerve. Surgery for removal of acoustic tumors often results in permanent loss of hearing due to the need to remove the cochlea to reach the tumor. If the tumor is small enough, however, a different surgical approach can be used that may spare hearing in that ear. During this latter type of surgery, monitoring of auditory function can be very helpful to the surgeon.

During surgical removal of an acoustic tumor or other mass that impinges on the VIIIth nerve, hearing is quite vulnerable. One potential problem is that the blood supply to the cochlea can be interrupted. Another is that the tumor can be intertwined with the nerve, resulting in damage to or severing of the nerve during tumor removal. Sometimes, however, hearing can be spared by carefully monitoring the nerve during the course of such a surgery.

Auditory evoked potential monitoring involves measurement of the compound action potential (AP) of the VIIIth nerve. This is the major component of the ECoG and corresponds to wave I of the ABR. The AP is usually measured using one of two approaches, ECoG or cochlear nerve action potential (CNAP) measures. Both approaches measure essentially the same function. The ECoG approach uses a needle electrode that is placed on the promontory outside of the cochlea. The CNAP approach uses a ball electrode that is placed directly on the VIIIth nerve. In either case, click stimuli are presented to the ear throughout surgery, and the latency and amplitude of the AP are assessed. Because the recording electrode is so close to the source of the potential, especially in the case of CNAP measurement, the function of the cochlea and VIIIth nerve can be assessed rapidly, providing valuable feedback to the surgeon about the effects of tumor manipulation or other surgical actions.

Summary

- An auditory evoked potential is a waveform that reflects the electrophysiologic function of a certain portion of the central auditory nervous system in response to sound.
- For audiologic purposes, it is convenient to group the AEPs into categories based loosely on the latency ranges over which the potentials are observed.
- The earliest of the evoked potentials, occurring within the first 5 msec following signal presentation, is referred to as an electrocochleogram (ECoG) and reflects activity of the cochlea and VIIIth nerve.
- The most commonly used evoked potential is referred to as the auditory brain stem response (ABR) and occurs

within the first 10 msec following signal onset. The ABR reflects neural activity from the VIIIth nerve to the midbrain.

■ The middle latency response (MLR) occurs within the first 50 msec following signal onset and reflects activity at or near the auditory cortex.

■ The late latency response (LLR) occurs within the first 250 msec following signal onset and reflects activity of the primary-auditory and association areas of the cerebral cortex.

■ One of the most important applications of auditory evoked potentials is the prediction of hearing sensitivity in infants and young children.

■ The ABR is the evoked-potential method of choice for infant hearing screening.

■ Another important application of evoked potentials is the diagnosis of disorders of the peripheral and central auditory nervous system.

■ Auditory evoked potentials are also useful in monitoring the function of the cochlea and VIIIth nerve during surgical removal of a tumor on or near the nerve.

OTOACOUSTIC EMISSIONS AUDIOMETRY

We tend to think of sensory systems as somewhat passive receivers of information that detect and process incoming signals and send corresponding neural signals to the cortex. We know that sound impinges on the tympanic membrane, setting the middle ear ossicles in motion. The stapes footplate, in turn, creates a disturbance of the fluid in the scala vestibuli, resulting in a traveling wave of motion that displaces the basilar membrane maximally at a point corresponding to the frequency of the signal. The active processes of the outer hair cells are stimulated, translating the broadly tuned traveling wave into a narrowly tuned potentiation of the inner hair cells. Inner hair cells, in turn, create neural impulses that travel through the VIIIth nerve and beyond.

The active processes of the outer hair cells make this sensory system somewhat more complicated than a passive receiver of information. These outer hair cells are stimulated in a manner that causes them to act on the signal that stimulates them. One by-product of that action is the generation of a replication or echo of the sound, which travels back out of the cochlea, through the middle ear, and into the ear canal. This echo is referred to as an otoacoustic emission or OAE.

Otoacoustic emissions are low-intensity sounds that are generated by the cochlea and emanate into the middle ear and ear canal. They are frequency specific in that emissions of a given frequency arise from the place on the cochlea's basilar membrane responsible for processing that frequency. OAEs are probably not essential to hearing, but rather are the by-product of active processing by the outer hair cell system. Of clinical interest is that OAEs are present when outer hair cells are healthy and absent when outer hair cells are damaged. Thus, OAE measures have tremendous potential for revealing, with exquisite sensitivity, the integrity of cochlear function.

Types of Otoacoustic Emissions

There are two broad categories of otoacoustic emissions, spontaneous OAEs (SOAEs) and evoked OAEs (EOAEs).

Spontaneous Otoacoustic Emissions

Spontaneous OAEs are narrow-band signals that occur in the ear canal without the introduction of an eliciting signal. Spontaneous emissions are present in 50–70% of all normal-hearing ears and absent in all ears at frequencies where sensorineural hearing loss exceeds approximately 30 dB. It appears that spontaneous OAEs originate from outer hair cells corresponding to that portion of the basilar membrane tuned to their frequency.

A sensitive, low-noise microphone housed in a probe is used to record spontaneous OAEs. The probe is secured into the external auditory meatus with some type of flexible cuff. Signals detected by the microphone are routed to a spectrum analyzer, which is a device that provides real-time frequency analysis of the signal. Usually the frequency range of interest is swept several times, and the results are signal averaged to reduce background noise. Spontaneous OAEs, when they occur, appear as peaks of energy along the frequency spectrum.

Because spontaneous OAEs are absent in many ears with normal hearing, clinical applications have not been forthcoming. Efforts to relate SOAEs to tinnitus have revealed a relationship in some, but not many subjects who have both. Other clinical applications

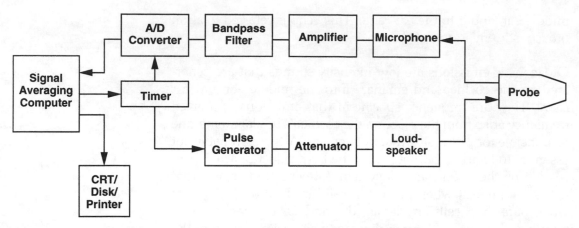

Figure 7-30. Schematic representation of the instrumentation used to elicit and measure transient-evoked OAEs.

await development. Evoked OAEs, in contrast, enjoy widespread clinical use.

Evoked Otoacoustic Emissions

Evoked OAEs occur during and after the presentation of a stimulus. That is, an EOAE is elicited by a stimulus. EOAEs bear a close resemblance to the eliciting signal, and thus the term *echo* has been employed to describe them. There are several classes of evoked OAEs, two of which have proven to be useful clinically, transient-evoked otoacoustic emissions (TEOAE) and distortion-product otoacoustic emissions (DPOAE).

TEOAEs are elicited by a transient signal or click. A schematic representation of the instrumentation used to elicit a TEOAE is shown in Figure 7–30. A probe is used to deliver the click signal and to record the response. The probe is secured into the external auditory meatus with some type of flexible cuff. Series of click stimuli are presented, usually at an intensity level of about 80–85 dB SPL. Output from the microphone is signal averaged, usually within a time window of 20 msec. In a typical clinical paradigm, alternating samples of the emission are placed into separate memory locations, so that the final result provides two traces of the response for comparison purposes.

TEOAEs occur about 4 msec following stimulus presentation and continue for about 10 msec. An example of a TEOAE is shown in Figure 7–31. Depicted here are two replications of the signal-

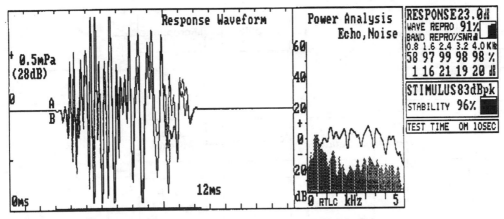

Figure 7-31. A transient-evoked OAE.

averaged emission, designated as A and B. Because a click is a broad-spectrum signal, the echo is similarly broad in spectrum. By convention, these waveforms are subjected to spectral analysis, the results of which are often shown in a graph depicting the amplitude-versus-frequency components of the emission. Also by convention, an estimate of the background noise is made by subtracting waveform A from waveform B, and a spectral analysis of the resultant waveform is plotted on the same graph. Another important aspect of TEOAE analysis is the reproducibility of the response. An estimate is made of how similar A is to B by correlating the two waveforms. This similarity or reproducibility is then expressed as a percentage, with 100% being identical. If the magnitude of the emission exceeds the magnitude of the noise, and if the reproducibility of the emission exceeds a predetermined level, then the emission is said to be present. If an emission is present, it is likely that the outer hair cells are functioning in the frequency region of the emission.

Distortion-product OAEs occur as a result of nonlinear processes in the cochlea. When two tones are presented to the cochlea, distortion occurs in the form of other tones that are not present in the two-tone eliciting signals. These distortions are combination tones, or harmonics, that are related to the eliciting tones in a predictable mathematical way. The two tones used to elicit the DPOAE are, by convention, designated f_1 and f_2. The most robust distortion product occurs at the frequency represented by the equation $2f_1 - f_2$. A schematic representation of the instrumentation used to elicit a DPOAE is shown in Figure 7–32. As with TEOAEs, a probe is used to deliver the tone pairs and to record the response. The probe is secured into the external auditory

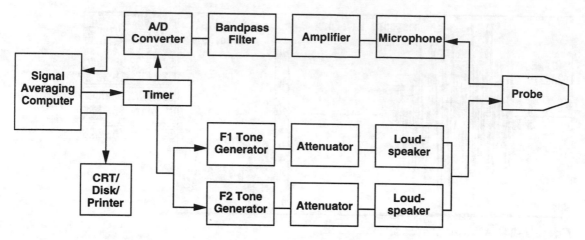

Figure 7-32. Schematic representation of the instrumentation used to elicit and measure distortion-product OAEs.

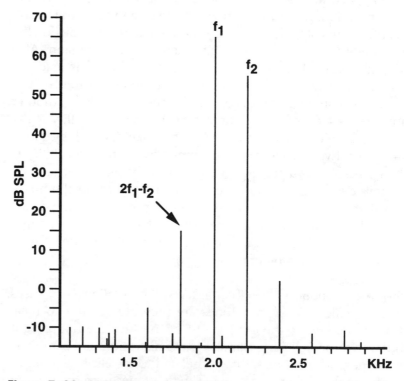

Figure 7-33. A distortion-product OAE.

meatus with a flexible cuff. Pairs of tones are presented across the frequency range to elicit distortion products from approximately 1000 to 6000 Hz. The tone pairs that are presented are at a fixed

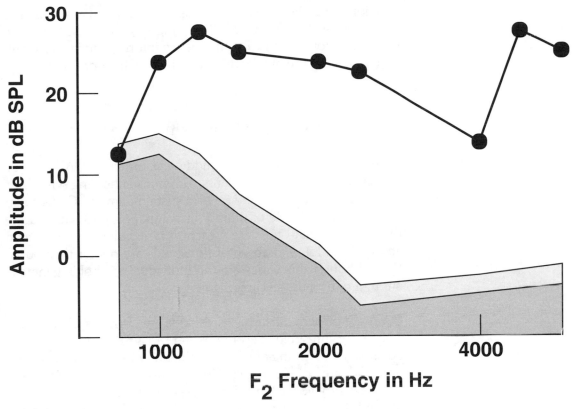

Figure 7-34. DPOAE amplitude as a function of frequency of the f_2 tone.

frequency and intensity relationship. Typically, the pairs are presented from low frequency to high frequency. As each pair is presented, measurements are made at the $2f_1 - f_2$ frequency to determine the amplitude of the DPOAE and also at a nearby frequency to provide an estimate of the noise floor at that moment in time. An example of a DPOAE is shown in Figure 7–33.

DPOAEs are typically depicted as the amplitude of the distortion product ($2f_1 - f_2$) as a function of frequency of the f_2 tone (Figure 7–34). The shaded area in this figure represents the estimate of background noise. If the amplitude exceeds the background noise, the emission is said to be present. If an emission is present, it is likely that the outer hair cells are functioning in the frequency region of the f_2 tone.

Results of TEOAE and DPOAE testing provide a measure of the integrity of outer hair cell function. Both approaches have been successfully applied clinically as objective indicators of cochlear function. TEOAEs are likely to be used when rapid assessment is necessary, such as in neonatal hearing screening. DPOAEs are more commonly used when frequency information is important, such as during the monitoring of cochlear function.

Relation to Hearing Sensitivity

Assuming normal outer and middle ear function, OAEs can be consistently recorded in patients with normal hearing sensitivity. Once outer hair cells of the cochlea sustain damage, OAEs begin to be affected. A rule of thumb for comparing OAEs to hearing thresholds is that OAEs are present if thresholds are better than about 30 dB HL and absent if thresholds are poorer than 30 dB HL. Although this varies among individuals, it holds generally enough to be a useful clinical guide.

OAEs are present if hearing thresholds are normal and disappear as hearing thresholds become poorer. As a result, OAEs tend to be used for screening of cochlear function rather than for prediction of degree of hearing sensitivity. Efforts to predict degree of loss have probably been most successful with use of DPOAEs. In general, though, they tell us more about the degree of hearing loss that a patient *does not have* than about the degree of loss that a patient has. For example, if a patient has a DPOAE amplitude of 10 dB SPL at 1000 Hz, it is likely that hearing sensitivity loss at that frequency does not exceed 20 dB HL. Although this information is quite useful, the absence of an OAE reveals little about degree of loss. Recent efforts to harness OAE technology to provide more information about hearing loss prediction have been encouraging, particularly with the use of DPOAEs. If patients have normal hearing or mild sensitivity loss, thresholds can be predicted with a fair degree of accuracy. However, presently OAEs are not generally applied as threshold tests.

Clinical Applications

OAEs are useful in at least four clinical areas:

1. infant screening
2. pediatric assessment
3. cochlear function monitoring
4. certain diagnostic cases

Infant Screening

OAEs are used most effectively as a screening measure, particularly in neonatal screening programs. Several test characteristics make OAEs particularly useful for this clinical application. First, the very nature of OAEs makes the technique an excellent one for screening. When present, OAEs provide an indicator of normal cochlear function or, at most, a mild sensitivity loss. When absent, OAEs provide an indicator that cochlear function is not normal, although degree of abnormality cannot be assessed. Second, measurement techniques have been simplified to an extent that screening can be carried out simply and rapidly. Third, OAEs are not affected by neuromaturation of the central auditory nervous system and can be obtained in newborns regardless of gestational age. The biggest drawback to OAE use is that outer and middle ear disorders often preclude our ability to measure an OAE. Thus, if an infant's ear canal is obstructed, or if the infant has otitis media, OAEs will not be recorded even though cochlear function may be normal. Despite this drawback, OAE measures now enjoy widespread use in infant hearing screening programs.

Pediatric Assessment

One of the most important applications of OAEs is as an additional part of the pediatric audiologic assessment battery. Prior to the availability of OAE measures, the audiologist relied on behavioral assessment and immittance audiometry in the initial pediatric hearing consultation. In a cooperative young child, behavioral measures could be obtained that provided adequate audiometric information. When these results were corroborated by SPAR testing, assessment was completed without the need for additional testing. Unfortunately, many young children are not altogether cooperative, and failure to establish audiometric levels by behavioral means usually led to AEP testing that required sedation. OAE measures have changed this approach dramatically.

In typical clinical settings, many of the children who undergo audiometric assessment have normal hearing sensitivity. They are usually referred for assessment due to some risk factor or concerns about speech and language development. As audiologists, we are interested in identifying these normal-hearing children quickly and getting them out of the system prior to the need for sedated AEP testing. That is, we are interested in concentrating the resources required to carry out pediatric AEP measures only on children with hearing impairment and not on normal-hearing children who cannot otherwise be tested. OAE measures have had a dramatic impact on our ability to identify normal-hearing children in a more cost- and time-efficient manner, which has led, in turn, to more efficient clinical application of AEP measures. With OAE testing, behavioral and immittance results can be cross-checked in a very efficient and effective way to identify normal hearing. If such measures show the presence of a hearing loss, then AEP testing can be implemented to confirm degree of impairment. On the other hand, if these measures show normal cochlear function, the need for additional testing is eliminated. Many audiologists have modified their pediatric protocols to initiate testing with OAEs followed by immittance and then by traditional speech and pure-tone audiometry. In many cases, the objective information about the peripheral auditory mechanism gained from OAEs and immittance measures, when results are normal, is sufficient to preclude additional testing.

Cochlear Function Monitoring

Ototoxic means it is poisonous to the ear.

Otoacoustic emission measures have also been used effectively to monitor cochlear function, particularly in patients undergoing treatment that is potentially **ototoxic**. Many drugs used as chemotherapy for certain types of cancer are ototoxic, as are some antibiotics used to control infections. Given in large enough doses, these drugs destroy outer hair cell function, resulting in permanent sensorineural hearing loss. Often, drug dosage can be adjusted during treatment to minimize these ototoxic effects. Thus, it is not unusual for patients undergoing chemotherapy or other drug treatment to have their hearing monitored before, during, and after the treatment regimen. High-frequency pure-tone audiometry is useful for this purpose. In addition, DPOAE testing is now being used as an early indicator of outer hair cell damage in these patients. The combination of pure-tone audiometry and DPOAE measures is quite accurate in determining when drugs are causing ototoxicity.

Diagnostic Applications

Otoacoustic emission can also be useful diagnostically. Some patients have hearing impairment that is caused by retrocochlear disorder, such as tumors impinging on VIIIth nerve or brain stem lesions affecting the central auditory nervous system pathways. Sometimes these patients will have measurable sensorineural hearing loss, but normal OAEs. In such cases, outer hair cell function is considered normal, and the hearing loss can be attributable to the neurologic diseases process. In other cases of neurologic disorder, OAEs are not normal, although the site of disorder is clearly beyond the cochlea. In these cases it is assumed that the lesion has affected the blood supply to the outer hair cells of the cochlea.

Otoacoustic emissions are also useful for evaluating patients with functional or nonorganic hearing loss. In a short period of time, the audiologist can determine whether the peripheral auditory system is functioning normally without voluntary responses from the patient. If OAEs are normal in such cases, their use can reduce the time and frustration often experienced with other measures in the functional test battery. Remember, however, that most functional hearing loss has some organicity as its basis, and OAEs are likely to simply reveal that fact.

One other aspect of otoacoustic emissions that is quite interesting from a diagnostic perspective is that the amplitude of a TEOAE is suppressed to a certain extent by stimulation of the contralateral ear. This *contralateral suppression* is a small but consistent effect that occurs when broad spectrum noise is presented to one ear and transient emissions are recorded in the other. The effect is mediated by the medial olivocochlear system, which is part of the auditory system's complex efferent mechanism. In some cases of peripheral and central auditory disorder, contralateral suppression is absent, so that the TEOAE is unaffected by stimulation of the contralateral ear. The use of contralateral suppression is promising as a tool for assessing auditory nervous system function.

Summary

- One by-product of the active processes of the cochlear outer hair cells is the generation of a replication or echo of a stimulating sound, which travels back out of the cochlea, through the middle ear, and into the ear canal. This echo is a low-intensity sound referred to as an otoacoustic emission or OAE.
- Evoked OAEs occur during and after the presentation of a stimulus. Two classes of evoked OAEs have proven to be useful clinically, transiently-evoked otoacoustic emissions (TEOAE) and distortion-product otoacoustic emissions (DPOAE).
- OAEs are useful in at least four clinical areas: infant screening, pediatric assessment, cochlear function monitoring, and certain diagnostic cases.

■ OAEs are used most effectively as a screening measure, particularly in neonatal screening programs.
■ One of the most important applications of OAEs is as an additional part of the pediatric audiologic assessment battery.
■ Otoacoustic emission measures have also been used effectively to monitor cochlear function, particularly in patients undergoing treatment that is potentially ototoxic.
■ Otoacoustic emission can also be useful diagnostically.

SUGGESTED READINGS

Berlin, C. I., Hood, L. J., Wen, H., Szabo, P., Cecola, R. P., Rigby, P., & Jackson, J. F. (1993). Contralateral suppression of non-linear click-evoked otoacoustic emissions. *Hearing Research, 71*, 1–11.

Ferraro, J. A. (1993). Electrocochleography. In J. T. Jacobson (Ed.), *Principles and applications in auditory evoked potentials* (pp. 101–122). Needham Heights, MA: Allyn and Bacon.

Fowler, C. G., & Wiley, T. L. (1997). *Acoustic immittance measures in clinical audiology.* San Diego: Singular Publishing Group.

Hall, J. W. (1992). *Handbook of auditory evoked responses.* Boston: Allyn and Bacon.

Kemp, D. T. (1978). Stimulated acoustic emissions from within the human auditory system. *Journal of the Acoustical Society of America, 64,* 1386–1391.

Kileny, P. R., & Niparko, J. K. (1993). Neurophysiologic intraoperative monitoring. In J. T. Jacobson (Ed.), *Principles and applications in auditory evoked potentials* (pp. 447–476). Needham Heights, MA: Allyn and Bacon.

Robinette, M. S., & Glattke, T. J. (Eds.). (1997). *Otoacoustic emissions: clinical applications.* New York: Thieme.

Stach, B. A., & Jerger, J. F. (1991). Immittance measures in auditory disorders. In J. T. Jacobson & J. L. Northern (Eds.), *Diagnostic audiology* (pp. 113–140). Austin, TX: Pro-Ed.

Stach, B. A., Jerger, J. F., & Penn, T. O. (1994). Auditory evoked potential testing strategies. In J. T. Jacobson (Ed.), *Principles and applications in auditory evoked potentials* (pp. 541–560). Needham Heights, MA: Allyn and Bacon.

8

Different Assessment Approaches for Different Populations

Although the overall goal of an audiological evaluation is to characterize hearing ability, the approach used to reach that goal can vary considerably across patients. The approach chosen to evaluate a patient's hearing is sometimes related to patient factors such as age and sometimes related to the reason that the patient has sought services or has been referred for services. For example, the strategy used for a patient who is seeking otologic care is different in some ways from the strategy used for a patient who is seeking audiologic care. In the former, emphasis is on determination of degree and site of disorder; in the latter, emphasis is on degree of impairment and prognosis for successful hearing aid use. Within these broad categories, the approach may also vary depending on a patient's age. Quantification of degree of hearing loss in a 2-year-old requires a different strategy than that in a 20-year-old. Similarly, testing an 80-year-old patient can require different techniques and an expanded approach from the testing of a 40-year-old. Finally, there are patients who exaggerate or feign hearing loss, requiring an entirely separate approach to assessment.

Although assessment must be adapted to the needs and expectations of individual patients, there are several broad categories of patients that present common challenges and can be approached in a similar clinical manner, including pediatric patients, those being assessed for otologic reasons, those being assessed for audiologic reasons, and patients with functional hearing loss.

OTOLOGIC REFERRALS

An otologist's evaluation of a patient, aimed at diagnosing and treating ear disease, often includes ancillary testing, such as imaging studies, laboratory tests, and audiologic evaluations. Audiologic assessment in this context serves to provide additional information to the physician to aid in diagnosis. In addition, because hearing loss is often a quantifiable consequence of auditory disorder, results can serve as a metric for the success or failure of treatment approaches.

In general, otologists are faced with three main categories of patients: those with outer or middle ear disorders, those with cochlear disorders, and those with neurologic disorders affecting the peripheral or central auditory nervous system.

Outer or Middle Ear Disorders

Evaluative Goals

Physicians who note the presence of an outer or middle ear disorder are likely to refer the patient for an audiologic consultation. For the audiologist, there are two primary goals in the assessment of outer and middle ear disorders:

1. investigation of the nature of the disorder and
2. assessment of the impact of that disorder on hearing sensitivity.

Audiologic determination of the nature of the disorder relates to the consequence that a disorder has on the *function* of the outer and middle ear structures. For example, excessive cerumen in the ear canal may or may not impede the transduction of sound to the tympanic membrane. Similarly, **tympanosclerosis** may or may not reduce the functioning of the tympanic membrane. The first goal is to determine whether these structural changes result in a disorder in function.

Tympanosclerosis is the formation of whitish plaques on the tympanic membrane, which can result in membrane stiffness.

The second goal of the evaluation is to determine whether and how much this disorder in function is causing a hearing loss. In some circumstances, a structural change in the outer and middle ear can result in outer or middle ear disorder without causing a measurable loss of hearing. For example, a tympanic membrane can be perforated, resulting in a disorder of eardrum function, without causing a significant conductive hearing loss. On the other hand, a similar perforation in the right location on the tympanic membrane can result in a substantial conductive hearing loss. Similarly, blockage of the Eustachian tube can result in significant negative pressure in the middle ear space that may result in hearing loss in one case but not in another.

In some cases, the referring physician may not be able to detect a structural change in the middle ear mechanism and will be referring the patient to rule out middle ear disorder as the cause of the patient's complaint. The approach in such cases is the same. First, you must assess the normalcy of middle ear function and then the degree to which any disorder is influencing hearing ability.

The importance of your assessment of hearing sensitivity in these cases cannot be overstated. If the patient has an outer or middle

Otosclerosis is the formation of new bone around the stapes and oval window, resulting in stapes fixation and conductive hearing loss.

ear disorder, the degree of hearing loss that it is causing will serve as an important metric of the success or failure of the medical treatment regimen. If the physician prescribes drugs to treat otitis media or performs surgery to overcome the effects of **otosclerosis**, the pure-tone audiogram will often be the metric by which the outcome of the treatment is judged. That is, the pretreatment audiogram will be compared to the post-treatment audiogram to evaluate the success of the treatment.

Test Strategies

Immittance audiometry is used to evaluate outer and middle ear function, and pure-tone audiometry is used to evaluate the degree of conductive component caused by the presence of middle ear disorder. In most cases, rudimentary speech audiometry will be carried out as a cross-check of pure-tone thresholds and as a gross assessment of suprathreshold word recognition ability.

Immittance Audiometry. The first step in the evaluation process is immittance audiometry. Because it is the most sensitive indicator of middle ear function, a full battery of tympanometry, static immittance, and acoustic reflex thresholds should be carried out. Results will provide information indicating whether a disorder is due to

- an increase in the mass of the middle ear mechanism,
- an increase or decrease in the stiffness of the middle ear system,
- the presence of a perforation of the tympanic membrane, or
- significant negative pressure in the middle ear space.

If all immittance results are normal, any hearing loss measured by pure-tone audiometry can be attributed to sensorineural hearing loss. If immittance results indicate the presence of a middle ear disorder, pure-tone audiometry by air- and bone-conduction must be carried out to assess the degree of conductive component of the hearing loss attributable to the middle ear disorder.

Pure-Tone Audiometry. Pure-tone audiometry is used to quantify the degree to which middle ear disorder is contributing to a hearing sensitivity loss. If immittance audiometry shows any abnormality in outer or middle ear function, then complete air- and bone-conduction audiometry must be carried out on both ears to determine the degree of conductive hearing loss.

It is important to carry out both air and bone conduction in order to quantify the extent of the conductive component. It is important to test both ears because the presence of conductive hearing loss requires the use of masking in the nontest ear and that ear cannot be properly masked without knowing its air- and bone-conduction thresholds.

Speech Audiometry. In cases of outer and middle ear disorder, the most important component of speech audiometry is determination of the speech recognition threshold as a cross-check of the accuracy of pure-tone thresholds. Many audiologists prefer to establish the SRT before carrying out pure-tone audiometry so that they have a benchmark for the level at which pure-tone thresholds should occur. Although this is good practice in general, it is particularly useful in the assessment of young children. SRTs can also be established by bone conduction, permitting the quantification of an air-bone gap to speech signals.

Assessment of word recognition is also often carried out, though more as a matter of routine than importance. Conductive hearing loss has a predictable influence on word-recognition scores, and if such testing is of value, it is usually only to confirm this expectation.

Illustrative Cases

Illustrative Case 8-1. Case 1 is a patient with bilateral, acute otitis media with effusion. The patient is a 4-year-old boy with a history of recurring upper-respiratory infections, often accompanied by otitis media. The upper-respiratory infection often interferes with Eustachian-tube functioning, thereby limiting pressure equalization of the middle ear space. The patient had been experiencing symptoms of a cold for the past 2 weeks and complained to his parents of difficulty hearing.

Immittance audiometry, shown in Figure 8–1A, is consistent with middle ear disorder, characterized by flat, Type B tympanograms, low static immittance, and absent crossed and uncrossed reflexes bilaterally. These results are consistent with an increase in the mass of the middle ear mechanism, a result that often indicates the presence of effusion in the middle ear space.

Results of pure-tone audiometry are shown in Figure 8–1B. Results show a mild conductive hearing loss bilaterally, with slightly

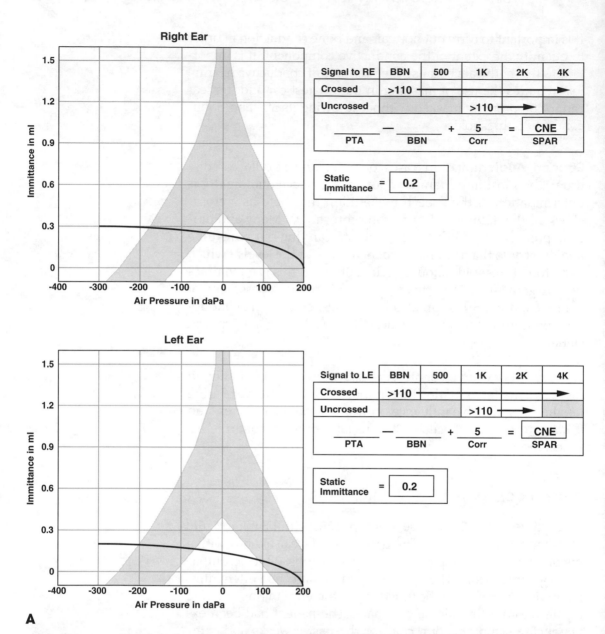

Figure 8-1. Hearing consultation results in a 4-year-old boy with a history of otitis media. Immittance measures (A) are consistent with an increase in the mass of the middle ear mechanism, secondary to otitis media with effusion. Pure-tone audiometric results (B) show a mild conductive hearing loss bilaterally, with slightly more loss in the left ear. Speech audiometric results (C) show excellent suprathreshold recognition of words and sentences once intensity level is sufficient to overcome the conductive hearing loss.

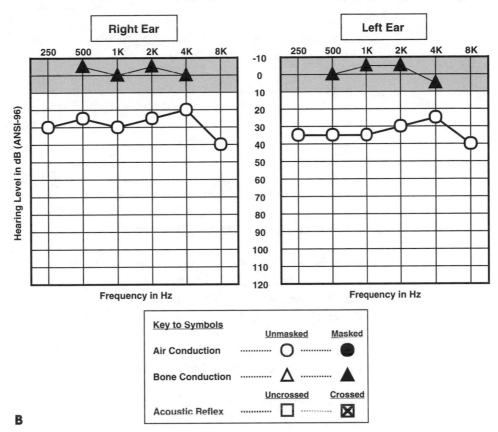

Right Ear
Left Ear

Key to Symbols

	Unmasked	Masked
Air Conduction	○	●
Bone Conduction	△	▲
	Uncrossed	Crossed
Acoustic Reflex	☐	☒

B

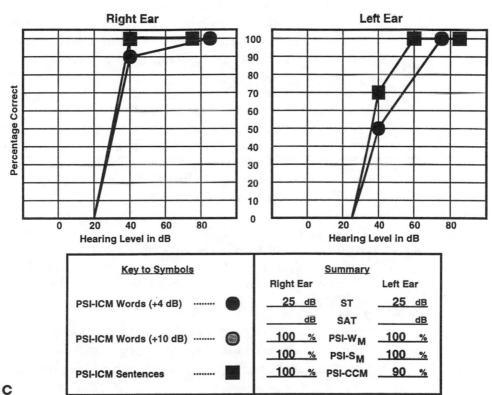

Right Ear
Left Ear

Key to Symbols

PSI-ICM Words (+4 dB) ········· ●

PSI-ICM Words (+10 dB) ········· ◉

PSI-ICM Sentences ········· ■

Summary

Right Ear		Left Ear
25 dB	ST	25 dB
dB	SAT	dB
100 %	PSI-W$_M$	100 %
100 %	PSI-S$_M$	100 %
100 %	PSI-CCM	90 %

C

more loss in the left ear. Bone conduction thresholds indicate normal cochlear function bilaterally.

Speech audiometric results, shown in Figure 8–1C, indicate speech thresholds that are consistent with pure-tone thresholds. In addition, suprathreshold understanding of words and sentences is excellent, as expected.

This child's ear problems have not responded well in the past to antibiotic treatment. The child's physician is considering the placement of pressure-equalization tubes into the eardrums to help overcome the effects of the Eustachian-tube problems.

Illustrative Case 8–2. Case 2 is a patient with bilateral otosclerosis, a bone disorder that often results in fixation of the stapes into the oval window. The patient is a 33-year-old woman who developed hearing problems during pregnancy. She describes her problem as a muffling of other people's voices. She also reports tinnitus in both ears that bothers her at night. There is a family history of otosclerosis on her mother's side.

Results of immittance audiometry, as shown in Figure 8–2A, are consistent with middle ear disorder, characterized by a Type A tympanogram, low static immittance, and absent crossed and uncrossed acoustic reflexes bilaterally. This pattern of results suggests an increase in the stiffness of the middle ear mechanism and is often associated with fixation of the ossicular chain.

Pure-tone audiometric results are shown in Figure 8–2B. The patient has a moderate, bilateral, symmetric, conductive hearing loss. As is typical in otosclerosis, the patient also has an apparent hearing loss by bone conduction at around 2000 Hz in both ears. This so-called Carhart's notch is actually the result of an elimination of the middle ear contribution to bone-conducted hearing rather than a loss in cochlear sensitivity.

Speech audiometric results show speech thresholds consistent with pure-tone thresholds. Suprathreshold speech recognition ability, as shown in Figure 8–2C, is normal once the effect of the hearing loss is overcome by presenting speech at higher intensity levels.

The patient is scheduled for surgery on her right ear. The surgeon will likely remove the stapes and replace it with a prosthesis. The result should be restoration of nearly normal hearing sensitivity.

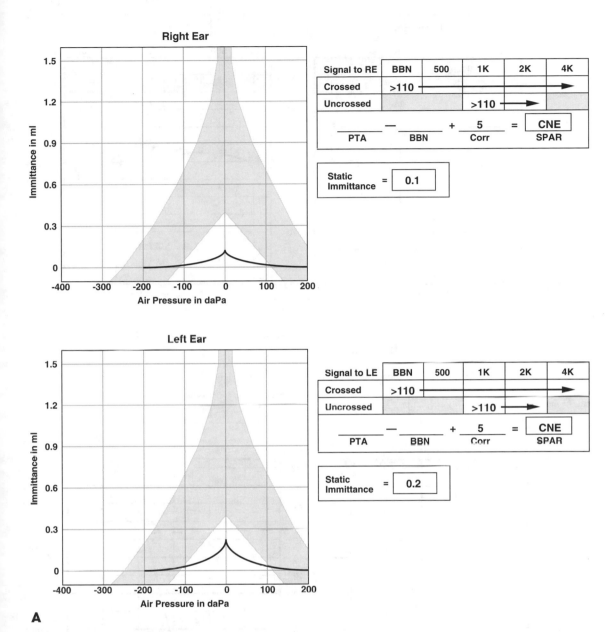

Figure 8-2. Hearing consultation results in a 33-year-old woman with otosclerosis. Immittance measures (A) are consistent with an increase in the stiffness of the middle ear mechanism, consistent with fixation of the ossicular chain. Pure-tone audiometric results (B) show a moderate conductive hearing loss with a 2000-Hz notch in bone-conduction thresholds bilaterally. Speech audiometric results (C) show excellent suprathreshold speech recognition once intensity level is sufficient to overcome the conductive hearing loss.

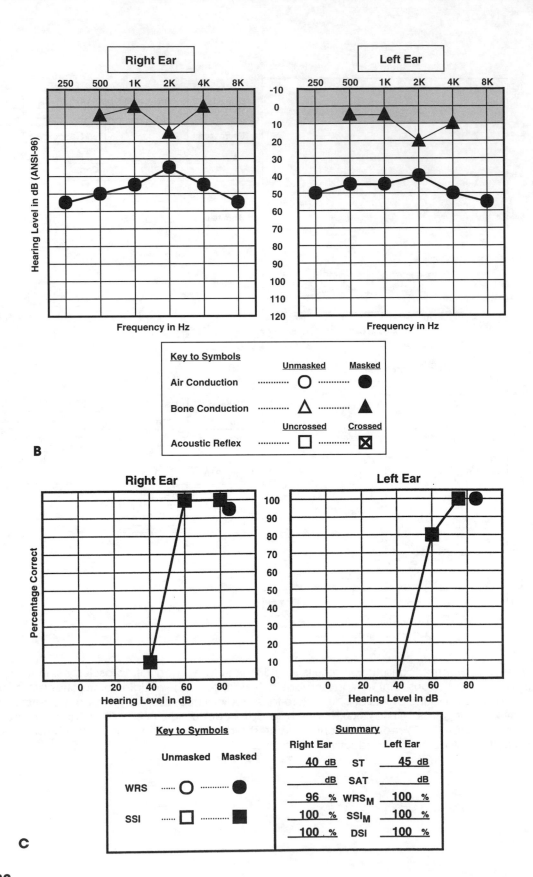

Right Ear

Left Ear

Hearing Level in dB (ANSI-96)

Frequency in Hz

Frequency in Hz

Key to Symbols

	Unmasked	Masked
Air Conduction	·········· ○ ··········	●
Bone Conduction	·········· △ ··········	▲
	Uncrossed	Crossed
Acoustic Reflex	·········· □ ··········	⊠

B

Right Ear

Left Ear

Percentage Correct

Hearing Level in dB

Hearing Level in dB

Key to Symbols

	Unmasked	Masked
WRS	······ ○ ··········	●
SSI	······ □ ··········	■

	Summary	
Right Ear		**Left Ear**
40 dB	ST	45 dB
dB	SAT	dB
96 %	WRS$_M$	100 %
100 %	SSI$_M$	100 %
100 %	DSI	100 %

C

Cochlear Pathology

Evaluative Goals

When an otologist refers a patient with a suspected cochlear disorder, the physician is interested in the answers to several questions, including:

- Is there a hearing loss and what is the extent of it?
- Is the loss truly of a cochlear nature or is there also a conductive component?
- Is the loss truly of a cochlear nature or is it retrocochlear?
- Is the loss fluctuating or stable?
- Could the loss be due to a treatable condition such as endolymphatic hydrops?

The goals of the audiologic evaluation, then, pertain to these questions. The first goal is to determine whether a middle ear disorder is contributing to the problem. The second goal is to determine the degree and type of hearing loss. The third goal is to scrutinize the audiologic findings for any evidence of retrocochlear disorder.

Test Strategies

Immittance audiometry is used to evaluate outer and middle ear function, to indicate the presence of cochlear hearing loss, and to assess the integrity of VIIIth nerve and lower auditory brain stem function. Pure-tone audiometry is used to evaluate the degree and type of hearing loss. Speech audiometry is used as a cross-check of pure-tone thresholds and as an estimate of suprathreshold word recognition ability.

Immittance Audiometry. A complete immittance battery will provide valuable information about the cochlear hearing loss. If a loss is truly cochlear in origin, then the tympanograms will be normal, static immittance will be normal, and acoustic reflex thresholds will be consistent with the degree of sensorineural hearing loss. For example, if a cochlear hearing loss is less than approximately 50 dB HL, then acoustic reflex thresholds to pure tones should be at normal levels. If the loss is greater than 50 dB, reflex thresholds will be elevated accordingly. In either case, a cochlear hearing loss will cause an elevation of the acoustic reflex thresholds to noise stimuli relative to pure-tone stimuli, resulting in a reduced **SPAR** value.

The **SPAR** test is designed to predict the presence or absence of cochlear hearing loss by comparing the difference between acoustic reflex thresholds elicited by pure tones and by broad-band noise.

If immittance audiometry suggests the presence of middle ear disorder, then any cochlear loss is likely to have a superimposed conductive component that must be quantified by pure-tone audiometry. If immittance audiometry is consistent with normal middle ear function, but acoustic reflexes are elevated beyond that which might be expected from the degree of sensorineural hearing loss, then suspicion is raised about the possibility of retrocochlear disorder.

Pure-Tone Audiometry. Pure-tone audiometry is used to quantify the degree of sensorineural hearing loss caused by the cochlear disorder. If all immittance measures are normal, then air-conduction testing must be completed on both ears. Bone conduction will not be necessary because outer and middle ear function are normal, and air-conducted signals will properly evaluate the sensitivity of the cochlea. If all immittance measures are not normal, then air- and bone-conduction thresholds must be obtained for both ears to assess the possibility of the presence of a mixed hearing loss. In either case, both ears must be tested, because the use of masking is likely to be necessary and cannot be properly carried out without knowledge of the air- and bone-conduction thresholds of the nontest ear.

Pure-tone audiometry is also an important measure for assessing symmetry of hearing loss. If a sensorineural hearing loss is asymmetric, in the absence of other explanations, suspicion is raised about the possibility of the presence of retrocochlear disorder.

There are other ways in which pure-tone audiometry can be useful in the otologic diagnosis of cochlear disorder. Some types of cochlear disorder are dynamic and may be treatable at various stages. One example is endolymphatic hydrops, a cochlear disorder caused by excessive accumulation of endolymph in the cochlea. In its active stage, otologists will attempt to treat it in various ways and will often use the results of pure-tone audiometry as both partial evidence of the presence of hydrops and as a means for assessing benefit from the treatment regimen.

Speech Audiometry. Speech audiometry is used in two ways in the assessment of cochlear disorder. First, speech reception thresholds are used as a cross-check of the validity of pure-tone thresholds in an effort to ensure the organicity of the disorder. Second, word-recognition and other suprathreshold measures are used to assess whether the cochlear hearing loss has an expected influence on speech recognition. That is, in most cases, suprathreshold speech-recognition ability is predictable from the degree and configuration of a sensorineural hearing loss if the loss is cochlear in origin. Therefore, if word-recognition scores are appropriate for the degree of hearing loss, then the results are consistent with a cochlear site of disorder. If scores are poorer than would be expected from the degree of hearing loss, then suspicion is aroused that the disorder may be retrocochlear in nature.

Otoacoustic Emissions. Otoacoustic emissions can be used in the assessment of sensorineural hearing loss as a means of verifying that there is a cochlear component to the disorder. For example, if the cochlea is disordered, OAEs are expected to be abnormal or absent. Although this does not preclude the presence of retrocochlear disorder, it does implicate the cochlea. Conversely, if OAEs are normal in the presence of a sensorineural hearing loss, a retrocochlear site of disorder is implicated.

Auditory Evoked Potentials. Auditory evoked potentials can be used for two purposes in the assessment of cochlear disorder. First, if there is suspicion that the hearing loss is exaggerated, evoked potentials can be used to predict the degree of organic hearing loss. Second, if there is suspicion that the disorder might be retrocochlear in nature, the auditory brain stem response can be used in an effort to differentiate a cochlear from a retrocochlear site.

Illustrative Cases

Illustrative Case 8-3. Case 3 is a patient with bilateral sensorineural hearing loss of cochlear origin, secondary to ototoxicity. The patient is a 56-year-old man with cancer who recently finished a round of chemotherapy with a drug regimen that included cisplatin.

Immittance audiometry, as shown in Figure 8–3A, is consistent with normal middle ear function bilaterally, characterized by Type A tympanograms, normal static immittance, and normal crossed and uncrossed acoustic reflex thresholds. You will note that the SPARs, or sensitivity prediction by acoustic reflexes, predict the presence of a sensorineural hearing loss, as they are below the score of 15, which is the lower limit for normal cochlear function.

Pure-tone audiometry is shown in Figure 8–3B. Results show bilaterally symmetric, high-frequency sensorineural hearing loss, progressing from mild levels at 2000 Hz to profound at 8000 Hz.

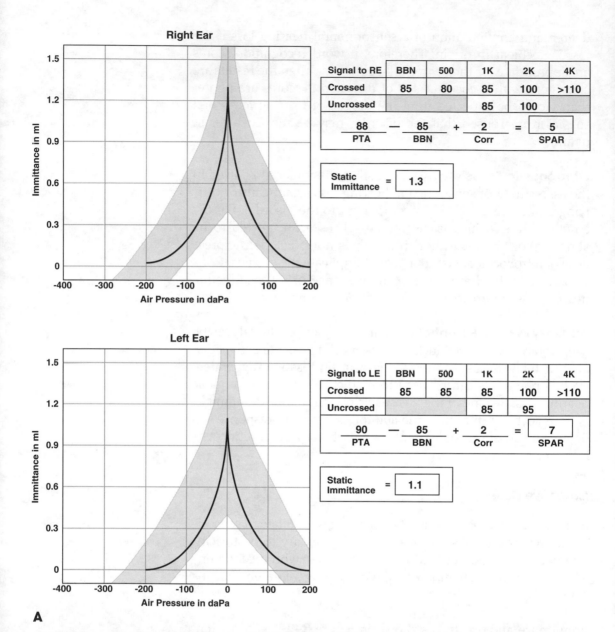

Right Ear

Signal to RE	BBN	500	1K	2K	4K
Crossed	85	80	85	100	>110
Uncrossed			85	100	

$$\underset{\text{PTA}}{88} - \underset{\text{BBN}}{85} + \underset{\text{Corr}}{2} = \underset{\text{SPAR}}{5}$$

Static Immittance = 1.3

Left Ear

Signal to LE	BBN	500	1K	2K	4K
Crossed	85	85	85	100	>110
Uncrossed			85	95	

$$\underset{\text{PTA}}{90} - \underset{\text{BBN}}{85} + \underset{\text{Corr}}{2} = \underset{\text{SPAR}}{7}$$

Static Immittance = 1.1

A

Figure 8–3. Hearing consultation results in a 56-year-old man with hearing loss resulting from ototoxicity. Immittance measures (A) are consistent with normal middle ear function. SPARs predict the presence of hearing loss. Pure-tone audiometric results (B) show a high-frequency sensorineural hearing loss bilaterally. Speech audiometric results (C) are consistent with the degree and configuration of the hearing loss.

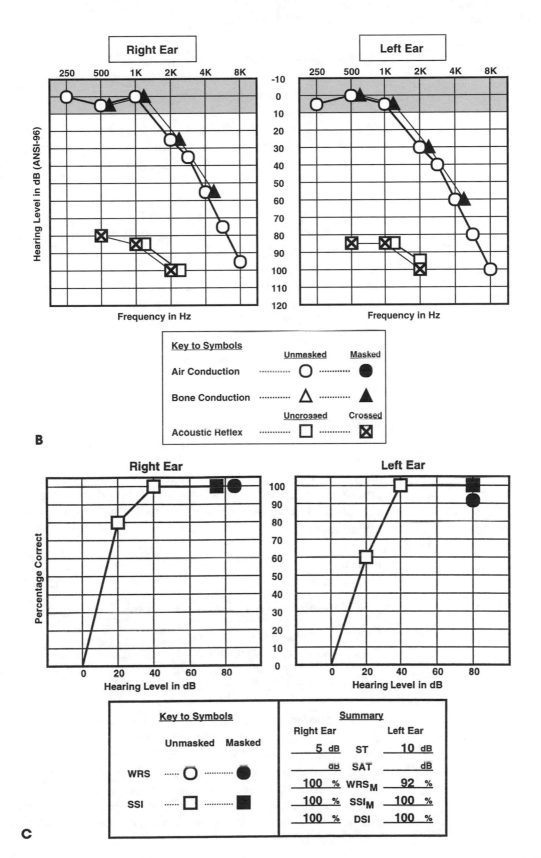

Further doses of chemotherapy would be expected to begin to affect the remaining high-frequency hearing and progress downward toward the low frequencies.

Speech audiometric results, as shown in Figure 8–3C, are consistent with the degree and configuration of cochlear hearing loss. First, the speech thresholds match the pure-tone thresholds. Second, the word recognition scores are consistent with this degree of hearing loss. You can compare these results with those that would be expected from the degree of loss by comparing them to Table 6–4 or by calculating the audibility index and predicting the score from that calculation.

This patient may well be a candidate for high-frequency amplification, if the hearing loss is causing a communication disorder for him. Caution should also be taken to monitor hearing sensitivity if the patient undergoes additional chemotherapy. He is at risk for additional hearing loss, and the physician may be able to alter the dosage of cisplatin to reduce the potential for further cochlear damage.

Illustrative Case 8–4. Case 4 is a patient with unilateral sensorineural hearing loss secondary to endolymphatic hydrops. The patient is a 45-year-old woman who, 2 weeks prior to the evaluation, experienced episodes of hearing loss, ear fullness, tinnitus, and severe vertigo. After several episodic attacks, hearing loss persisted. A diagnosis of Ménière's disease was made by her otolaryngologist.

Immittance audiometry, as shown in Figure 8–4A is consistent with normal middle ear function bilaterally, characterized by Type A tympanograms, normal static immittance, and normal crossed and uncrossed reflex thresholds.

Pure-tone audiometry is shown in Figure 8–4B. Results show a moderate, rising, sensorineural hearing loss on the left ear and normal hearing sensitivity on the right.

Speech audiometric results, shown in Figure 8–4C, were normal for the right ear. On the left, although speech thresholds agree with the pure-tone thresholds, suprathreshold speech-recognition scores are very poor for the left ear. This performance is significantly reduced from what would normally be expected from a cochlear hearing loss. These results are unusual for cochlear hearing loss, except in cases of Ménière's disease, where they are characteristic.

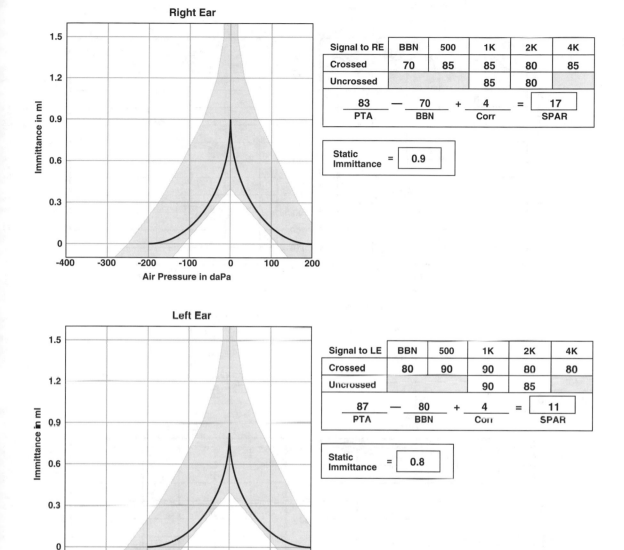

Figure 8-4. Hearing consultation results in a 45-year-old woman with hearing loss secondary to endolymphatic hydrops. Immittance measures (A) are consistent with normal middle ear function. SPARs predict the presence of hearing loss in the left ear. Pure-tone audiometric results (B) show normal hearing sensitivity on the right and a moderate, rising sensorineural hearing loss on the left. Speech audiometric results (C) show that speech-recognition ability on the left ear is poorer than would be predicted from the degree and configuration of hearing loss. Auditory brain stem response results (D) show that both the absolute and interpeak latencies are normal and symmetric, consistent with normal VIIIth nerve and auditory brain stem function.

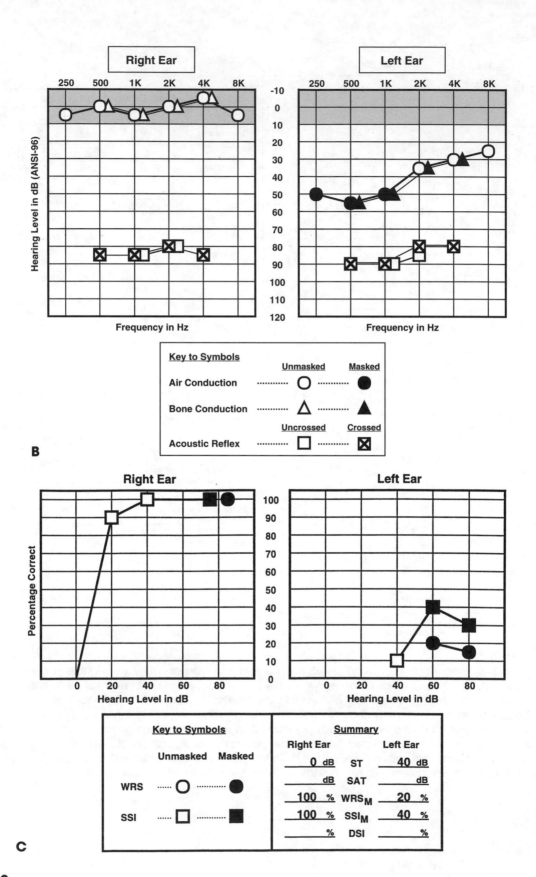

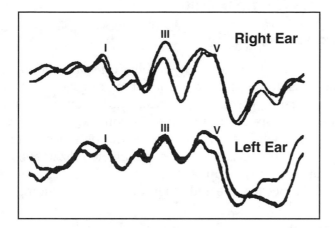

	Latency Wave V	Interwave Intervals		
		I-III	III-V	I-V
RE	5.8	2.0	2.0	4.0
LE	5.8	2.0	2.0	4.0

Click Level: 90 dB nHL

D

Because of the unilateral nature of the disorder, the physician was interested in ruling out an VIIIth nerve tumor as the causative factor. Results of an auditory brain stem response assessment are shown in Figure 8–4D. Both the absolute and interpeak latencies are normal and symmetric, supporting the diagnosis of cochlear disorder.

The physician may recommend a course of diuretics or steroids and may recommend a change in diet and stress level for the patient. From an audiologic perspective, the patient is not a good candidate for amplification because of the normal hearing in the right ear and because of the exceptionally poor speech recognition ability in the left. Presenting amplified sound to an ear that distorts this badly is unlikely to result in a favorable reaction. Monitoring of hearing is indicated to assess any changes that might occur in the left ear.

Retrocochlear Pathology

Evaluative Goals

Sometimes the patient history or physical examination will lead the otologist to suspect that a patient might have a retrocochlear disorder. In most cases, the physician will be concerned about the presence of a space-occupying lesion on the VIIIth nerve. This often occurs when a patient reports the presence of unilateral hearing loss, unilateral tinnitus, unexplained dizziness, or other neurologic symptoms. In such cases, the physician is interested in several aspects of the audiologic evaluation, including:

Unilateral pertains to one side only; **bilateral** pertains to both sides.

Symmetric means there is a similarity between two parts; **asymmetric** means there is a dissimilarity between two parts.

■ Is there a hearing loss, and what is the extent of it?
■ Is the loss **unilateral** or **asymmetric**?
■ Is speech understanding asymmetric or poorer than predicted from the hearing loss?
■ Are acoustic reflexes normal or elevated?
■ Is there other evidence of retrocochlear disorder?

One goal of the audiologic evaluation is to determine the degree and type of hearing loss. Another goal is to scrutinize the audiologic findings for any evidence of retrocochlear disorder. Often a third goal is to assess the integrity of the VIIIth nerve and auditory brain stem with electrophysiologic measures.

Test Strategies

Immittance audiometry is used to evaluate outer and middle ear function and to assess the integrity of the VIIth and VIIIth cranial nerves and lower auditory brain stem function. Pure-tone audiometry is used to evaluate the extent of any hearing asymmetry. Speech audiometry is used as a cross-check of pure-tone thresholds, as an estimate of suprathreshold speech recognition ability, as a measure of hearing symmetry, and as an assessment of any abnormality of hearing under adverse listening conditions. Electroacoustic and electrophysiologic measures are used in an effort to assess integrity of the cochlea, VIIIth nerve, and auditory brain stem.

Immittance Measures. A complete immittance battery may provide valuable information about the nature of a retrocochlear hearing disorder. Assuming normal middle ear function, the absence of crossed and uncrossed reflexes measured from the same ear may be indicative of facial nerve disorder on that side. The absence of crossed and uncrossed reflexes when the eliciting signal is presented to one ear may be indicative of VIIIth nerve disorder on that side.

If the disorder is truly cochlear in origin, the tympanograms will be normal, static immittance will be normal, and acoustic reflex thresholds will be consistent with the degree of sensorineural hearing loss. Immittance audiometry is also important in assessing middle ear function in cases of suspected retrocochlear disorder, because middle ear disorder and any resultant conductive hearing loss can affect interpretation of other audiometric measures.

Pure-Tone Audiometry. Pure-tone audiometry is used to quantify the degree of sensorineural hearing loss caused by the retrocochlear disorder. If all immittance measures are normal, only air-conduction testing must be completed on both ears. Bone conduction will not be necessary because outer and middle ear function is normal, and air-conducted signals will properly evaluate the sensitivity of the cochlea. If all immittance measures are not normal, air- and bone-conduction thresholds must be obtained for both ears to assess the possibility of the presence of a mixed hearing loss. In either case, both ears must be tested, because the use of masking is likely to be necessary and cannot be properly carried out without knowledge of the air- and bone-conduction thresholds of the nontest ear.

Pure-tone audiometry is also an important measure for assessing symmetry of hearing loss. If a sensorineural hearing loss is asymmetric in the absence of other explanations, suspicion is raised about the possibility of the presence of retrocochlear disorder.

Speech Audiometry. Speech audiometry is used in two ways in the assessment of retrocochlear disorder. First, as usual, speech reception thresholds are used as a cross-check of the validity of pure-tone thresholds in an effort to ensure the organicity of the disorder. Second, word recognition and other suprathreshold measures are used to assess whether speech recognition is poorer than would be expected from the amount of hearing loss. That is, in most cases of cochlear disorder, suprathreshold speech-recognition ability is predictable from the degree and configuration of a sensorineural hearing loss. However, if speech-recognition ability is poorer than would be expected from the degree of hearing loss, suspicion is aroused that the disorder may be retrocochlear in nature.

Suprathreshold speech audiometric measures are very important in the assessment of patients suspected of retrocochlear disorder.

Often such a disorder will escape detection of simple measures of word recognition presented in quiet. One useful technique is to obtain performance-intensity functions by testing word recognition ability at several intensity levels and looking for the presence of rollover of the function. Rollover, as you will recall, is the unexpectedly poorer performance as intensity level is increased, a phenomenon associated with retrocochlear disorder. Another useful technique is to evaluate speech recognition in background competition. Although those with normal neurologic systems will perform well on such measures, those with retrocochlear disorder are likely to perform more poorly than would be predicted from their hearing sensitivity loss.

Otoacoustic Emissions. Otoacoustic emissions can be used in the assessment of retrocochlear disorder, although the results are often equivocal. If a hearing loss is caused by a retrocochlear disorder due to the disorder's effect on function of the VIIIth nerve, otoacoustic emissions may be normal despite the hearing loss. That is, the loss is caused by neural disorder, and the cochlea is functioning normally. However, in some cases a retrocochlear disorder can affect function of the cochlea, presumably by interrupting its blood supply, resulting in a hearing loss and abnormality of otoacoustic emissions. Thus, in the presence of a hearing loss and normal middle ear function, the absence of OAEs indicates either cochlear or retrocochlear disorder. On the other hand, in the presence of a hearing loss, the preservation of OAEs suggests that the disorder is retrocochlear in nature.

Auditory Evoked Potentials. If suspicion of a retrocochlear disorder exists and if that suspicion is enhanced by the presence of audiometric indicators, it is quite common to assess the integrity of the auditory nervous system directly with the auditory brain stem response. The ABR is a sensitive indicator of the integrity of VIIIth nerve and auditory brain stem function. If it is abnormal, there is a very high likelihood of retrocochlear disorder.

In recent years, imaging techniques have improved to the point that structural changes in the nervous system can sometimes be identified before those changes have a functional influence. Thus, the presence of a normal ABR does not rule out the presence of a neurologic disease process. It simply indicates that the process is without apparent functional consequence. The presence of an abnormal ABR, however, remains a strong indicator of neurologic disorder and can be very helpful to the physician in the diagnosis of retrocochlear disease.

Illustrative Cases

Illustrative Case 8-5. Case 5 is a patient with an VIIIth nerve tumor on the left ear. The tumor is diagnosed as a cochleovestibular schwannoma. The patient is a 42-year-old man with a 6-month history of left-ear tinnitus. His health and hearing histories are otherwise unremarkable.

Immittance audiometry, as shown in Figure 8–5A is consistent with normal middle ear function bilaterally, characterized by Type A tympanograms, normal static immittance, and normal right crossed and right uncrossed reflex thresholds. Left crossed and left uncrossed reflexes are absent, consistent with some form of afferent abnormality on the left, in this case an VIIIth-nerve tumor.

Pure-tone audiometric results are shown in Figure 8–5B. The patient has normal hearing sensitivity on the right ear and a mild, relatively flat sensorineural hearing loss on the left.

Speech audiometric results, shown in Figure 8–5C, are normal on the right ear but abnormal on the left. Although maximum speech-recognition scores are normal at lower intensity levels, the performance-intensity function demonstrates significant rollover, or poorer performance at higher intensity levels. This rollover is consistent with retrocochlear site of disorder.

Results of an auditory brain stem response assessment are shown in Figure 8–5D. Right ear results are normal. Left ear results show delayed latencies and prolonged interpeak intervals. These results are also consistent with retrocochlear site of disorder.

This patient had surgery to remove the tumor. Because the tumor was relatively small and the hearing relatively good, the surgeon opted to try a surgical approach to remove the tumor *and* preserve hearing. Hearing was monitored throughout the surgery, and postsurgical audiometric results showed that hearing was effectively preserved.

Illustrative Case 8-6. Case 6 is a patient with auditory complaints secondary to multiple sclerosis. The patient is a 34-year-old woman. Two years prior to her evaluation, she experienced an episode of diplopia, or double vision, accompanied by a tingling sensation and weakness in her left leg. These symptoms gradually subsided and reappeared in slightly more severe form a year later. Ultimately, she was diagnosed with multiple sclerosis.

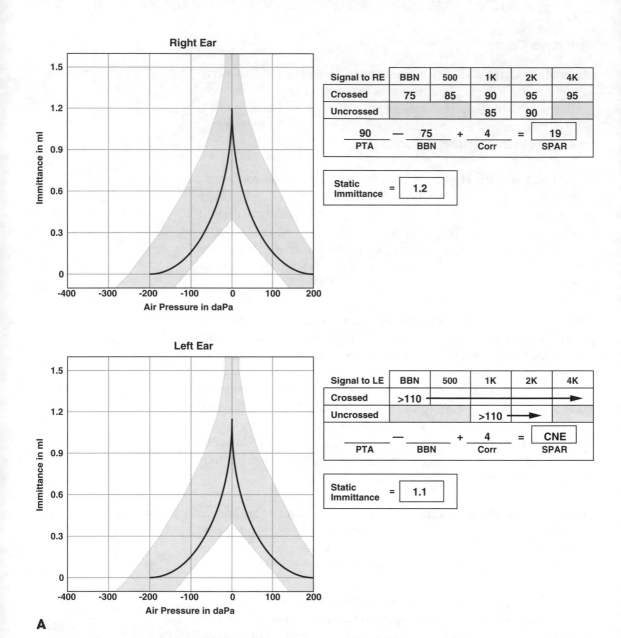

Figure 8–5. Hearing consultation results in a 42-year-old man with a left VIIIth nerve tumor. Immittance measures (A) are consistent with normal middle ear function. Left crossed and left uncrossed reflexes are absent, consistent with left afferent disorder. Pure-tone audiometric results (B) show normal hearing sensitivity on the right and a mild, relatively flat sensorineural hearing loss on the left. Speech audiometric results (C) show rollover of the performance-intensity functions on the left ear. Auditory brain stem response results (D) show delayed latencies and prolonged interpeak intervals on the left ear, consistent with retrocochlear site of disorder.

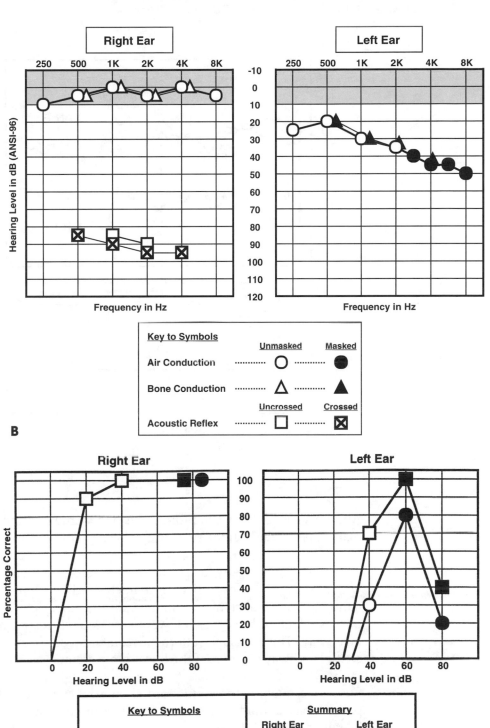

347

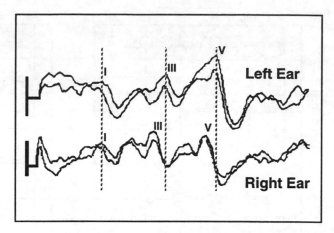

	Latency Wave V	Interwave Intervals		
		I-III	**III-V**	**I-V**
RE	5.9	1.9	2.0	3.9
LE	6.5	2.5	2.0	4.5

Click Level: 90 dB nHL

D

Among various other symptoms, she had vague hearing complaints, particularly in the presence of background noise.

Immittance audiometry, as shown in Figure 8–6A is consistent with normal middle ear function, characterized by a Type A tympanogram, normal static immittance, and normal right and left uncrossed reflex thresholds. However, crossed reflexes are absent bilaterally. This unusual pattern of results is consistent with a central pathway disorder of the lower brain stem.

Pure-tone audiometric results are shown in Figure 8–6B. The patient has a mild low-frequency sensorineural hearing loss bilaterally.

Speech thresholds match pure-tone thresholds in both ears. However, suprathreshold speech-recognition performance is abnormal in both ears. Although speech-recognition scores are normal when words are presented in quiet, they are abnormal when sentences are presented in the presence of competition, as

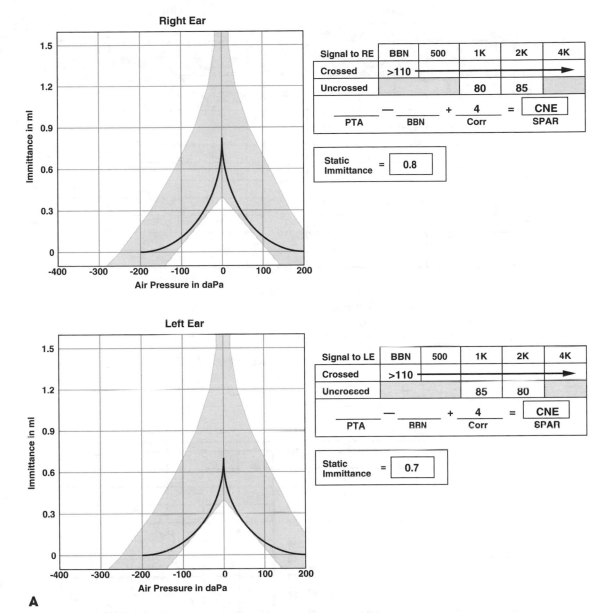

Right Ear

Signal to RE	BBN	500	1K	2K	4K
Crossed	>110	→			
Uncrossed			80	85	

$$\frac{\quad\quad}{\text{PTA}} - \frac{\quad\quad}{\text{BBN}} + \frac{4}{\text{Corr}} = \boxed{\begin{matrix}\text{CNE}\\ \text{SPAR}\end{matrix}}$$

Static Immittance = 0.8

Left Ear

Signal to LE	BBN	500	1K	2K	4K
Crossed	>110	→			
Uncrossed			85	80	

$$\frac{\quad\quad}{\text{PTA}} - \frac{\quad\quad}{\text{BBN}} + \frac{4}{\text{Corr}} = \boxed{\begin{matrix}\text{CNE}\\ \text{SPAR}\end{matrix}}$$

Static Immittance = 0.7

A

Figure 8-6. Hearing consultation results in a 34-year-old woman with multiple sclerosis. Immittance measures (A) are consistent with normal middle ear function. However, left crossed and right crossed reflexes are absent, consistent with brain stem disorder. Pure-tone audiometric results (B) show mild low-frequency sensorineural hearing loss bilaterally. Speech audiometric results (C) show that word recognition in quiet is normal, but sentence recognition in competition is abnormal. Auditory brain stem response results (D) show no identifiable waves beyond Wave I on the left and significant prolongation of the Wave I–V interpeak interval on the right.

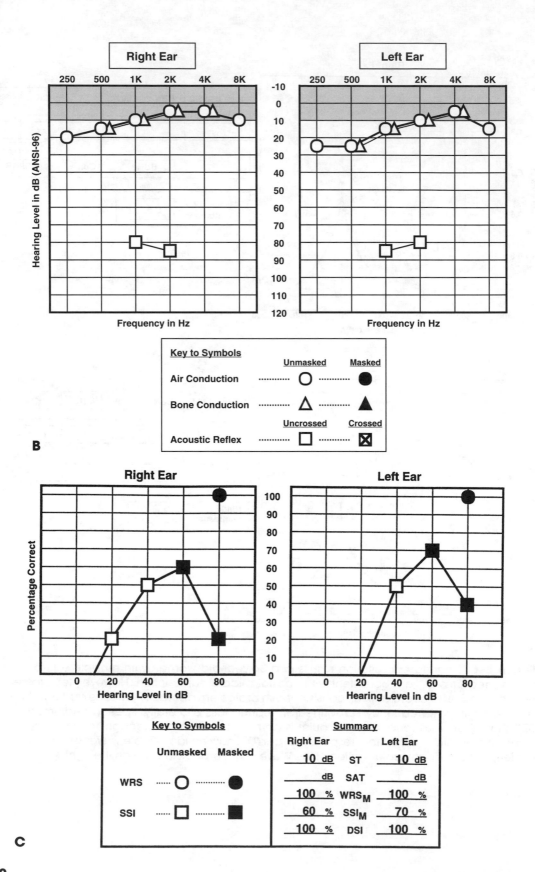

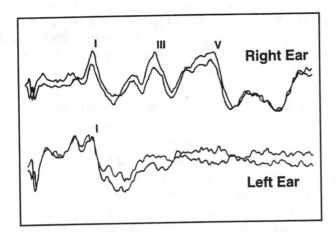

	Latency Wave V	Interwave Intervals		
		I-III	III-V	I-V
RE	6.6	2.3	2.3	4.6
LE	CNE	CNE	CNE	CNE

Click Level: 80 dB nHL

D

shown in Figure 8–6C. These results are consistent with retro-cochlear pathology.

Auditory evoked potentials are also consistent with abnormality of brain stem function. Figure 8–6D shows auditory brain stem responses for both ears. On the left, no waves were identifiable beyond component Wave I, and on the right, absolute latencies and interpeak intervals were significantly prolonged.

Multiple sclerosis is commonly treated with chemotherapy in an attempt to keep it in its remission stage. Although the patient's auditory complaints were vague and subtle, she was informed of the availability of certain assistive listening devices that could be used if she was experiencing substantive difficulty during periods of exacerbation of the multiple sclerosis.

ADULT AUDIOLOGIC REFERRALS

An audiologist's evaluation of a patient is aimed at diagnosing and treating hearing impairments that are caused by a diseased or disordered auditory system. The purpose of the evaluation is to quantify the degree and nature of the hearing impairment, assess its impact on a patient's communication ability, and plan and provide prosthetic and rehabilitative treatment for the impairment.

In some patients referred for audiologic purposes, the absence of active disease process has been determined. For example, some referrals for audiologic assessment are from otolaryngologists or other physicians who have ruled out the presence of active or medically treatable conditions. In other cases, the referral is a self-referral or emanates from some source other than the medical community. In both cases, the audiologic assessment is carried out with vigilance for indicators of medically treatable conditions. The focus, however, is on the impact of the hearing loss on the individual's communication ability.

In general, audiologists are faced with two main categories of adult patients, those who are younger and have significant vocational communication demands and those who are older and have more complex auditory problems. Of course, age is not necessarily a factor, so that some of the older adults may fit into the younger category and vice versa. However, often the approach that is appropriate for patients who are elderly is different from that necessary for those who are younger, and the distinction seems worth making.

Younger Adults

Evaluative Goals

The main goals of the audiologic evaluation of adult patients are to assess the degree and type of hearing loss and to assess the impact that the hearing loss has on their communicative function. An important subgoal is to maintain vigilance for indicators of underlying conditions that might require medical attention.

Test Strategies

Immittance audiometry is used to evaluate outer and middle ear function, to indicate the presence of cochlear hearing loss, and to assess the integrity of VIIIth nerve and lower auditory brain stem function. Pure-tone audiometry is used to evaluate the degree and type of hearing loss. Speech audiometry is used as a cross-check of pure-tone thresholds and as an estimate of supra-threshold word recognition ability. Both pure-tone and speech audiometric measures are used as prognostic indicators for the successful use of hearing aid amplification. Hearing handicap assessment is used to quantify the impact that the hearing impairment is having on communication ability.

Immittance Measures. A complete immittance battery is an important first step in the audiologic evaluation. It is important to assess the integrity of middle ear function for several reasons. If it is abnormal, proper medical referrals may need to be made, depending on the initial referral source. Also, results will direct the audiologist as to the need for bone-conduction testing. Should a middle ear disorder cause a conductive hearing loss, the degree of the conductive component is likely to influence hearing aid fitting.

Immittance audiometry also provides valuable information about the cochlear hearing loss. If a loss is truly cochlear in origin, the tympanograms will be normal, static immittance will be normal, and acoustic reflex thresholds will be consistent with the degree of sensorineural hearing loss. A cochlear hearing loss will also cause an elevation of the acoustic reflex thresholds to noise stimuli relative to pure-tone stimuli, resulting in a reduced SPAR value. This information serves as an important cross-check of the organicity of the hearing loss.

Finally, immittance audiometry allows an assessment of the integrity of the auditory nervous system. If immittance audiometry is consistent with normal middle ear function, but acoustic reflexes are elevated beyond a level that might be expected from the degree of sensorineural hearing loss, suspicion is raised about the possibility of retrocochlear disorder.

Pure-Tone Audiometry. Pure-tone audiometry is used to quantify the degree of conductive, sensorineural, or mixed hearing loss caused by the auditory disorder. If all immittance measures are normal, only air-conduction testing is necessary. Bone conduction testing will not be necessary because outer and middle ear function are normal, and air-conducted signals will properly evaluate the sensitivity of the cochlea. If all immittance measures are not normal, air- and bone-conduction thresholds must be obtained for both ears to assess the possibility of the presence of a conductive or mixed hearing loss.

Correctly or incorrectly, the audiogram itself has become the single most important metric in an audiologic evaluation. Nearly all estimates of hearing impairment, disability, and handicap begin with this measure of hearing sensitivity as their basis. Gain, frequency response, and sometimes output limitations of hearing aids are also estimated based on the result of pure-tone audiometry.

Pure-tone audiometry is also an important measure for assessing symmetry of hearing loss. If a sensorineural hearing loss is asymmetric, in the absence of other explanations, then suspicion is raised about the possibility of the presence of retrocochlear disorder.

Speech Audiometry. Speech audiometry is used in several ways in the audiologic assessment of hearing disorder. First, speech reception thresholds are used as a cross-check of the validity of pure-tone thresholds in an effort to ensure the organicity of the disorder.

Second, word-recognition and other suprathreshold measures are used to assess whether the hearing loss has an expected influence on speech recognition. That is, in most cases, suprathreshold speech recognition ability is predictable from the degree and configuration of a hearing loss if the loss is due to conductive or cochlear disorders. If not, then suspicion is aroused that the disorder may be retrocochlear in nature.

Third, speech recognition measures are used for assessing the amount of impairment caused by a hearing loss and for assessing prognosis for successful hearing aid use. If a patient's speech recognition ability is significantly reduced, he or she is likely to have greater impairment and reduced success with conventional hearing aid amplification.

Hearing Handicap Assessment. One final important aspect of the audiologic evaluation is an assessment of the impact that a hearing loss has on self-perception of handicap. If the hearing loss is perceived to be handicapping, motivation for treatment and rehabilitation will be significantly higher than if the hearing loss is perceived to have little influence on communication. Thus, hearing handicap assessment tools can be useful as prognostic indicators of hearing aid success. In addition, they can be used before and after intervention as a way of quantifying benefit received from the treatment.

Illustrative Case

Illustrative Case 8-7. Illustrative Case 7 is a patient with a history of exposure to excessive noise. The patient is a 54-year-old man with bilateral sensorineural hearing loss that has progressed slowly over the past 20 years. He has a positive history of noise exposure, first during military service and then at his workplace. In addition, he is an avid hunter. The patient reports that he has used hearing protection on occasion in the past, but has not done so on a consistent basis. He was having his hearing tested at the urging of family members who were having increasing difficulty communicating with him.

Immittance audiometry, as shown in Figure 8–7A, is consistent with normal middle ear function, characterized by a Type A tympanogram, normal static immittance, and normal crossed and uncrossed reflex thresholds bilaterally.

Pure-tone audiometric results are shown in Figure 8–7B. The patient has a bilateral, fairly symmetric, high-frequency sensorineural hearing loss. The loss is greatest at 4000 Hz.

Speech audiometric results, as shown in Figure 8–7C, are consistent with the degree and configuration of cochlear hearing loss. First, the speech thresholds match the pure-tone thresholds. Second, the word-recognition scores, although reduced, are consistent with this degree of hearing loss.

The patient also completed a hearing handicap assessment. Results showed that he has communication problems a significant proportion of the time that he spends in certain listening environments, especially those involving background noise.

The hearing loss is sensorineural in nature, resulting from exposure to excessive noise over long periods of time. It is not amenable to surgical or medical intervention. Because the patient is experiencing significant communication problems due to the hearing loss, he is a candidate for hearing aid amplification. A hearing aid consultation was recommended.

Older Adults

Evaluative Goals

The goals in evaluating older adults are similar to those in younger adults. However, the complexity of auditory disorders

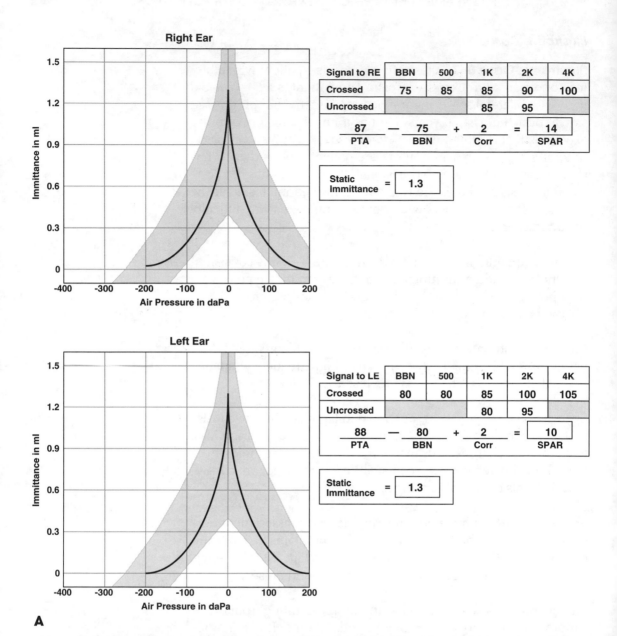

Right Ear

Signal to RE	BBN	500	1K	2K	4K
Crossed	75	85	85	90	100
Uncrossed			85	95	

$$\frac{87}{\text{PTA}} - \frac{75}{\text{BBN}} + \frac{2}{\text{Corr}} = \frac{14}{\text{SPAR}}$$

Static Immittance = 1.3

Left Ear

Signal to LE	BBN	500	1K	2K	4K
Crossed	80	80	85	100	105
Uncrossed			80	95	

$$\frac{88}{\text{PTA}} - \frac{80}{\text{BBN}} + \frac{2}{\text{Corr}} = \frac{10}{\text{SPAR}}$$

Static Immittance = 1.3

A

Figure 8-7. Hearing consultation results in a 54-year-old man with noise-induced hearing loss. Immittance measures (A) are consistent with normal middle ear function. Pure-tone audiometric results (B) show high-frequency sensorineural hearing loss bilaterally, greatest at 4000 Hz. Speech audiometric results (C) are consistent with the degree and configuration of cochlear hearing loss.

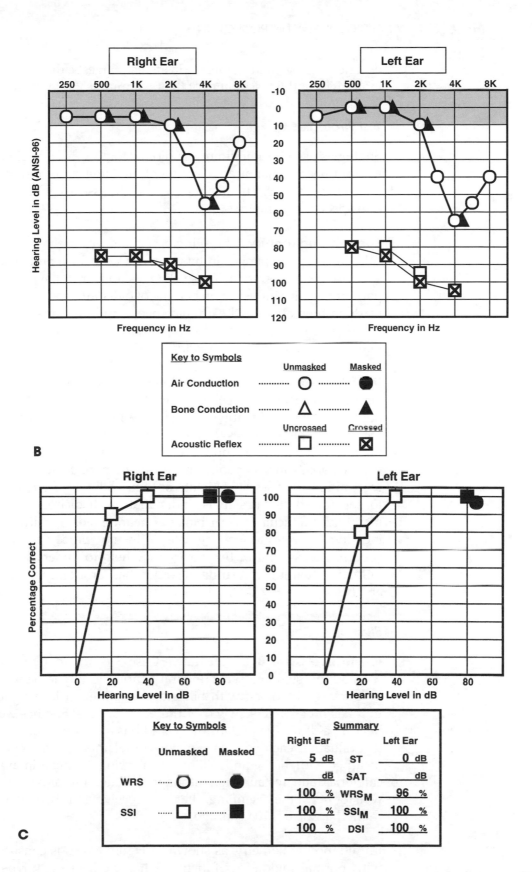

357

experienced by many older individuals suggests the need for more rigor in the assessment of their communication function.

Test Strategies

Strategies used for immittance audiometry, pure-tone audiometry, and hearing handicap assessment are similar to those used for younger adults. The major difference in assessment strategy is in speech audiometry.

Speech Audiometry. The aging of the auditory mechanism results in complex changes in function of the cochlea and central auditory nervous system. These changes appear to have an important negative influence on hearing of older individuals, particularly in their ability to hear rapid speech and to hear speech in the presence of background competition. Assessment of older individuals should include quantification of such changes.

In addition to routine speech audiometric measures, speech recognition in background competition should be assessed. If a patient has difficulty identifying speech under fairly easy listening conditions, the prognosis for successful use of conventional hearing aids is likely to be reduced. Older individuals may also have reduced ability in using both ears. Assessment of dichotic speech recognition provides an estimate of their ability to use two ears to separate different signals. Individuals with dichotic deficits may find it difficult to wear binaural hearing aids. Finally, older individuals seem to have greater difficulty processing rapid speech. Assessment of this ability may help to understand the influence that their hearing disorder has on communication ability.

Illustrative Case

Illustrative Case 8–8. Illustrative Case 8 is an elderly patient with a long-standing sensorineural hearing loss. The patient is a 78-year-old woman with bilateral sensorineural hearing loss that has progressed slowly over the past 15 years. She has worn hearing aids for the past 10 years, and has an annual audiologic re-evaluation each year. Her major complaints are in communicating with her grandchildren and trying to hear in noisy cafeterias and restaurants. Although her hearing aids worked well for her at the beginning, she is not receiving the benefit from them that she did 10 years ago.

Immittance audiometry, as shown in Figure 8–8A, is consistent with normal middle ear function, characterized by a Type A

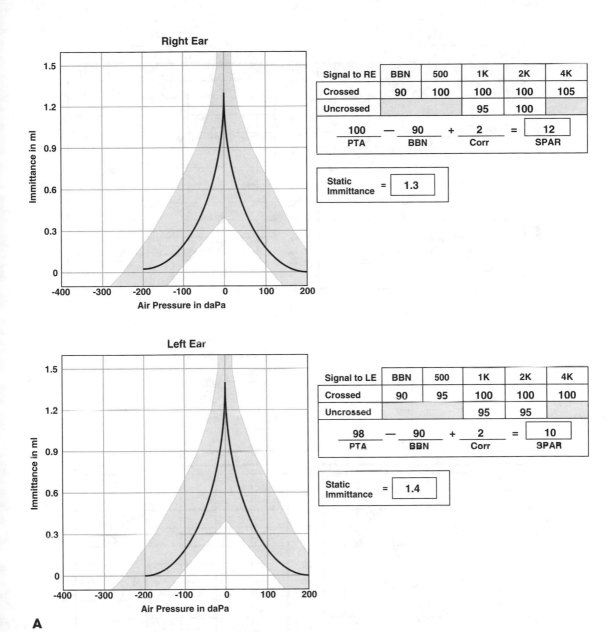

Right Ear

Signal to RE	BBN	500	1K	2K	4K
Crossed	90	100	100	100	105
Uncrossed			95	100	

$$\underset{\text{PTA}}{100} - \underset{\text{BBN}}{90} + \underset{\text{Corr}}{2} = \underset{\text{SPAR}}{\boxed{12}}$$

Static Immittance = $\boxed{1.3}$

Left Ear

Signal to LE	BBN	500	1K	2K	4K
Crossed	90	95	100	100	100
Uncrossed			95	95	

$$\underset{\text{PTA}}{98} - \underset{\text{BBN}}{90} + \underset{\text{Corr}}{2} = \underset{\text{SPAR}}{\boxed{10}}$$

Static Immittance = $\boxed{1.4}$

A

Figure 8–8. Hearing consultation results in a 78-year-old woman with long-standing, progressive hearing loss. Immittance measures (A) are consistent with normal middle ear function. Pure-tone audiometric results (B) show bilateral, symmetric, moderate, sensorineural hearing loss. Speech audiometric results (C) show reduced word recognition in quiet, consistent with the degree and configuration of cochlear hearing loss. Sentence recognition in competition is substantially reduced, as is dichotic performance.

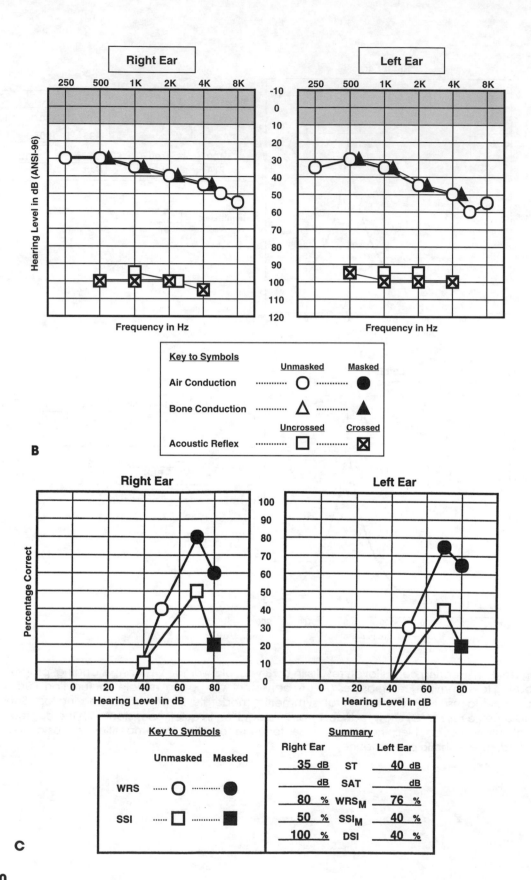

Right Ear

| | 250 | 500 | 1K | 2K | 4K | 8K |

Left Ear

Hearing Level in dB (ANSI-96)

Frequency in Hz

Key to Symbols

	Unmasked	Masked
Air Conduction	○	●
Bone Conduction	△	▲
	Uncrossed	Crossed
Acoustic Reflex	☐	⊠

B

Right Ear

Left Ear

Percentage Correct

Hearing Level in dB

Key to Symbols

	Unmasked	Masked
WRS	○	●
SSI	☐	■

Summary

Right Ear		Left Ear
35 dB	ST	40 dB
dB	SAT	dB
80 %	WRS$_M$	76 %
50 %	SSI$_M$	40 %
100 %	DSI	40 %

C

tympanogram, normal static immittance, and normal crossed and uncrossed reflex thresholds bilaterally.

Pure-tone audiometric results are shown in Figure 8–8B. The patient has a bilateral, symmetric, moderate, sensorineural hearing loss. Hearing sensitivity is slightly better in the low frequencies than in the high frequencies.

Speech audiometric results are consistent with those found in older patients. Speech thresholds match pure-tone thresholds. Word-recognition scores are reduced, but not below a level predictable from the degree of hearing sensitivity loss. However, speech recognition in the presence of competition is substantially reduced, as shown in Figure 8–8C, consistent with the patient's age. She also shows evidence of a dichotic deficit, with reduced performance in the left ear.

Results of the hearing handicap assessment show that she has communication problems a significant proportion of the time in most listening environments, especially those involving background noise.

The patient currently uses hearing aid amplification with some success, especially in quiet environments. Output of the hearing aids showed them to be functioning as expected. This patient may benefit from additional amplification systems known as assistive listening devices, and a consultation to discuss these alternatives was recommended.

PEDIATRIC AUDIOLOGIC REFERRALS

An audiologist's evaluation of an infant or child is aimed first at identifying the existence of an auditory disorder and then quantifying the degree of impairment resulting from the disorder. Once the degree and nature of the hearing impairment have been quantified, the goal is to assess its impact on the child's communication ability and plan and provide prosthetic and rehabilitative treatment for the impairment.

In general, the audiologist is faced with three main challenges in the assessment of infants and children. The first challenge is to identify children who are at risk for hearing loss and need further evaluation. Infant hearing screening may take place shortly after birth, and pediatric hearing screening is likely to occur at the time of enrollment in school. The goal here is to identify, as early as possible, children with hearing loss of a magnitude sufficient to interfere with speech and language development or academic achievement.

The second challenge is to determine if the children identified as being at risk for auditory disorder actually have a hearing loss and, if so, to determine the nature and degree of the loss. The goal here is to differentiate outer and middle ear disorder from cochlear disorder and to quantify the resultant conductive and sensorineural hearing loss.

The third challenge is to assess the hearing ability of preschool and early school-age children suspected of having central auditory processing disorders. The goal here is to try to identify the nature and quantify the extent of suprathreshold hearing deficits in children who generally have normal hearing sensitivity but exhibit hearing difficulties.

Infant Screening

Evaluative Goals

The goal of an infant hearing screening program is to identify infants who are at risk for significant sensorineural hearing loss and require further audiologic testing. The challenge of any screening program is to both capture all children who are at risk and, with similar accuracy, identify those children who are normal or not at risk. Several methods have been employed in an effort to meet this challenge, some with more success than others.

Test Strategies

Prenatal pertains to the time period before birth.
Perinatal pertains to the period around the time of birth, from the 28th week of gestation through the 7th day following delivery.

Two test strategies are used in infant screening: (a) identifying children at risk and (b) identifying children who have normal hearing. Efforts to identify children who are at risk involve mainly an evaluation of **prenatal, perinatal**, and parental factors that place a child at greater risk for having sensorineural hearing loss. It might also be argued that a failed screening is also a risk factor and that any screening efforts are aimed at determining risk in this manner. Some screening programs combine these two ideas and only screen the hearing of children who meet certain risk criteria. Such an approach tries to maximize the screening effort by only screening a limited sample of children that is likely to have a disproportionate amount of hearing loss.

Another perspective on the screening strategy is to view it as a way, not of identifying those who might have significant hearing loss, but of identifying those who have normal hearing. That is, most newborns have normal hearing. **The incidence of hearing loss** at birth is approximately **2 per 1000 births**. Thus, if you were attempting to screen the hearing of all newborns, you might want to develop strategies that focus on identifying those who are normal, leaving the remainder to be evaluated with a full audiologic assessment.

The incidence of hearing loss in newborns is **2 per 1000 births**.

Consensus on how to screen the hearing of infants, although emerging, has not yet been reached. An explanation of the various techniques can be found in Chapter 7. A summary of the benefits and challenges of these techniques as they relate specifically to the screening process follows.

Risk Factors. Several factors have been identified as placing a newborn at risk for sensorineural hearing loss. A list of those factors was delineated previously in Table 5–1. For many years, such factors have been used as a way of reducing the number of children whose hearing needed to be screened or to be monitored carefully over time. Applying risk factors has been successful in at least one important way. The percentage of the general population of newborns who have risk factors is reasonably low, and the relative proportion of those who actually have hearing loss is fairly high. Conversely, the number of infants in the general population who do not have risk factors is high, and the proportion with hearing loss is relatively much lower. So if you were to concentrate your efforts on one population, it makes sense to focus on the smaller, at-risk population, because your return on investment of time and resources would be much higher.

The major problem with using risk factors alone is that there are probably as many children with significant sensorineural hearing loss who fall into the at-risk category as there are children who do not appear to have any risk factors. Thus, although the prevalence of hearing loss in the at-risk population is significantly higher than in the nonrisk population, the numbers of children are the same. Thus, limiting your screening approach to this population would identify only about half of those with significant sensorineural hearing loss.

Behavioral Screening. Early efforts to screen hearing involved the presentation of relatively high-level acoustic signals and the observation, in one manner or another, of outward changes in an infant's behaviors. Typical behaviors that can be observed include alerting movements, cessation of sucking, changes in breathing, and so on.

In some areas, a behavioral screening approach is still used, usually in combination with risk-factor screening. Although successful in identifying some babies with significant sensorineural hearing loss, the approach has proven to be less than adequate when viewed on the basis of its test characteristics. From that perspective, too many infants with significant hearing loss pass the screening, and too many infants with normal hearing sensitivity fail the screening. Applied to a specific high-risk population and carried out with sufficient care, the approach might be useful. Applied generally to the newborn population, this approach does not meet screening standards.

Auditory Brain Stem Response Screening. For a number of years, measurement of the auditory brain stem response has been used successfully in the screening of newborns. Initial application of this technology was limited mainly to the neonatal intensive care unit, where risk factors were greatest. The cost of the procedure and the skill level of the audiologist needed to carry out such testing simply precluded its application to wider populations. Nevertheless, its accuracy in identifying children with significant sensorineural hearing loss made it an excellent tool for screening hearing.

Limitations to using the ABR for screening purposes are few. One is the cost of widespread application as described above. Another is the occasional problem of electrical interference with other equipment, which is especially challenging in an environment such as an intensive care unit. One other limitation is that, due to neuromaturational delays, especially in infants who are at risk, the auditory brain stem response may not be fully formed at birth, despite normal cochlear hearing function. Thus an infant might fail an ABR screening and still have normal hearing sensitivity. The other side of that coin is that the ABR is quite good at not missing children who have significant hearing loss.

Automated ABR strategies have now been implemented which address the issue of widespread application of the technology for infant screening. These automated approaches are designed to be easy to administer and result in a "Pass" or "No-Pass" decision. Automation allows the procedure to be administered by technical and support staff in a routine manner that can be applied to all newborns.

Otoacoustic Emissions Screening. In general, otoacoustic emissions are present in ears with normally functioning cochleas and absent in ears with more than mild sensorineural hearing losses. In many ways, OAE measurement appears to be an excellent strategy for infant hearing screening. First, with few exceptions, if otoacoustic emissions are normal, there is a very high likelihood that the infant's outer, middle, and inner ears are functioning appropriately. Thus, the technique is very useful in identifying infants who have normal hearing. Second, the response is absent when hearing disorders are present, making it useful in identifying those who need additional assessment.

Limitations to using OAEs for screening purposes are few, but important. One is that they are more easily recorded in quieter environments. This can be challenging in a noisy nursery. Another is that the technique is susceptible to obstruction in sound transmission of the outer and middle ears. Thus, an ear canal of a newborn that is not **patent** or contains fluid, as many do, will result in the absence of an OAE, even if cochlear function is normal. The result is similar for middle ear disorder. This susceptibility to these peripheral influences can make OAE screening challenging, resulting in too many normal children failing the screen.

When something is open or unobstructed it is **patent**.

Advances in noise-reduction and testing strategies have made infant OAE measurement a viable and useful screening technique. Children who pass the screen are quite likely to have normal auditory function. Those who fail can either be rescreened or referred for further audiologic assessment.

Combined Approaches. There are advantages and disadvantages to all of these screening techniques. Most of the disadvantages can be overcome by combining techniques in a systematic way (see the Clinical Note on pages 366–367). Many centers have combined the use of OAE screening and automated ABR screening in a manner that takes advantage of the strengths of both. For example, in some centers, well-babies are screened with OAEs and infants in the NICU are screened with ABR. Rescreening of infants who do not pass the original screen is completed with one or the other technology. In other centers, all infants are screened with one technique, and all those who do not pass are rescreened with the other. Such combined strategies help to reduce the problems of over-referral for additional testing.

Protocols for Infant Hearing Screening

The use of OAEs and automated ABR have had a major impact on our ability to screen the hearing of newborns. Each technique has its challenges, however, and that has led to different approaches being used among hospitals or even different approaches within a hospital in its different nurseries.

At least two major factors influence the approach that is used. The first is noise. In general, OAEs are more adversely affected by acoustic noise than ABRs. Because OAE responses are small amplitude acoustic events, they are difficult to record in a noisy room. In contrast, ABRs are more adversely affected by electrical noise than OAEs. Because ABR responses are small amplitude electrical events, they are difficult to record in a room with excessive electrical noise.

The second factor is noncochlear auditory system disorder. Remember, screening is aimed at identifying those with significant sensorineural hearing loss, not those with other types of auditory disorder. OAEs are adversely affected by the presence of outer or middle ear disorder, whereas ABRs are rather immune to these disorders unless they cause substantial conductive hearing loss. Conversely, ABRs are adversely affected by neuromaturational delays, whereas OAEs will be unaffected by any delays in brain stem maturation.

These tradeoffs have prompted audiologists to integrate both OAE and ABR testing into the screening process. One approach is shown in the top left figure. Here, OAEs are used as the first line of screening; those who do not pass are rescreened with OAEs; those who do not pass the rescreening are referred for testing by ABR. A second approach is shown in the top right figure. Here, newborns are screened initially with OAEs, and those who do not pass are rescreened with automated ABR; those who do not pass rescreening are referred for a complete audiological evaluation. A third approach is shown in the bottom figure. Here, newborns are screened initially with automated ABR; those who do not pass are rescreened with OAEs. In general, the third approach usually results in the fewest referrals for additional testing.

The approach to screening may change as a function of the type of nursery in which screening is done. In a quiet well-baby nursery, OAEs may work well as the initial screening technique. In a noisy NICU, automated ABR may be the initial measure of choice.

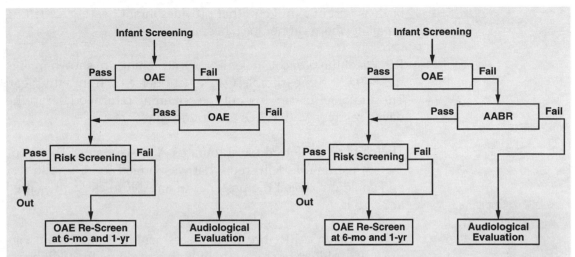

Infant hearing screening approach with OAE used for both the initial screening and rescreening.

Infant hearing screening approach with OAE used for the initial screening and AABR used for rescreening.

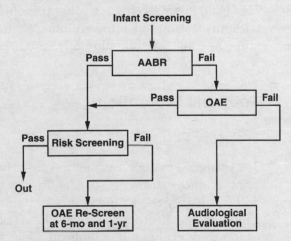

Infant hearing screening approach with AABR used for the initial screening and OAE used for rescreening.

Illustrative Case

Illustrative Case 8–9. Illustrative Case 9 is an infant born in a well-baby nursery. She was the product of a normal pregnancy and delivery. There is no reported family history of hearing loss, and the infant does not fall into any of the risk-factor categories for hearing loss. She was tested within the first 24 hours after birth as part of a program that provides infant hearing screening for all newborns at her local hospital.

Results of the otoacoustic emissions screening are shown in Figure 8–9A. No measurable OAEs were detected from either ear. The audiologists carrying out the screening returned later in the day to rescreen with OAEs and found similar results.

The child was referred for automated ABR screening. The automated instrument delivered what was judged to be a valid test and could not detect the presence of an ABR to clicks presented at 35 dB HL.

Results of an ABR threshold assessment are shown in Figure 8–9B. ABRs were recorded in both ears down to 60 dB by air conduction. No responses could be recorded by bone conduction at equipment limits of 40 dB. These results predict the presence of a moderate, primarily sensorineural hearing loss bilaterally.

This child is not likely to develop speech and language normally without hearing aid intervention. Ear impressions were made, and a hearing aid evaluation was scheduled.

Pediatric Evaluation

Evaluative Goals

The goals of a pediatric evaluation are to (a) identify the existence of an auditory disorder, (b) identify the nature of the disorder, and (c) identify the nature and extent of the hearing impairment caused by the disorder. Although these goals are not unlike those of the adult evaluation, infants and young children present special challenges in reaching them.

A child who has been referred for an audiologic consultation has usually been screened in one manner or another and determined to be at risk for hearing impairment. Infants are usually referred because they have failed a hearing screening or have some other known risk factor for hearing loss. Young children are usually referred either because their speech and language are not developing normally or because they have otologic disease and a physician is interested in understanding its effect on hearing. Older children are usually referred because of an otologic problem, because they have failed a school screening, or because they are suspected of having central auditory processing disorder.

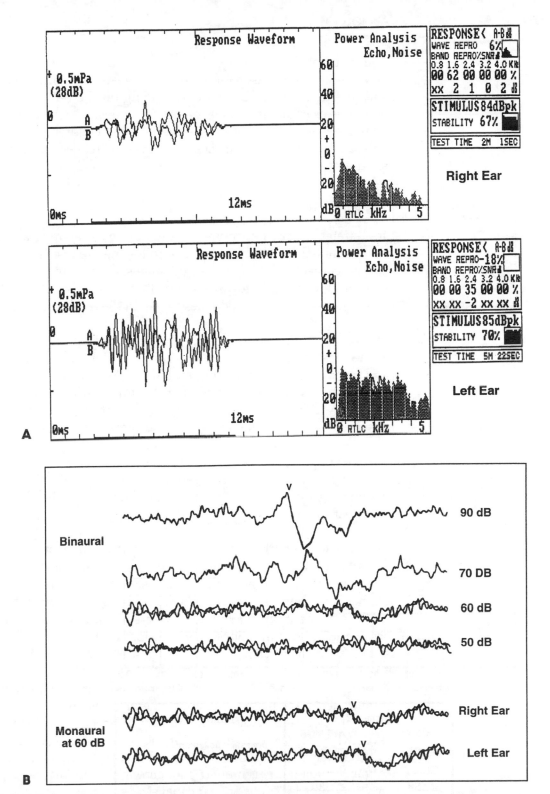

Figure 8-9. Results of otoacoustic emissions screening (A) in a newborn. No measurable OAEs were detected from either ear. Results of ABR threshold assessment (B) in the same newborn. ABRs were recorded in both ears down to 60 dB, consistent with a moderate sensorineural hearing loss.

369

The goals of the evaluation for each of these groups will vary depending on the reason for referral and the nature of the referral source. The approach can vary depending on the nature of the goal. For example, in young infants, the question is usually an audiologic one, not an otologic one. In young children, it can be either. In older children, it might not even be related to hearing sensitivity, but rather to suprathreshold auditory ability.

Test Strategies

Test strategies vary depending on the nature of the referral and the functional age of the child. The following are test strategies as a function of chronologic age guidelines. Because the relationship of chronologic age to functional age varies from child to child, there may be considerable overlap in these age categories.

In most clinical settings, despite whatever screening might have led to a referral, many if not most children who are evaluated end up having normal hearing sensitivity. As unusual as it may seem, much of a pediatric audiologist's time is spent evaluating children with normal hearing. As such, test strategies tend to be designed around quickly identifying normal-hearing children so that resources can be committed to evaluating children who truly have hearing impairment. So the process of pediatric assessment may begin with more of a screening approach, again aimed at eliminating from further testing those individuals who do not require it.

Infants 0 to 6 Months. Infants are usually referred for audiologic consultation because they failed a hearing screening or because they have been identified as being at risk for hearing loss. Many of these patients have normal hearing. Thus, the approach to their assessment is usually one of rescreening, followed by assessment and confirmation of hearing loss in those who fail the screening. A diagram of the approach is shown in Figure 8–10.

A productive approach to the initial rescreening is to combine immittance audiometry, otoacoustic emissions measurement, and behavioral observation audiometry in an effort to identify those with normal hearing. Otoacoustic emissions can be carried out routinely in this population to assess cochlear function. Immittance audiometry is more challenging in this population than in adults, mostly because of ear canal size.

Results of immittance testing appear to be more valid with use of a higher frequency probe tone than is customary in use for older

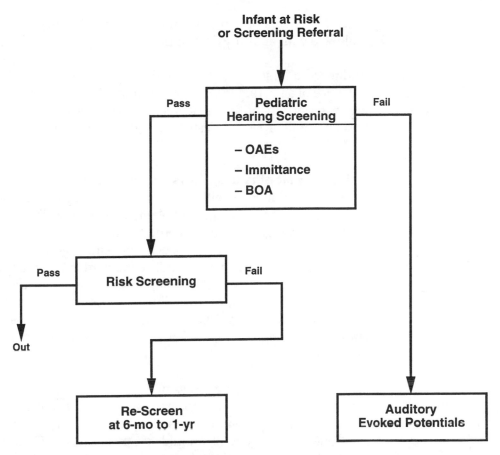

Figure 8-10. Hearing consultation model for infants age 0 to 6 months. The model begins with screening, followed by rescreening, and then by assessment of hearing sensitivity in those who do not pass the screening.

children and adults. Nevertheless, immittance testing can give a general impression of the integrity of middle ear function at this age.

Behavioral observation audiometry involves the controlled presentation of signals in a **sound field** and careful observation of the infant's response to those signals. Minimal response levels to signals across a frequency range can be determined with a fair degree of accuracy and reliability, even in young infants.

Sound field is an area or room into which sound is introduced via a loudspeaker.

The combination of OAEs, immittance audiometry, and behavioral audiometry should determine the need for additional audiologic testing. If an infant is found to have normal cochlear and middle ear function, the child passes the hearing screening, and no further testing is required. If the child does not pass the screening, then a hearing loss may exist, and the child should be evaluated with auditory evoked potentials.

Auditory brain stem response audiometry is used to verify the existence of a hearing loss, help determine the nature of the hearing loss, and quantify the degree of loss. Judicious use of ABR measures will provide an estimate of the type, degree, and slope of the hearing loss.

Children 6 Months to 2 Years. Young children are usually referred to an audiologist either as part of an otologic evaluation of middle ear disorder or for audiologic consultation because the parents or caregivers are concerned about hearing loss or the child has failed to develop speech and language as expected. Many of these patients have middle ear disorder, and many have normal hearing. Thus, the first step in their assessment is again almost a screening approach, followed by assessment and confirmation of middle ear disorder and hearing loss in those who fail the screening. A diagram of the approach is shown in Figure 8–11.

A useful way to begin the assessment is by measuring otoacoustic emissions. If emissions are normal, the middle ear mechanism is normal. If a sensorineural hearing loss exists, it is no more than a mild one and, in general, should not preclude speech and language development. If otoacoustic emissions are absent, the cause of that absence must be explored, because the culprit could be anything from mild middle ear disorder to profound sensorineural hearing loss.

Immittance audiometry is an important next step in the evaluation process. If otoacoustic emissions are normal, prediction of hearing loss by acoustic reflexes can be used as a cross-check for normal hearing sensitivity. If emissions are abnormal, immittance audiometry can shed light as to whether their absence is due to middle ear disorder. If immittance measures indicate middle ear disorder, the absence of otoacoustic emissions is equivocal in terms of predicting hearing loss.

In the absence of otoacoustic emissions information, immittance audiometry is a good beginning. Normal immittance measures suggest that any hearing problem that might be detected is due to sensorineural rather than conductive impairment. Normal immittance measures also allow assessment of acoustic reflex thresholds as a means of screening hearing sensitivity. If prediction of hearing level by acoustic reflexes suggests normal hearing

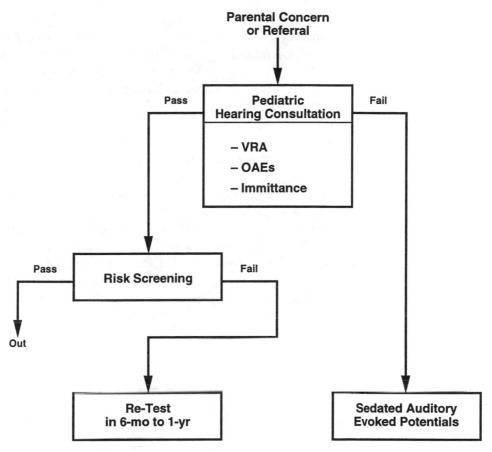

Figure 8–11. A pediatric hearing consultation model for assessing children age 6 months to 2 years. The model begins with screening, followed by assessment of middle ear function and hearing sensitivity in those who do not pass the screening.

sensitivity, the audiologist has a head start in knowing what might be expected from behavioral audiometry. Similarly, if the prediction is that a hearing loss might be present, the audiologist is so alerted. Abnormal immittance measures indicating middle ear disorder suggest that any hearing problem that might be detected has at least some conductive component. The conductive component may be the entire hearing loss or it may be superimposed on a sensorineural hearing loss. Immittance audiometry provides no insight into this issue. If immittance measures are abnormal, little or no information can be gleaned about hearing sensitivity

Depending on a child's functional level, behavioral thresholds can often be obtained by **visual reinforcement audiometry (VRA).** VRA is a technique in which the child's behavioral re-

Visual reinforcement audiometry (VRA) is an audiometric technique used in pediatric assessment in which an appropriate response to a signal presentation, such as a head turn toward the speaker, is rewarded by the activation of a light or lighted toy.

sponse to a sound, usually a head turn toward the sound source, is conditioned by reinforcement with some type of visual stimulus. Careful conditioning and a cooperative child may permit the establishment of threshold or near-threshold levels to speech and tonal signals. A typical approach is to obtain speech thresholds in a sound field, followed by thresholds to as many **warble-tone** stimuli as possible. If a young child will wear earphones, and many *will* tolerate insert earphones, ear-specific information can be obtained to assess hearing symmetry.

A **warble tone** is a frequency-modulated pure tone used in sound field testing.

As in any testing of children, the assessment becomes somewhat of a race against time, as attention is not a strong point at this age. Although the goal of behavioral audiometry is to obtain hearing threshold levels across the audiometric frequency range in both ears, this can be a fairly lofty goal for some children. The approach and the speed at which information can be gathered is the art of testing this age group. It is probably far better to understand hearing in the sound field, which in general reflects hearing in the better ear, and have an estimate of hearing symmetry than to have a complete audiogram in one ear only.

In many children of this age group, a definitive assessment can be made of hearing ability by the combined use of OAEs, immittance measures, and behavioral audiometry, especially if hearing is normal. However, in some cases, due to the need to confirm a hearing loss or because the child was not cooperative with such testing, auditory evoked potentials are used to predict hearing sensitivity. Specifically, the auditory brain stem response is measured to verify the existence of a hearing loss, help determine the nature of the hearing loss, and quantify the degree of loss. Judicious use of ABR measures will provide an estimate of the type, degree, and slope of hearing loss in both ears and may be the only reliable measure attainable in some children of this age group.

You will recall that ABR measures require that a patient be still or sleeping throughout the evaluation. Children in this younger age group, and, indeed, some children up to 4 or 5 years of age, can seldom be efficiently tested in natural sleep. Therefore, pediatric ABR assessment is often carried out while the child is under mild sedation. Sedation techniques vary, and all pose an additional challenge to evoked potential measurement. However, once the child is properly sedated, the ABR measures provide the best confirmation available of the results of behavioral audiometry.

Children Older than 2 Years. Not unlike their younger counterparts, children in this age group are usually referred to an audiologist either as part of an otologic evaluation of middle ear disorder or for audiologic consultation because the parents or caregivers are concerned about hearing loss or the child has failed to develop speech and language as expected. Many of these patients have middle ear disorder and many have some degree of hearing impairment.

Otoacoustic emissions can be used very effectively as an initial screening tool in this population. Normal emissions indicate a middle ear mechanism that is functioning properly and suggest that any sensorineural hearing impairment that might exist would be mild in nature. Absent otoacoustic emissions are consistent with either middle ear disorder or some degree of sensorineural hearing loss.

Immittance audiometry in this age group, as in all children, can provide a large amount of useful information. If tympanograms, static immittance, and acoustic reflexes are normal, middle ear disorder can be ruled out, and a prediction can be made about the presence or absence of sensorineural hearing loss. Combined with the results of OAE testing, the audiologist will begin to have an accurate picture of hearing ability, especially if all results are normal. If immittance audiometry is abnormal, the nature of the middle ear disorder will be apparent, but no predictions can be made about hearing sensitivity.

At this age, children can often be tested with **conditioned play audiometry**, in which the reinforcer is some type of play activity, such as tossing blocks in a box or putting pegs in a board. Usually under earphones, the typical first step is to establish speech recognition or speech awareness thresholds, depending on language skills, in both ears. Speech awareness thresholds can be obtained by conditioning the child to respond to the presence of the examiner's voice. Speech recognition thresholds are obtained in the youngest children by, for example, pointing to body parts; in young children, by pointing to pictures presented in a **closed-set** format; and in older children by having them repeat familiar **spondaic words**. The next step is to try to establish pure-tone thresholds at as many frequencies as possible. Behavioral bone conduction thresholds are also attainable in this age group. Again, a successful strategy is to begin with speech thresholds and move to pure-tone thresholds.

Conditioned play audiometry is an audiometric technique used in pediatric assessment in which a child is conditioned to respond to a stimulus by engaging in some game, such as dropping a block in a bucket, when a tone is heard.

Closed-set means the choice is from a limited set; multiple choice.

A **spondee** is a two-syllable word spoken with equal emphasis on each syllable.

If reliable behavioral thresholds can be obtained, especially in combination with immittance and OAE measures, results of the audiologic evaluation will provide the necessary information about type and degree of hearing loss. Unfortunately, even in children of this age group, and especially in the 2- to 3-year-old group, cooperation for audiometric testing is not always assured, and reliability of results may not be acceptable. In these cases, auditory evoked potentials can be used either to establish hearing levels or to confirm the results of behavioral testing. Again in children of this age, judicious use of ABR measures will provide an estimate of the type, degree, and slope of the hearing loss. Once again as well, sedation is likely to be needed in order to obtain useful evoked potential results.

The Cross-Check Principle. There is a principle in pediatric testing that is worth learning early and demanding of yourself throughout your professional career. The principle is the cross-check principle of pediatric audiometry. The cross-check principle simply states that *no single test result obtained during pediatric assessment should be considered valid until you have obtained an independent cross-check of its validity.* Stated another way, if you rely on one audiometric measure as *the* answer in your assessment of young children, you will probably misdiagnose children during your career. Conversely, if you insist on an independent cross-check of your results, the odds against such an occurrence improve dramatically.

Practically, we do not use the cross-check principle when we are screening hearing. Here we simply assume a certain percentage of risk of being wrong. Such is the nature of screening. However, if a child has been referred to you for an audiologic evaluation because of a suspected hearing loss, then you have a professional obligation to be correct in your assessment. That is not always easy, and it is certainly not always efficient, but if you do not get the answer right, then who does? Perhaps an example will serve to illustrate this point.

The patient was 18 months old and enrolled in a multidisciplinary treatment program for pervasive delays in development. The speech-language pathologist suspected a hearing loss because of the child's behavior. A very experienced audiologist evaluated the child. Immittance measures showed patent pressure-equalization tubes in both ears, placed recently due to chronic middle ear disorder. No other information could be obtained from immittance testing because of the tubes. Results of visual-reinforcement audiometry to warble tones presented in a sound field showed thresholds better than 20 dB HL across the frequency range. The audiologist concluded that hearing was normal in at least one ear and dismissed the speech-language pathologist's concern about hearing. Six months later, the speech-language pathologist asked the audiologist to evaluate again, certain that the audiologist was incorrect the first time. On re-evaluation, immittance testing showed normal tympanograms, normal static immittance, and no measurable acoustic reflexes. OAEs were absent. Behavioral measures continued to suggest no more than a mild hearing loss. ABR testing revealed a profound sensorineural hearing loss. Behavioral testing in this case was misleading, due probably to undetectable parental cueing of the child in the sound field.

This is just one of many examples of misdiagnosis that could have been prevented by insisting on a cross-check. In this case, results of behavioral audiometry were incorrect. There are also examples of cases in which ABR measures were absent due to brain stem disorder even though hearing sensitivity was normal or cases in which OAEs were normal but hearing was not. Although these cases are rare, and test results usually agree, they happen often enough that the best clinicians take heed. The solution is really rather simple. If you always demand from yourself a cross check, then you can be confident in your results.

Illustrative Case

Illustrative Case 8–10. Illustrative Case 10 is a young child with a fluctuating, mild-to-severe sensorineural hearing loss bilaterally. The patient is a 4 year-old girl. The hearing loss appears to be caused by CMV or cytomegalic inclusion disease, a viral infection usually transmitted in utero. There is no family history of hearing loss and no other significant medical history.

Immittance audiometry, as shown in Figure 8–12A, is consistent with normal middle ear function, characterized by a Type A tympanogram, normal static immittance, and normal crossed and uncrossed reflex thresholds bilaterally. SPAR predicts sensorineural hearing loss bilaterally.

Otoacoustic emissions are present in the right ear in the 1000 Hz frequency region, but absent at higher frequencies. OAEs are absent in the left ear, as shown in Figure 8–12B.

Air-conduction pure-tone thresholds were obtained via play audiometry and are shown in Figure 8–12C. The patient responded consistently by placing pegs in a pegboard.

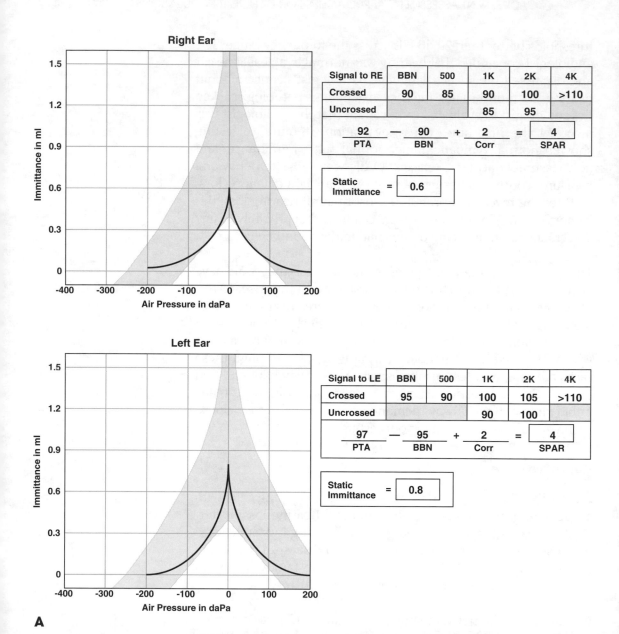

Right Ear

Signal to RE	BBN	500	1K	2K	4K
Crossed	90	85	90	100	>110
Uncrossed			85	95	

$$\underset{\text{PTA}}{92} - \underset{\text{BBN}}{90} + \underset{\text{Corr}}{2} = \underset{\text{SPAR}}{4}$$

Static Immittance = 0.6

Left Ear

Signal to LE	BBN	500	1K	2K	4K
Crossed	95	90	100	105	>110
Uncrossed			90	100	

$$\underset{\text{PTA}}{97} - \underset{\text{BBN}}{95} + \underset{\text{Corr}}{2} = \underset{\text{SPAR}}{4}$$

Static Immittance = 0.8

A

Figure 8-12. Hearing consultation results in a 4-year-old child with hearing loss secondary to CMV infection. Immittance measures (A) are consistent with normal middle ear function. SPARs predict sensorineural hearing loss bilaterally. Distortion-product otoacoustic emissions results (B) show that OAEs are present in the lower frequencies on the right ear, but absent at higher frequencies. OAEs are absent on the left. Pure-tone audiometric results (C) show bilateral sensorineural hearing loss.

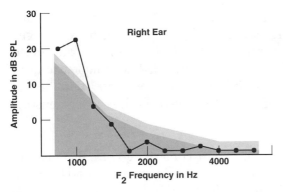

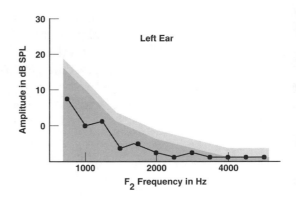

B

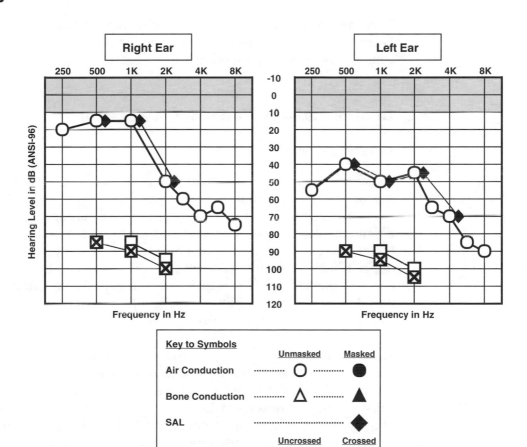

C

Key to Symbols

	Unmasked	Masked
Air Conduction	○	●
Bone Conduction	△	▲
SAL		◆
	Uncrossed	Crossed
Acoustic Reflex	□	⊠

Bone-conduction thresholds could not be obtained conventionally because the child had difficulty responding to tones presented to the bone vibrator in the presence of masking noise presented to an earphone. However, the SAL technique was used to estimate the amount of air-bone gap. Bone conduction thresholds estimated by the SAL test showed the loss to be sensorineural in nature.

Speech audiometric results were consistent with the hearing loss. Speech thresholds matched pure-tone thresholds. Word-recognition scores were good, despite the degree of hearing loss.

This child is a candidate for hearing aid amplification and will likely benefit substantially from hearing aid use. A hearing aid consultation was recommended.

Central Auditory Processing Assessment

Evaluative Goals

Diagnosis of CAPD is challenging because there is no biologic marker. That is, it cannot be identified "objectively" with MRI scans or blood tests. Instead, its diagnosis relies on operational definitions, based mostly on results of speech audiometry. Basing the diagnosis solely on behavioral measures such as these can be difficult because interpretation of the test results can be influenced by nonauditory factors such as language delays, attentional deficits, and impaired cognitive functioning. Thus, one important evaluative goal is to separate CAPD from these other disorders.

The importance of this evaluative goal cannot be overstated. One of the main problems with CAPD measures is that too many children who do not have CAPD fail some of the tests. This results in a large number of false-positive test results, which not only burdens the health-care system with children who do not need further testing, but also muddles the issue of CAPD and its contribution to a child's problems. The reason that so many children who do not have CAPD fail these tests is that nonauditory factors influence the interpretation of results.

This problem has been illustrated clearly in a number of studies. For example, in one study children who were considered to be hyperactive and have attention deficit disorders were evaluated with several speech audiometric tests of auditory processing ability and a battery of tests aimed at measuring attention ability.

Both the CAPD test battery and the attention test battery were administered before and after the children were medicated with stimulants to control hyperactivity. Results showed that most of the children improved on the CAPD test battery following stimulant administration. What these results showed is that the CAPD tests are very sensitive to the effects of attention. Stated another way, children who have attention disorders often perform poorly on these CAPD measures even if they do not have CAPD, because they cannot attend to the task thoroughly enough for the auditory system to be evaluated. As a result, the effects of auditory processing disorder cannot be separated from the effects that attention deficits have on a child's ability to complete these particular test measures.

What this study and others suggest is that, if our clinical goal is to test exclusively for CAPD, then the influences of attention, cognition, and language skills must be controlled during the evaluation process.

Test Strategies

Well-controlled speech audiometric measures, in conjunction with auditory evoked potential measures, can be powerful diagnostic tools for assessing CAPD. Although there is no single gold standard against which to judge the effectiveness of CAPD testing, it can be operationally defined on the basis of behavioral and electrophysiologic test results.

Speech Audiometry. There are several speech audiometric measures of central auditory processing disorders. Most of them evolved from adult measures that were designed to aid in the diagnosis of neurological disease in the pre-MRI era. The application of many of these adult measures to the pediatric population has not been altogether successful, largely because of a lack of control over linguistic and cognitive complexity in applying them to young children.

Speech audiometric approaches have been developed that have proven to be valid and reliable. When they are administered under properly controlled acoustic conditions, with materials of appropriate language age and testing strategies that control for the influences of attention and cognition, these measures permit a diagnosis with reasonable accuracy in most children.

Perhaps an example of a successful testing strategy will illustrate the challenges and some of the ways to solve them. One example

Table 8–1. An example of a CAPD test battery.

Test Parameter	Younger Children	Older Children
Monaural word recognition	PSI-ICM words	PB word lists
Monaural sentence recognition	PSI-ICM sentences	SSI
Dichotic speech recognition	PSI-CCM	DSI
Auditory evoked potentials	MLR/LLR	MLR/LLR

Note: PSI-ICM: Pediatric Speech Intelligibility test with ipsilateral competing message; PSI-CCM: Pediatric Speech Intelligibility test with contralateral competing message; PB: phonetically-balanced; SSI: Synthetic Sentence Identification test; DSI: Dichotic Sentence Identification test; MLR: middle latency response; LLR: late latency response

The difference in dB between a sound of interest and background noise is called the **signal-to-noise ratio** (S/N).

Redundancy is the abundance of information available to the listener due to the substantial informational content of a speech signal and the capacity of the central auditory nervous system.

Dichotic refers to different signals presented simultaneously to each ear; **monotic** refers to different signals presented to the same ear.

of a CAPD test battery is summarized in Table 8–1. The strategy used with this test battery is to vary several parameters of the speech testing across a continuum in order to "sensitize" the speech materials or to make them more difficult. The parameters include intensity, **signal-to-noise ratio, redundancy** of informational content, and **monotic** versus **dichotic** performance.

Suppose we are testing a young child. We might choose to use the *Pediatric Speech Intelligibility* (PSI) test. In this test, words are presented with a competing message in the same ear at various signal-to-noise ratios (S/Ns) or message-to-competition ratios (MCRs). Testing at a better ratio provides an easier listening condition to ensure that the child knows the vocabulary, is cognitively capable of performing the task, and can attend adequately enough to complete the procedure. Then the ratio is made more difficult to challenge the integrity of the auditory nervous system. At the more difficult MCR, a performance-intensity (PI) function is obtained to evaluate for "rollover" of the function, or poorer performance at higher intensity levels. This assessment in the intensity domain is also designed to assess auditory nervous system integrity.

Both words and sentences are usually presented with competition in the same ear and the opposite ear. The word-versus-sentence comparison is used to assess the child's ability to process speech signals of different redundancies. The same-ear versus opposite-ear competition comparison is used to assess the difference between monotic and dichotic auditory processing ability.

An illustration of the results of these test procedures and how they serve to control the nonauditory influences is shown in the

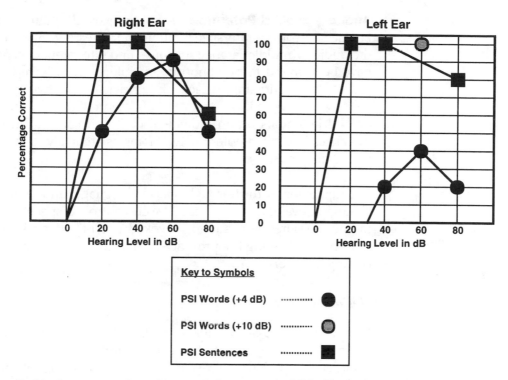

Figure 8–13. Speech audiometric results in a young child with central auditory processing disorder. Results of the Pediatric Speech Intelligibility (PSI) test illustrate how assessment procedures can be used to control for nonauditory influences on test interpretation.

speech audiometric results in Figure 8–13. The patient is a 4-year 1-month-old child who was diagnosed with CAPD. Hearing sensitivity is within normal limits in both ears. However, speech audiometric results are strikingly abnormal. In the right ear, the PI functions for both words and sentences show rollover. Rollover of these functions cannot be explained as attention, linguistic, or cognitive disorders because such disorders are not intensity-level dependent. In other words, language, cognition, or attention deficits are not present at one intensity level and absent at another. In addition, in the left ear, there is a substantial discrepancy between understanding of sentences and understanding of words. This is obviously not a language problem, because, at 60 dB HL, the child understands all of the sentences correctly and, at an easier listening condition, the child identifies all of the words correctly. The child is clearly capable of doing the task linguistically and cognitively. Thus, use of PI functions, various S/Ns, and word-versus-sentence comparisons permits the assessment of auditory processing ability in a manner that reduces the likelihood of nonauditory factors influencing the interpretation of test results.

Auditory Evoked Potentials. Auditory evoked potentials may be used to corroborate speech audiometric testing. Specifically, the auditory middle latency response and late latency response have been found to be abnormal in children who have CAPD. Although encouraging, a lack of sufficient normative data on young children reduces the ease of interpretation of auditory evoked potentials on an individual basis at this point in time. Advances in evoked potential technologies are likely to enhance CAPD diagnosis.

In conjunction with thorough speech, language, and neuropsychological evaluations, the use of well-controlled speech audiometric measures and auditory evoked potentials can be quite powerful in defining the presence or absence of an auditory processing disorder.

Illustrative Case

Illustrative Case 8–11. Illustrative Case 11 is a young child with normal hearing sensitivity but with central auditory processing disorder. The patient is a 6-year-old girl with a history of chronic otitis media. Although her parents have always suspected that she had a hearing problem, previous screening results were consistent with normal hearing sensitivity. Previous tympanometric screening results showed either Type B tympanograms during periods of otitis media or normal tympanograms during times of remission from otitis media.

Immittance audiometry, as shown in Figure 8–14A is consistent with normal middle ear function, characterized by a Type A tympanogram, normal static immittance, and normal crossed and uncrossed reflex thresholds bilaterally.

Pure-tone audiometric results are shown in Figure 8–14B. Hearing sensitivity is normal in both ears.

Speech audiometry reveals a different picture. Results are shown in Figure 8–14C. For both ears, the pattern is one of rollover of the performance-intensity functions for both word recognition and sentence recognition in the presence of competition. In addition, she shows a dichotic deficit, with poor performance in her left ear. These results are consistent with central auditory processing disorders.

Auditory evoked potentials provide additional support for the diagnosis. Although ABRs are present and normal bilaterally,

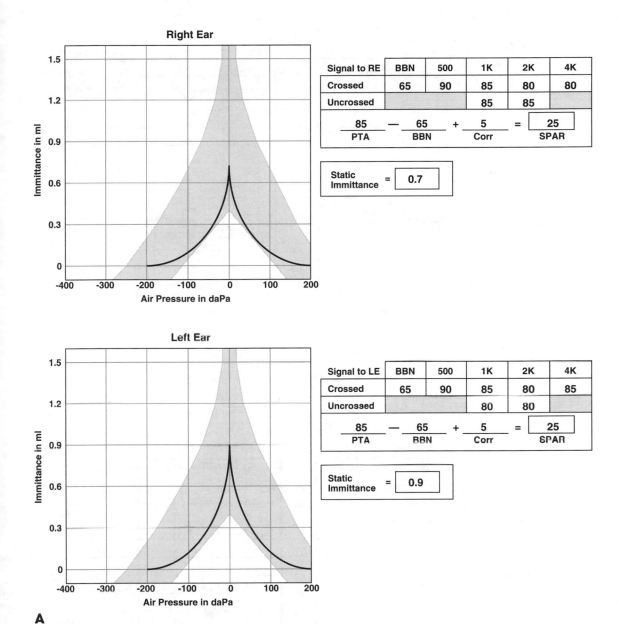

Right Ear

Signal to RE	BBN	500	1K	2K	4K
Crossed	65	90	85	80	80
Uncrossed			85	85	

$$\frac{85}{\text{PTA}} - \frac{65}{\text{BBN}} + \frac{5}{\text{Corr}} = \boxed{\frac{25}{\text{SPAR}}}$$

Static Immittance = 0.7

Left Ear

Signal to LE	BBN	500	1K	2K	4K
Crossed	65	90	85	80	85
Uncrossed			80	80	

$$\frac{85}{\text{PTA}} - \frac{65}{\text{BBN}} + \frac{5}{\text{Corr}} = \boxed{\frac{25}{\text{SPAR}}}$$

Static Immittance = 0.9

A

Figure 8-14. Hearing consultation results in a 6-year-old girl with central auditory processing disorder. Immittance measures (A) are consistent with normal middle ear function. Pure-tone audiometric results (B) show normal hearing sensitivity in both ears. Speech audiometric results (C) show significant rollover of PI functions for both word and sentence recognition. Results also show a dichotic deficit, with poorer performance on the left ear.

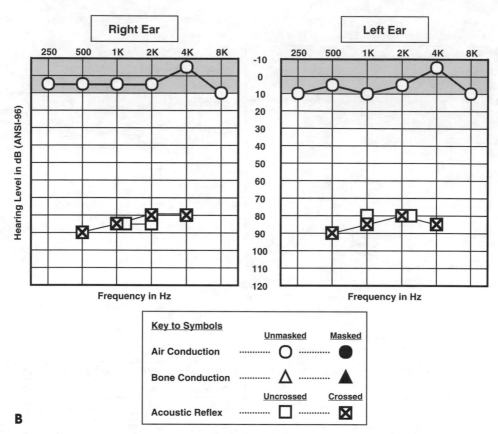

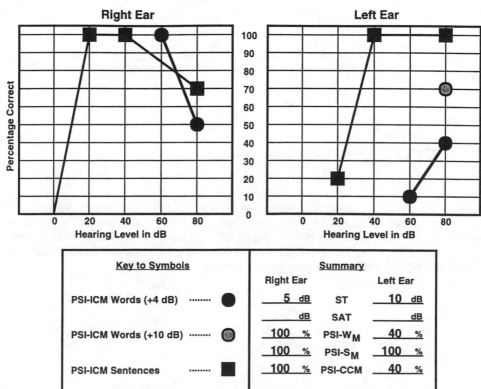

middle- and late-latency responses are not measurable in response to signals presented to either ear.

This child is likely to experience difficulty in noisy and distracting environments. She may be at risk for academic achievement problems if her learning environment is not structured to be a quiet one. The parents were provided with information about the nature of the disorder and the strategies that can be used to alter listening environments in ways that will be useful to this child. The patient will be re-evaluated periodically, especially during the early academic years.

FUNCTIONAL HEARING LOSS

Exaggerated, functional, or nonorganic hearing loss is a timeless audiologic challenge. Functional hearing loss is the exaggeration or feigning of hearing impairment. In many cases, particularly in adults, an organic hearing loss exists but is willfully exaggerated, usually for compensatory purposes. In other cases, often secondary to trauma of some kind, the entire hearing loss will be willfully feigned.

Adults and children feign hearing loss for different reasons. Adults are usually seeking secondary or financial gain. For example, an employee may be applying for worker's compensation for hearing loss secondary to exposure to excessive sound in the workplace. Or someone discharged from the military may be seeking compensation for hearing loss from excessive noise exposure. Although most patients have legitimate concerns and provide honest results, a small percentage tries to exaggerate hearing loss in the mistaken notion that they will receive greater compensation. There are also those who have been involved in an accident or altercation and are involved in a lawsuit against an insurance company or someone else. Occasionally such a person will think that feigning a hearing loss will lead to greater monetary award. In either case of functional hearing loss, the patient is wasting valuable professional resources in an attempt to reap financial gain. Although these cases are always interesting and challenging to the audiologist, the clinical approach changes from one of caregiving to something a little more direct.

Children with functional hearing loss often are using hearing impairment as an excuse for poor performance in school or to gain attention. The idea may have emerged from watching a classmate or sibling getting special treatment for having a hearing impairment or it may be secondary to a bout of otitis media and the consequent parental attention paid to the episode. The challenge is to identify this functional loss before the child begins to realize the secondary gains inherent in having hearing loss. This is challenging business. Children feigning hearing loss need support. Their parents, on the other hand, may not be overly pleased to learn that they have taken time off of work and spent money to discover that their child was faking a hearing loss. Counseling is an important aspect following the discovery of functional hearing loss in a child.

Regardless of the reason for functional hearing loss, the role of the audiologist is (a) to detect that a functional component exists and (b) to resolve the true hearing sensitivity.

Indicators of Functional Hearing Loss

The evaluation of functional hearing loss begins with identification of the existence of the disorder. There are several indicators of the existence of a functional component, some of which are audiometric and some of which are nonaudiometric.

Nonaudiometric Indicators

Careful observation of a patient from the very beginning of the evaluation can often provide indications of the likelihood of a functional component to a hearing loss. For example, as a general rule, patients with functional hearing loss are late for appointments. Perhaps the thought is that the later they are, the more rushed will be the evaluation, and the greater the likelihood that their malingering will not be detected. For whatever reasons, many patients with functional hearing loss will be late. It seems important to point out that the argument is not transitive. That is, clearly, not everyone who is late has a functional hearing loss. Nevertheless, those who have functional hearing loss are often late.

Other signs of functional hearing loss can also be detected early. Patients with functional hearing loss will often exhibit behaviors that are exaggerated compared to what might be expected from someone with an organic loss. For example, patients with true hearing impairment are usually alert in the waiting room because of concern that they will not hear their appointment being called. Those with functional hearing loss may overexaggerate to the point that they will appear to struggle when they are being identified in the waiting room. This exaggeration may continue throughout the process of greeting the patient and taking a case history. Experienced audiologists understand how individuals with true hearing impairment function in the world. For example, they seldom bring attention to themselves by purposefully raising their voices or by cupping their hands behind their ears. Those feigning hearing loss are likely to not handle this type of communication very subtly. As another example, the case history process is full of context that allows patients with true hearing impairment to answer questions reasonably routinely and graciously. Patients with functional hearing loss will often struggle inappropriately with this task.

Other behaviors that are often attributable to patients with functional hearing loss are excessive impatience, tension, and irritability.

One other nonaudiometric indicator that is not subtle but suprisingly often overlooked is the reason for the referral and evaluation. Is the patient having a hearing evaluation for compensation purposes? This is a question that should be asked. Again, many who are will have legitimate hearing loss and will be forthcoming during the audiologic evaluation. But if compensation or litigation is involved, the audiologist must be alert to the possibility of functional hearing loss.

Audiometric Indicators

There are also several audiometric indicators of the presence of functional hearing loss. First, and perhaps most obvious, the amateur malingerer will display substantial variability in response to pure-tone audiometry. However, the more malingerers are tested, the more consistent their responses become. An experienced malingerer will not demonstrate variability in responding.

One important audiometric indicator is a disparity between the **speech recognition threshold** and pure-tone thresholds. In patients who are feigning or exaggerating hearing loss, the speech recognition threshold is usually significantly better than pure-tone thresholds. Thus, it is important to begin testing with the SRT and then evaluate whether the pure-tone thresholds match up appropriately.

The threshold level for speech recognition, expressed as the lowest intensity level at which 50% of spondaic words can be identified is called the **speech recognition or speech reception threshold.**

These and other indicators alert the experienced audiologist to the possibility of functional hearing loss:

- variability in response to pure-tone audiometry
- lack of correspondence of SRT to pure-tone thresholds
- bone conduction poorer than air conduction
- very flat audiogram
- lack of a **shadow curve** in unilateral functional loss
- air-conduction pure-tone thresholds poorer than acoustic reflex thresholds
- half-word spondee responses during speech recognition threshold testing
- rhyming word responses on word recognition testing
- unusual pattern of word recognition scores on performance-intensity functions
- normal sensitivity prediction by acoustic reflexes in the presence of an apparent hearing sensitivity loss
- normal otoacoustic emissions measures in the presence of an apparent hearing sensitivity loss

A **shadow curve** appears on an audiogram during unmasked testing of an organic, unilateral hearing loss; thresholds for the test ear occur at levels equal to the interaural attenuation.

Assessment of Functional Hearing Loss

If functional hearing loss is suspected but not confirmed, audiometric measures should be carried out to confirm the existence of a functional component. Once functional hearing loss is confirmed, several strategies can be used to determine the true nature of hearing sensitivity.

Strategies to Detect Exaggeration

Sometimes a patient will feign complete deafness in one or both ears and behavioral audiometric measures will not be available to judge the validity of responding. The most useful tools to detect functional hearing losses in these cases are the sensitivity prediction by acoustic reflexes and the use of otoacoustic emissions. If the results of these measures are normal, then functional loss has been detected and the search for true thresholds can begin. It is just that simple in patients who are truly malingering. The problem is that most feigned hearing loss is actually a functional overlay on an existing hearing loss. In such cases, both reflex predictions and OAEs will indicate the presence of hearing loss, and the functional component will not be detectable.

In cases where a patient is feigning complete bilateral loss, simple clinical strategies can be used to determine that the loss is functional. One is to attempt to elicit a startle response by presenting an unexpected, high-intensity signal into the audiometric sound field. Another is to present some form of an unexpected comment through the earphones and watch for the patient's reaction. There are also some older formalized tests that were championed in the days before electrophysiologic measures. For example, one test, the *Lombard voice intensity test,* made use of the fact that a person's voice increases in intensity when masking noise is presented to both ears. In this case, the patient was asked to read a passage. Vocal level was monitored while white noise was introduced into the earphones. Any change in vocal level would indicate that the patient was perceiving the white noise and feigning the hearing loss. Another example is the *delayed auditory feedback test.* This test made use of the fact that patients' speech becomes dysfluent if the perception of their own voice is delayed by a certain amount. That is, patients were asked to read a passage. A microphone recorded the speech and delivered it back into the patients' ears with a carefully controlled time delay. Any change in fluency would indicate that the patients were hearing their own voices and feigning a hearing loss.

In cases where the patient is feigning a complete unilateral hearing loss, the best strategy to detect the malingering is the *Stenger test.* A detailed description of procedures for carrying out the Stenger test is presented in the following Clinical Note. Briefly, the test is based on the Stenger principle, which states that only the louder of similar sounds presented simultaneously to both ears will be perceived. For example, if you have normal hearing, and I simultaneously present a 1000-Hz tone to your right ear at 30 dB HL and to your left ear at 40 dB HL, you will only perceive the sound in your left ear. In the Stenger test, a tone is presented to the good ear at a level at which the patient responds. The signal in the poorer ear is raised until the patient stops responding. Patients who are feigning a hearing loss will stop responding as soon as they perceive sound in the suspect ear, unaware that sound is also being presented to the good ear at a perceptible level. The Stenger test is so simple, valid, and reliable that many audiologists use it routinely in any case of unilateral hearing loss just to be sure of its authenticity.

Strategies to Determine "True" Thresholds

Once a functional hearing loss has been detected, the challenge becomes one of determining actual hearing sensitivity levels. Sometimes this is very simply a matter of reinstructing the patient. Thus, the first step is to make patients aware that you have detected their exaggeration, provide them with a reasonable "face-saving" explanation for why they may have been having difficulty with the pure-tone task, reinstruct them, and re-

The Stenger Test: A Good Clinical Friend

A good clinical rule to live by: If a patient has a unilateral hearing loss or significant asymmetry, always do a Stenger test.

The Stenger test is a simple and fast technique for verifying the organicity of a hearing loss. If the hearing loss is organic, you will have wasted a minute of your life verifying that fact. If the hearing loss is feigned or exaggerated, you will have rapid verification of the presence of a functional component.

The Stenger test is easy to do. A form is provided on the next page to make it even easier.

Either speech or pure-tone stimuli are presented simultaneously to both ears. Initially, the signal is presented to the good ear at a comfortable, audible level of about 20 dB SL and to the poorer ear at 20 dB below the level of the good ear. The patient will respond, because the patient will hear the signal presented to the good ear. Testing proceeds by increasing the intensity level of the signal presented to the poorer ear. If the loss in the poorer ear is organic, the patient will continue to respond to the signal being presented to the good ear. This is a negative Stenger. If the loss is functional, the patient will stop responding when the loudness of the signal in the poorer ear exceeds that in the good ear, because the signal will only be heard in the poorer ear due to the Stenger principle. Because you are still presenting an audible signal to the good ear, you know that the patient is not cooperating. This is a positive Stenger, indicative of functional hearing loss.

Stenger Test
Recording Form

Name:_____ Age:_____ Date:_____

Pure-Tone

Voluntary Thresholds

Right Ear: _____ Frequency:_____

Left Ear: _____

Presentation Level		Response
Better Ear	Test Ear	+ correct − no response
_____	_____	_____
_____	_____	_____
_____	_____	_____
_____	_____	_____
_____	_____	_____
_____	_____	_____
_____	_____	_____
_____	_____	_____
_____	_____	_____
_____	_____	_____
_____	_____	_____
_____	_____	_____

Stenger is: positive
             negative

Speech

Voluntary Thresholds

Right Ear: _____

Left Ear: _____

Presentation Level		Response
Better Ear	Test Ear	+ correct − no response
_____	_____	_____
_____	_____	_____
_____	_____	_____
_____	_____	_____
_____	_____	_____
_____	_____	_____
_____	_____	_____
_____	_____	_____
_____	_____	_____
_____	_____	_____
_____	_____	_____
_____	_____	_____

Stenger is: positive
             negative

Clinical form for recording results of the Stenger test.

establish pure-tone thresholds. Some patients will immediately recant and begin cooperating. Others will not.

For those who continue to exaggerate their hearing levels, there are several behavioral strategies that can be used. Children are the easiest under these circumstances, and some of the approaches to children work remarkably well with some adults. One particularly useful strategy in children is the *yes-no* test. For this test, children are instructed to indicate that they hear a tone by saying "yes" and that they do not hear the tone by saying "no." In most cases, you will be able to track the "no" responses all the way down to the real threshold level. Another useful technique is to have the child "count the beeps" while presenting groups of two or more tones at each intensity level. As threshold approaches, the child will begin counting incorrectly, but will continue to respond.

In adults, one of the more productive approaches is to use a variable *ascending-descending strategy* to try to bracket the threshold. Many audiologists will adhere strictly to an ascending approach so that the patient does not have too many opportunities to judge suprathreshold loudness levels. If a patient is feigning a unilateral hearing loss, the Stenger test can be used to predict threshold levels generally, as described in the Clinical Note on page 392.

In patients who simply will not cooperate, accurate pure-tone threshold levels might not be attainable despite considerable toil on the part of the audiologist. Many audiologists feel that their time is not being well spent by trying to establish a behavioral audiogram in patients who will not cooperate. Those audiologists are likely to stop testing fairly early in the evaluation process and move immediately to assessment by auditory evoked potentials. The strategy is a good one in terms of resource utilization because, most likely, the patient will be undergoing evoked potential testing anyway. The art of audiometric testing in this case is to know quickly when you have reached a point at which additional testing will not yield additional results.

If valid and reliable behavioral thresholds cannot be obtained, current standard of care is to use auditory evoked potentials to predict the audiogram. Three approaches are commonly used. One approach is to establish ABR thresholds to clicks as a means of predicting high-frequency hearing and 500-Hz tone bursts as a means of predicting low-frequency hearing. The advantages to this approach are that testing can be completed quickly and the patient can be sleeping during the procedure. The disadvantages are that the audiogram is predicted in broad frequency categories, and low-frequency tone-burst ABRs can be difficult to record.

Another approach is to establish late latency response (LLR) thresholds to pure tones across the audiometric frequency range. The advantage of this approach is that an electrophysiologic audiogram can be established with frequency-specific stimuli. The disadvantage is that the procedure is rather time consuming.

A third approach is to combine ABR and LLR testing. ABR threshold to clicks provides an estimate of high-frequency sensitivity, and LLR threshold to 500-Hz pure tones provides a prediction of low-frequency sensitivity.

Regardless of the test strategy, auditory evoked potentials are now commonly used as the method of choice for verifying and documenting hearing thresholds in cases of functional hearing loss.

Illustrative Case

Illustrative Case 8–12. Illustrative Case 12 is a patient who complains of a hearing loss in his right ear following an automobile accident. The patient is a 30-year-old man with an otherwise unremarkable health and hearing history. Two months prior to the evaluation, he was involved in an automobile accident. He reports that he sustained injuries to his neck and head and that a blow to the right side resulted in a significant loss of hearing in that ear.

Immittance audiometry, as shown in Figure 8–15A is consistent with normal middle ear function bilaterally, as characterized by a Type A tympanogram, normal static immittance, and normal crossed and uncrossed reflex thresholds. SPAR results predict normal hearing sensitivity bilaterally.

Pure-tone audiometry shows normal hearing sensitivity in the left ear. Results from the right ear show responses that were generally inconsistent in the 80 to 100 dB range. Air conduction thresholds are above or close to acoustic reflex thresholds. Admitted thresholds are shown in Figure 8–15B. Bone-conduction thresholds are also inconsistent and suggest the presence of an air-bone gap in the poorer ear and a bone-air gap in the normal ear.

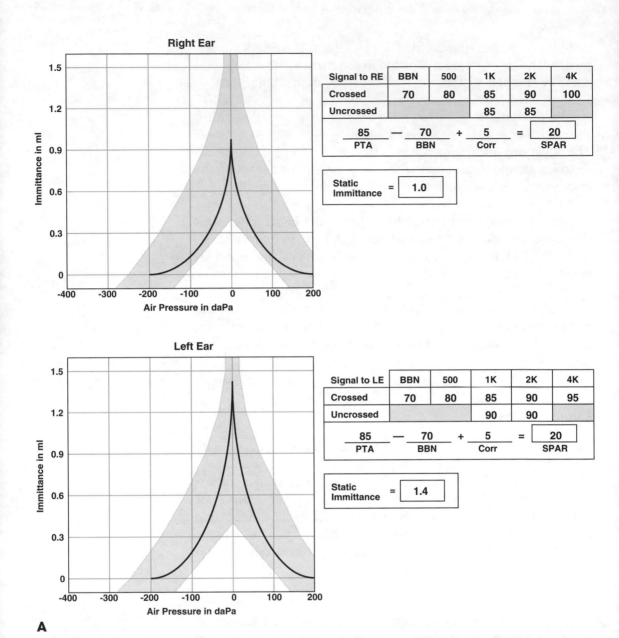

Right Ear

Signal to RE	BBN	500	1K	2K	4K
Crossed	70	80	85	90	100
Uncrossed			85	85	

$$\underset{\text{PTA}}{85} - \underset{\text{BBN}}{70} + \underset{\text{Corr}}{5} = \underset{\text{SPAR}}{20}$$

Static Immittance = 1.0

Left Ear

Signal to LE	BBN	500	1K	2K	4K
Crossed	70	80	85	90	95
Uncrossed			90	90	

$$\underset{\text{PTA}}{85} - \underset{\text{BBN}}{70} + \underset{\text{Corr}}{5} = \underset{\text{SPAR}}{20}$$

Static Immittance = 1.4

A

Figure 8–15. Hearing consultation results in a 30-year-old man with functional hearing loss. Immittance measures (A) are consistent with normal middle ear function. SPARs predict normal hearing sensitivity bilaterally. Pure-tone audiometric measures (B) yielded responses that were inconsistent and considered to be at suprathreshold levels. Distortion-product otoacoustic emissions (C) are present bilaterally.

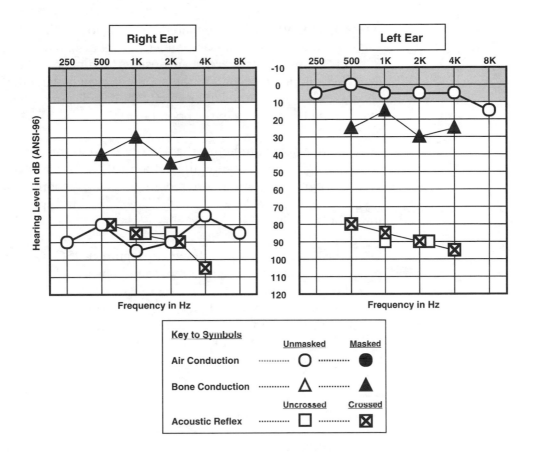

Key to Symbols

	Unmasked	Masked
Air Conduction	⚪	⚫
Bone Conduction	△	▲

	Uncrossed	Crossed
Acoustic Reflex	▢	⊠

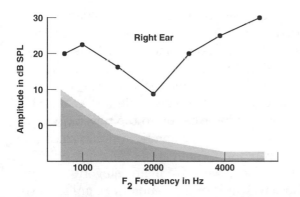

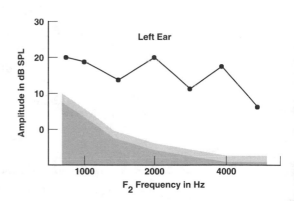

C

As is customary in cases of unilateral hearing loss, a Stenger test was carried out to verify the authenticity of behavioral thresholds. Results of a speech Stenger test are positive for functional hearing loss. Presentation of signals to the poorer ear resulted in interference with hearing in the better ear at 20 dB, indicating no more than a mild hearing loss in the poorer ear.

Speech thresholds are better than the pure-tone thresholds by 20 dB, bringing into question the authenticity of either measure. Word-recognition testing resulted in unusual responses with rhyming words at levels at or below admitted pure-tone thresholds.

Otoacoustic emissions are shown in Figure 8–15C. OAEs are present bilaterally, indicating at most a mild hearing loss.

The patient was confronted with the inconsistencies of the test results, but no reliable behavioral thresholds could be obtained. He was scheduled for evoked potential audiometry but did not return for the evaluation.

SUMMARY

- Although the overall goal of an audiological evaluation is to characterize hearing ability, the approach used to reach that goal can vary considerably across patients.
- The approach chosen to evaluate a patient's hearing is sometimes related to patient factors such as age and sometimes related to the reason that the patient has sought services or been referred for services.
- Audiologic assessment of otologic referrals is aimed at providing additional information to the physician to aid in diagnosis or to provide a metric for the success or failure of medical or surgical treatment.
- Audiologists are faced with two main categories of adult patients, those who are younger and have significant vocational communication demands and those who are older and have more complex auditory problems.
- The audiologist is faced with three main challenges in the assessment of infants and children.
- The first challenge in pediatric assessment is to identify children who are at risk for hearing loss and need further evaluation.
- The second challenge in pediatric assessment is to determine if the children identified as being at risk for auditory

disorder actually have a hearing loss and, if so, to determine the nature and degree of the loss.

■ The third challenge in pediatric assessment is to evaluate the hearing ability of preschool and early school-age children suspected of having central auditory processing disorders.

■ Regardless of the reason for functional hearing loss, the role of the audiologist is to detect that a functional component exists and to resolve the true hearing sensitivity.

SUGGESTED READINGS

Hayes, D., & Northern, J. L. (1996). *Infants and hearing.* San Diego: Singular Publishing Group.

Jacobson, J. T., & Northern, J. L. (Eds.). (1991). *Diagnostic audiology.* Austin, TX: Pro-Ed.

Musiek, F. E., Baran, J. A., & Pinheiro, M. L. (1994). *Neuroaudiology case studies.* San Diego: Singular Publishing Group.

Northern, J. L., & Downs, M. P. (1991). *Hearing in children* (4th ed.). Baltimore: Williams and Wilkins.

Reporting and Referring

Once an audiologic evaluation is completed, the results need to be reported to the referral source, patients, and others. In addition, referrals may need to be made based on testing outcomes. This section covers some of the strategies and challenges in the reporting and referring process.

REPORTING

One important aspect in the provision of health care is the reporting of results of an evaluation or treatment outcome. The challenge of reporting is to describe what was found or what was done in a clear, concise, and consistent manner. The actual nature of a report can vary greatly depending on the setting and the referral source to whom a report is most likely written.

Confusion about the most appropriate approach to reporting can result because of two common misconceptions about the process of reporting. One misconception is that every aspect of the evaluation or treatment needs to be reported in some manner. In audiology, this can lead to the creation of some very busy forms, packed with all manner of information, that are then passed on to the referral in the hope that the information they are seeking will be included somewhere. Another misconception is that a report needs to be generated that describes the nature of the case and the nature of testing in elaborate detail. An analogy here is the scientific journal article that is all introduction and procedure, with very few results and conclusions. Although sometimes appropriate for articles, the approach does little to help the communication process involved in clinical report writing.

Audiology reports are generally of two types. The type of report is usually dictated by the setting, and in some cases both types are used within a setting based on the nature of the referral source. One type of report is the *audiogram report*. The audiogram report usually consists of an audiogram, a table of other audiometric information, and space at the bottom for summary and impressions. The audiogram report is often used for inpatient reporting in hospital settings, where the results are added to the patient's chart and constitute the medical record. The audiogram report is also often used in otolaryngology offices, where the audiometric evaluation is one component of the medical evaluation and is used to supplement the medical report generated by the physician. The great challenge in creating an appropriate audiogram report is to be thorough, since this may constitute the entirety of the audiologic record in a medical chart, while at the same time being clear and concise. Certain necessary information must be included, but it needs to be presented in a way that promotes communication between the audiologist and the consumers of the report.

The other common type of audiologic report is the *letter report.* This report is often dictated or computer-generated. It is meant to either stand on its own or to accompany an audiogram and other test-result forms. The report in this case serves as the summary of results and a statement of disposition of the patient. When written appropriately it can be sent to a patient, a referral source, a school, or other interested parties without supporting documentation. It can also be used as a cover letter for supporting documentation when the report is sent to referral sources or others who might understand what an audiogram, an immittance form, or a latency-intensity function represents. The great challenge in creating an appropriate letter report is to say enough, but not too much. The letter should state clearly the outcome of test results and the recommendations or other disposition related to the patient. In most cases, it should *not* serve as a lengthy description of the patient or the test procedures used to reach the outcome conclusions.

Reporting of test results can be a relatively simple and efficient process, or it can be quite burdensome. The most important aspect of report writing is to write for the reader, not for yourself, the medical record, your colleagues, and so on. The purpose is to communicate, not to impress or obfuscate. A list of do's and don't's for report writing can be found in the Clinical Note on the next page. These should serve as general guidelines for the generation of the majority of reports that you write. Remember that the reader is busy and wants your professional interpretation and impression. Three of the more important do's are: (a) be clear, (b) be concise, and (c) be consistent.

Report Destination

The primary reason for report writing is to communicate results to the referral source. Thus, the primary destination of any report is back to the referral source. In fact, as a rule, your only obligation as a professional is to report back to the referral source, as that person has requested a consultation from you.

The patient may also request a copy of the report or that a copy be sent to additional health care providers, schools, and so on. It

Report Writing Do's and Don't's

The following are some tips on report writing:

Do:
- Be clear
- Be concise
- Be consistent
- Be descriptive
- Summarize
- State outcomes clearly
- State recommendations clearly
- State disposition clearly
- Write for the reader
- Provide all relevant information
- Provide only relevant information
- Include lengthy information as a supplement

Don't:
- ■ Write long reports
- ■ Rehash case history to the referral source
- ■ Report every aspect of the evaluation process
- ■ Describe the nature of the case in elaborate detail
- ■ Describe the nature of testing in elaborate detail
- ■ Be interpretive unless clearly noted
- ■ Use audiologic jargon
- ■ Recommend audiologic re-evaluation without a reason

is customary and appropriate to address a letter report to the referral source, with additional copies "cc'd" to the other requested parties. On occasion, there are circumstances under which an additional report is written to an individual or institution as a service to the patient. It is appropriate to write such a report, as long as in doing so, the lines of referral are not breached. The concept of referral lines is introduced later in this chapter.

Nature of the Referral

Reporting of audiometric test results should be done in a clear enough manner that the report can be generally understood, regardless of the nature of the referral source. That is, the type and severity of the hearing loss are described the same whether the report is being sent to a parent or an otolaryngologist. However, conclusions and recommendations may vary considerably depending on the referral source.

Reports to the medical community must be short and to the point. But even within that community there is often a need for different levels of explanation, particularly of the disposition of the patient. For example, the **otolaryngologist** will understand the steps that must be taken if the audiologist indicates that the patient is a candidate for hearing aid use. The **oncologist** may not. Reports to school personnel may include an explanation of the consequences of a hearing impairment. This same explanation might be unnecessary for, or certainly underutilized by, the medical community.

An **otolaryngologist** is a physician specializing in the diagnosis and treatment of diseases of the ear, nose, and throat.

An **oncologist** is a physician specializing in the diagnosis and treatment of cancer.

One of the important challenges in reporting, then, is to develop a strategy that combines consistency in the basic reporting of results with the flexibility to adapt the implications and conclusions to meet the expectations of the reader.

Information to be Communicated

The goal of any report is to communicate the outcome of your evaluation and/or treatment. Reporting is just that simple. If you always strive to describe your results succinctly and to provide the referral source, patient, or parent with essential information and a clear understanding of what to do next, you will have succeeded in writing an effective report.

One of the biggest challenges in report writing is to provide *all* relevant information while *only* reporting relevant information. Although this concept seems simple, it is often ignored under the dubious notion that thoroughness rather than succinctness is of paramount importance. If you ascribe to such a notion, you would probably think that it is useful to provide a complete description of a patient's health history, the nature and manner of the tests that you carried out, the possible consequences of the results, and a myriad of recommendations related to the outcome. Indeed, such an approach is not uncommon in educational models or in circumstances in which a patient is undergoing prolonged treatment or is being referred from one professional to another for continuation of treatment. Although such an approach might be appropriate under those circumstances, it is seldom appropriate in audiological settings.

One of the most useful ways to judge the appropriateness of the information that you are communicating in a report is to put yourself in the reader's shoes. As a reader, you probably lack one of two things, time or technical expertise. In either case, your interest in lengthy, detailed reports will be limited. Perhaps some examples will make this clear.

Suppose for a moment that you are a physician. You refer a patient to the audiologist to determine the extent to which the fluid that you have observed behind the tympanic membrane is causing an auditory disorder. What might you want to know? You would probably want to know whether or not middle ear disorder is detected by immittance measures and, if so, what the nature of the results is. You would also probably want to know the degree of hearing loss that the disorder is creating and the nature of the hearing loss, for example, whether it is a conductive or mixed hearing loss. Finally, you would want to know if speech perception measures or any other auditory measures suggest any evidence of additional cochlear or retrocochlear disorder. This is all information that would help you as a physician make appropriate decisions about diagnosis and treatment, and it should be summarized in a report. Okay, so what don't you care about? First, you don't care to hear about the patient's medical history. Why? Because you already know all about it. Second, you probably do not want to hear about the nuances of the audiologic tests that were carried out. Although important to the audiologist and imperative for the audiologic records, their descriptions serve simply as extraneous information that obscures the results and conclusions of the audiologist's evaluation or treatment. Third, you are probably not interested at this point in getting recommendations about nonmedical or nonsurgical intervention strategies.

Let us use another example. Suppose this time that you are the patient. You have decided to see the audiologist because your hearing impairment has reached a point at which you feel that hearing aid use might be appropriate. You would like a report for your records, and you would like to have a copy sent to your family physician for hers. What do you care about? You are probably interested in a report describing the degree and type of hearing loss you have in both ears. You are also probably interested in written recommendations about the prognosis for pursuing hearing aid use. What don't you care about? Well, you don't care to read about your own medical history. You already know that. You also don't care about the specifics of the auditory tests. You simply want words to describe your problem and a cogent statement of the plans to fix it.

What, then, should be communicated in a report? What are the best strategies for doing so? As a general rule, the report should be a summary of evaluative outcomes. What is the hearing like in the right ear? The left ear? Where do we go from here? As another general rule, the report should not be a description of the testing that was done nor a description of the specific test results, except as they support the evaluative outcome. These are two

important points. First, there is very seldom any reason to describe audiometric tests in a report. If the report is going to a
referral source, it is safe to assume that the person receiving the
report is familiar with the testing or does not care about the
details. In most cases, an audiometric summary is sent with a
report and provides all the details that anyone might want to see.
Second, most audiometric test results are supportive of the general outcome and do not need to be described. For example, if a
patient has a mild sensorineural hearing loss and normal middle
ear function, there is no reason to describe pure-tone air conduction results, bone-conduction results, the tympanogram, acoustic
reflexes, speech audiometry, and so on. Simply stating the outcome is sufficient in a vast majority of cases.

For audiologic evaluations, a report usually consists of a brief
summary of testing outcomes, an audiogram form with more
specific information, and additional supplemental information as
necessary.

The Report

An audiologic report typically includes a description of the audiometric configuration, type of hearing loss, status of middle ear
function, and recommendations. Under certain circumstances, it
might also include case history information, speech audiometric
results, auditory electrophysiologic results, and a statement about
site of the auditory disorder.

Case History. Occasionally, but rarely, a description of relevant
information from the case history might be useful in the initial
portion of a report. In most cases, it can be considered superfluous. Reports written to referral sources do not need a summary
of why a patient was evaluated because the referral source would
obviously know, being the source of the referral. Similarly, a report written to a patient seldom requires this information, because, clearly, the patient already knows all of this information.

Nevertheless, there are times when a succinct statement can be
made about some aspect of a patient's medical or communication
history that might be new or relevant information to the person
receiving the report. For example, for a patient who has suspected
hearing loss secondary to noise exposure, a report might include
a summary of relevant noise-exposure information.

The key to judging the need for case history information lies in
the nature of the referral source and the people or institutions to
whom the report is being sent. In the vast majority of cases,

reports are being sent either to the referral source, the patient, or the patient's parents. In most of these cases, a summary of relevant history is superfluous.

Type of Hearing Loss. If a hearing loss exists, it should be described as conductive, sensorineural, or mixed. If it is conductive at some frequencies and sensorineural at others, it should be considered a mixed hearing loss.

Degree and Configuration of Hearing Loss. Most audiologists describe degree of hearing loss as falling into one of several categories, minimal, mild, moderate, moderately severe, severe, or profound. If the audiometric pattern or configuration is that of a flat loss, the loss is often described simply as, for example, a moderate hearing loss. If the loss is not relatively flat, it is usually described by its configuration as either rising, sloping, high-frequency, or low-frequency, depending on its shape.

Describing the degree and configuration of hearing loss is not an exact science, and it should not be treated as such. Rather, the goal should be to put the audiogram into words that can be conveyed with relative consistency to the patient and among health-care professionals. To describe a hearing loss as a mild sensorineural loss at 500 Hz, moderately sloping mixed hearing loss in the mid-frequencies, and moderately severe sensorineural hearing loss in the high frequencies, although perhaps accurate, is not very useful. Providing the words *moderate, mixed hearing loss* is probably much more useful to all who might read the report.

Terminology that can be used to consistently describe type, degree, and configuration of hearing loss is shown in Table 9–1. These codes and descriptors are part of a computer-based reporting strategy that will be described later in this chapter.

Change in Hearing Status. When a patient has been evaluated a second or third time, it is important to include a statement of comparison to previous test results. This should be done even if the results have not changed. A simple statement such as, *hearing sensitivity is unchanged/has decreased/has improved since the previous evaluation on (date),* will suffice and will be an important contribution to the report.

Middle Ear Function. It is often important to state the status of middle ear function based on results of immittance audiometry, even if that status is normal. Much of the direction and course of treatment relates to whether or not the function is normal.

Table 9-1. Report-writing terminology used to describe type and degree of hearing loss and audiometric configuration.

Code	Descriptor
NH	Normal hearing.
NHS	Normal hearing sensitivity.
CMI	Mild conductive hearing loss.
CMIR	Mild, rising conductive hearing loss.
CMIL	Mild, low-frequency conductive hearing loss.
CMO	Moderate conductive hearing loss.
CMOR	Moderate, rising conductive hearing loss.
CMOL	Moderate, low-frequency conductive hearing loss.
CS	Severe conductive hearing loss.
MMI	Mild mixed hearing loss.
MMIR	Mild, rising mixed hearing loss.
MMIS	Mild, sloping mixed hearing loss.
MMO	Moderate mixed hearing loss.
MMOR	Moderate, rising mixed hearing loss.
MMOS	Moderate, sloping mixed hearing loss.
MS	Severe mixed hearing loss.
MSR	Severe, rising mixed hearing loss.
MSS	Severe, sloping mixed hearing loss.
MP	Profound mixed hearing loss.
SNMI	Mild sensorineural hearing loss.
SNMIR	Mild, rising sensorineural hearing loss.
SNMIL	Mild, low-frequency sensorineural hearing loss.
SNMIS	Mild, sloping sensorineural hearing loss.
SNMIH	Mild, high-frequency sensorineural hearing loss.
SNMO	Moderate sensorineural hearing loss.
SNMOR	Moderate, rising sensorineural hearing loss.
SNMOL	Moderate, low-frequency sensorineural hearing loss.
SNMOS	Moderate, sloping sensorineural hearing loss.
SNMOH	Moderate, high-frequency sensorineural hearing loss.
SNS	Severe sensorineural hearing loss.
SNSR	Severe, rising sensorineural hearing loss.
SNSL	Severe, low-frequency sensorineural hearing loss.
SNSS	Severe, sloping sensorineural hearing loss.
SNSH	Severe, high-frequency sensorineural hearing loss.
SNP	Profound sensorineural hearing loss.
SUNCH	Sensitivity is essentially unchanged since the previous evaluation on (date).
SDEC	Sensitivity is decreased since the previous evaluation on (date).
SIMP	Sensitivity is improved since the previous evaluation on (date).

When middle ear function is normal, it should be stated directly without a delineation of immittance results.

When middle ear function is abnormal, the nature of the immittance results should be described. It is useful to limit the description of the disorder to a few categories that can be conveyed consistently to the referral source. Once the disorder is described, the specific immittance results that characterized the disorder can be delineated. In general, middle ear disorders fall into one of five categories:

■ an increase in the mass of the middle ear system, characterized by a Type B tympanogram, low static immittance, and absent acoustic reflexes, often caused by otitis media with effusion and impacted cerumen;

■ an increase in the stiffness of the middle ear system due to fixation of the ossicular chain, characterized by a Type A tympanogram, low static immittance, and absent acoustic reflexes, often caused by otosclerosis;

■ a decrease in the stiffness of the middle ear system due to disruption of the ossicular chain, characterized by a Type A tympanogram, high static immittance, and absent acoustic reflexes, often caused by some form of trauma;

■ significant negative pressure in the middle ear space, characterized by a Type C tympanogram, caused by Eustachian tube dysfunction; and

■ perforation of the tympanic membrane, characterized by a large equivalent volume and absent reflexes, often caused by tympanic membrane rupture secondary to otitis media or to trauma.

In describing these results, only the description of the type of middle ear disorder and the immittance results should be described. The underlying cause of the disorder is a medical diagnosis and is the purview of the physician. The audiologist's task is to identify and describe the disorder, not its cause.

Terminology that can be used to consistently describe immittance-measurement outcomes is shown in Table 9–2. These codes and descriptors are part of a computer-based reporting strategy that will be described later in this chapter.

Sometimes middle ear function will be normal, but acoustic reflex measures will be elevated, consistent with sensorineural hearing loss or retrocochlear disorder. When the reflex results might be useful to the referral source in helping to diagnose such a disorder, then they should be described. Otherwise, they simply confirm the description of the type of hearing loss and are probably redundant.

Speech Audiometric Results. Results of speech audiometry are seldom useful to describe in a report. As a general rule, con-

Table 9-2. Report-writing terminology used to describe results of immittance measurements.

Code	Descriptor
IMPNORM	Acoustic immittance measures are consistent with normal middle ear function.
TYMPNORM	Acoustic immittance measures yield a normal, type A, tympanogram.
IMPABN	Acoustic immittance measures indicate middle ear disorder.
IMPDIS	Acoustic immittance measures indicate middle ear disorder. The combination of a deep, type A tympanogram and abnormal acoustic reflex thresholds is consistent with discontinuity of the ossicular chain.
IMPFIX	Acoustic immittance measures indicate middle ear disorder. The combination of a shallow, type A tympanogram and abnormal acoustic reflex thresholds is consistent with fixation of the ossicular chain.
IMPNEGB	Acoustic immittance measures indicate middle ear disorder. The tympanogram is type C, with the compliance peak at -*** daPa, indicating significant negative pressure in the middle ear space.
IMPOM	Acoustic immittance measures indicate middle ear disorder. The combination of a type B tympanogram, low static compliance, and absent acoustic reflexes indicates significant increase in the mass of the middle ear mechanism.
IMPERF	Acoustic immittance measures are consistent with a perforation of the tympanic membrane.
IMPPE	Acoustic immittance measures are consistent with a patent pressure equalization tube.
IMPWAX	Acoustic immittance measures are consistent with excessive cerumen in the ear canal.
ARTABN	Acoustic immittance measures indicate middle ear disorder. The tympanogram is normal, but acoustic reflex thresholds are abnormally elevated.
IMPCONS	Acoustic immittance measures are consistent with a history of otologic surgery.
IMPCHL	Acoustic immittance measures yield a type A tympanogram. Acoustic reflexes are absent consistent with the severity of the hearing loss.
IMPFLUC	Acoustic immittance measures yield a type A tympanogram and high static compliance. Acoustic reflexes could not be measured due to excessive compliance fluctuation.
IMPMOVE	Acoustic immittance measures yield a type A tympanogram. Acoustic reflexes could not be measured due to patient movement during the test.
IMPSEAL	Acoustic immittance measures could not be completed due to an inability to maintain an airtight seal.
IMPSURG	Acoustic immittance measures were not carried out due to history of otologic surgery.
IMPNO	Acoustic immittance measures were not carried out at the referring physician's request.
TARABN	Acoustic immittance measures yield a type A tympanogram, but acoustic reflex thresholds are abnormally elevated.

ventional speech audiometric measures are consistent with results of pure-tone audiometry. That is, the speech recognition threshold is reflective of the pure-tone average, and speech recognition scores are consistent with the degree and configuration of hearing loss. As long as they are included on the audiogram form, there is no real need to describe them in a report, because the information they provide is redundant and, thus,

Table 9–3. Report-writing terminology used to describe results of speech audiometry.

Code	Descriptor
SPAGE	Decreased speech understanding performance is consistent with the patient's age.
SPPBROL	Speech audiometric results show significant rollover of the PI-PB function.
SSIROL	Speech audiometric results show significant rollover of the PI-SSI function.
PBSSIROL	Speech audiometric results show significant rollover of the PI-PB and PI-SSI functions.
PBSSIDIS	Speech audiometric results show significant discrepancy in performance for words (PB) versus performance for sentences (SSI).
SPDEP	Speech audiometric results are significantly depressed for both PI-PB and PI-SSI functions.
SSIDEP	Speech audiometric results are significantly depressed for the PI-SSI function.

contributes little to the overall summary of results that you are trying to convey.

Sometimes speech audiometric results are poorer than would be expected from the results of pure-tone audiometry. In such cases, the results may be important to the diagnosis and should be included in a report. Here again, rather than providing a specific score on a test, the results should be summarized in a meaningful way. Statements such as *word recognition scores were poorer than expected for the degree of hearing loss* or *speech audiometric measures showed abnormal rollover of the performance-intensity function* serve to alert the informed reader to potential retrocochlear involvement without burdening the report with details.

Terminology that can be used to consistently describe speech-audiometric results is shown in Table 9–3. These codes and descriptors are part of a computer-based reporting strategy that will be described later in this chapter.

When advanced speech audiometric measures are used to assess central auditory function, the same general rules apply. If results are normal, there is no need to describe them in a report. If results are abnormal, they should be described generally without details of the test procedures or too much specific information about test scores. Often, the report will be accompanied by an audiometric form that contains enough detail for readers with specific knowledge. Those without specific knowledge will not benefit from this information regardless of its availability, so it is even more important to summarize the information in a succinct and meaningful way in the body of the report.

Electrophysiologic Results. A variety of strategies are used to describe the results of auditory electrophysiologic measures. As a general rule, the more complicated the technology, the more compelled the writer seems to be to burden the reader with details of the testing itself. Again, however, you have the opportunity to treat this testing as any other audiometric measure by simply describing the outcome in your report. The details of how you reached that decision are better left as supplementary documentation for those who might understand it.

When auditory evoked potentials are used to predict hearing sensitivity, the results can be summarized in a standard audiologic report. If results are consistent with normal hearing sensitivity, then a statement such as *auditory brain stem response predicted hearing sensitivity to be within normal limits* will suffice. If results are consistent with a hearing loss, then the report should state that these measures predict a mild, moderate, or severe, sensorineural or conductive hearing loss. A latency-intensity function might be sent along with the report to provide more detail for the curious reader.

When auditory evoked potentials are used diagnostically, the same rules apply. A general statement should be made about the overall outcome of the testing. When results are normal, a statement should be made that *absolute and interpeak intervals are within normal limits* and that these *results show no evidence of VIIIth nerve or auditory brain stem response abnormality.* When results are abnormal, they should also be described generally as, for example, the absence of a measurable response, a prolongation of wave I–V interpeak interval, a significant asymmetry in absolute latency of wave V, and so on. The results should then be summarized by stating that they are consistent with VIIIth nerve or auditory brain stem response abnormality.

Terminology that can be used to consistently describe electrophysiologic test results is shown in Table 9–4. These codes and descriptors are part of a computer-based reporting strategy that will be described later in this chapter.

To some readers, the details of these evoked potential measures are important. They are interested in electrode montage, click

Table 9–4. Report-writing terminology used to describe results of auditory electrophysiologic measures.

Code	Descriptor
ABRNORM1	Auditory brainstem response (ABR) audiometry shows well-formed responses to click stimuli at normal absolute latencies and interwave intervals. There is no evidence of eighth nerve or auditory brainstem pathway disorder.
ABRNORM2	Auditory brainstem response (ABR) audiometry shows well-formed responses to click stimuli at normal absolute latencies and interwave intervals.
ABRNORM3	Auditory brainstem response (ABR) audiometry shows well-formed responses to click stimuli at intensity levels consistent with normal hearing sensitivity in the 1000 Hz to 4000 Hz frequency range. In addition, absolute and interwave latencies are age appropriate.
ABRHL	Auditory brainstem response (ABR) audiometry shows responses to click stimuli down to **** dB nHL. This is consistent with a **** hearing loss in the 1000 Hz to 4000 Hz frequency range. In addition, interwave latencies are age appropriate.
ABRCL	Auditory brainstem response (ABR) audiometry shows responses to click stimuli down to **** dB nHL by air conduction, and down to **** dB nHL by bone conduction. This is consistent with a **** hearing loss in the 1000 Hz to 4000 Hz frequency range. In addition, interwave latencies are age appropriate.
ABRABN	Auditory brainstem response (ABR) audiometry shows abnormal responses to click stimuli. Both the absolute latency of wave V and the I to V interwave interval are significantly prolonged.
ABRCHL	Auditory brainstem response (ABR) audiometry shows responses to click stimuli at absolute latencies consistent with peripheral sensitivity loss. There is no evidence of eighth nerve or auditory brainstem disorder.
ECOG	Electrocochleography shows an SP/AP ratio of ***%, which is within the limits of normal.
MLRNORM	In addition, middle latency and late latency responses are normal.
LLRNORM	Late latency response is normal.
TOAENORM	Transient-evoked otoacoustic emissions are present, suggesting normal cochlear function.
TOAEABN	Transient-evoked otoacoustic emissions are absent.
DPNORM	Distortion-product otoacoustic emissions are present, suggesting normal cochlear function.
DPABN	Distortion-product otoacoustic emissions are absent.

rate, stimulus polarity, EEG filtering, etc. For these individuals, a summary containing this information as well as the waveforms may be useful. Most readers, however, are only interested in the outcome and your professional opinion about it. In a report, there is no need to burden this latter group because of the interests of the former. The report should summarize and make conclusions. Supplemental information can always be attached.

Site of Disorder. In general, there is no need to make a statement about site of disorder in a report. A conductive hearing loss is related to outer or middle ear disorder, and a sensorineural hearing loss is related to cochlear disorder. Occasionally, however, the audiologist will find it useful to give an overall impression of the possible site of disorder. This is particularly useful if the referral source is trying to differentiate a cochlear disorder from a retrocochlear disorder or if the referral source is interested in knowing the status of central auditory processing ability.

Any statement of site of disorder should be based on an overall impression of results of the test battery. If an VIIIth nerve tumor is suspected as the cause of an auditory disorder and the referral source is interested in the audiologist's opinion, the report should state that the pattern of test results is consistent with cochlear disorder or consistent with retrocochlear disorder, depending on test outcomes. It should be emphasized that the site would be assumed to be cochlear and that a statement about cochlear site would be unnecessary unless there is some concern about retrocochlear disorder. In some cases, there is no *a priori* concern about retrocochlear disorder, but various audiometric measures suggest otherwise. In such cases, it is imperative that the audiologist make a statement about the pattern of test results.

The same general ideas hold for assessment of central auditory processing ability. If no concern is expressed, and routine testing is normal, no statement about site of disorder is necessary. However, if a diagnosis can be made based on routine testing, the report should state that the overall pattern of results is consistent with central auditory disorder. Additionally, if a patient is referred for evaluation of central auditory function, the reports should state that the pattern of test results is consistent with central auditory processing disorder or that there is no evidence of such disorder, depending on test outcomes.

Terminology that can be used to consistently describe site of disorder is shown in Table 9–5.

Table 9-5. Report-writing terminology used to describe site of auditory disorder.

Code	Descriptor
SITECOCH	The overall pattern of results is most consistent with cochlear site.
NOTCOCH	Speech audiometric results cannot be explained on the basis of age or degree of hearing sensitivity loss.
SITEVIII	The overall pattern of results is most consistent with retrocochlear site.
SITECAPD	The overall pattern of results is consistent with central auditory processing disorder.
SITEWIMP	These results, while not definitive, suggest the possibility of central auditory pathway disorder.
SITENEG	There is no evidence of central auditory disorder.

Recommendations. The recommendations section of a report is generally the first section that is read by the reader. As in all other aspects of the report, recommendations should be clear, concise, and consistently stated. Recommendations generally fall into one of four categories:

- ■ no recommendations,
- ■ recommendations for re-evaluation,
- ■ recommendations for additional testing, or
- ■ recommendations for referral.

Sometimes there is no consequence to the audiometric test results, and no recommendations are necessary. For example, a patient with symptoms of dizziness may be referred to the audiologist to rule out cochlear contribution to the dizziness. All pure-tone, immittance, and speech audiometric measures may be normal if the cochlea is not involved. As another example, a child may fail a school hearing screening because the testing was carried out in too noisy an environment. Results of the audiometric evaluation may be normal. What do you conclude? What do you recommend? Nothing. You simply state that *no audiologic recommendations are indicated at this time.*

Occasionally there is a need to recommend audiologic re-evaluation. For example, if a child is undergoing medical treatment for otitis media, and you discover a conductive hearing loss, you may want to recommend that the child return for audiologic re-evaluation following the completion of medical management as a means of ensuring that there is no residual hearing loss that needs to be managed. As another example, if a patient is exposed to damaging noise levels at work or recreationally, periodic re-evaluation is an appropriate recommendation. In these cases, the recommendation of re-evaluation is appropriate and important.

Unfortunately, the recommendation of audiologic re-evaluation is often overused. Particularly in pediatric assessment, there is a tendency on the part of some audiologists to recommend re-evaluation at some future point in time because sufficient clinical data could not be obtained during the current evaluation. In this case, the too-often used recommendation for re-evaluation in 6 months simply means that the clinician hopes that either the child grows up or the clinician's skills improve in the interim. A recommendation for re-evaluation should not serve as a substitute for completion of testing in the immediate future.

Another common recommendation is for additional testing. For example, if behavioral testing could not be completed on a child or a patient with functional hearing loss due to a lack of cooperation, the audiologist may recommend additional testing with auditory evoked potentials.

Recommendations are also quite commonly made for referral purposes. The patient may be referred for a hearing aid consultation, cochlear-implant evaluation, speech-language evaluation, medical consultation, otologic consultation, and so on. Although the audiologist must always be cognizant of the rules of referral as discussed later in the chapter, the responsibility for making appropriate referral recommendations is an important one.

Terminology that can be used to provide consistent recommendations is shown in Table 9–6.

The Audiogram and Other Forms

Under most circumstances it is customary to send an audiogram with a report. Because the audiogram has been a standard way to express hearing sensitivity for many years, it is widely recognized and generally understood by referral sources. As stated earlier, two strategies predominate, one the use of an audiogram report and the other the use of a letter report with an audiogram and other forms attached.

The *audiogram report* is typically an audiogram, a table of information, and a summary at the bottom. It often serves as the medical record in a hospital or physician's office. As such, it is

Table 9-6. Report-writing terminology used to describe recommendations.

Code	Descriptor
HANR	Hearing aid use is not recommended.
HAENEG	In view of the relatively mild sensitivity loss, hearing aid use is not recommended.
HAEQ	In view of the audiometric configuration, the prognosis for successful hearing aid use is only marginal.
HAENO	In view of the audiometric configuration, the prognosis for successful hearing aid use is unfavorable. Therefore, a hearing aid evaluation is not recommended.
HAEPOS	In view of the significant sensitivity loss, we recommend a hearing aid evaluation to assess the potential for successful use of amplification.
HAEPEND	In view of the significant sensitivity loss, we recommend a hearing aid evaluation to assess the potential for successful use of amplification, pending medical clearance.
CIREC	In view of the significant sensitivity loss, we recommend a cochlear implant evaluation.
RECALD	We recommend the use of an assistive listening device.
DEFER	Rehabilitative recommendations are deferred pending otologic consultation.
NOTINT	The patient is not interested in pursuing amplification at this time.
EMHAE	Ear impressions were made, and a hearing aid evaluation was scheduled.
HASUC	The patient reports successful hearing aid use.
HAOK	Electroacoustic analysis of the patient's hearing aid shows it to be functioning properly and providing adequate gain for the degree of hearing loss.
HASOK	Electroacoustic analysis of the patient's hearing aids show them to be functioning properly and providing adequate gain for the degree of hearing loss.
RECUSE	We recommend continued use of current amplification.
NOISPRO	We recommend the use of ear protection in noisy environments.
OTOCON	We recommend otologic consultation for evaluation of middle ear disorder.
MEDCON	We recommend medical consultation for evaluation of middle ear disorder.
RECRE	We recommend audiologic re-evaluation following completion of medical management.
RECMON	We recommend continued monitoring of hearing.
RECABR	This pattern of test results suggests retrocochlear disorder. We recommend further evaluation by auditory evoked potentials.
RECAEP	We recommend evoked potential audiometry to further assess hearing sensitivity.
NOREC	No audiologic recommendations are indicated at this time.
PASSSCREEN	This child passed our hearing screening measures. No further audiologic recommendations are indicated at this time.
FAILSCREEN	This child failed our hearing screening measures. We recommend further assessment by evoked potential audiometry.
PEDINORM	Although results are limited on a child of this young age, the overall pattern suggests normal hearing sensitivity and normal middle ear function bilaterally.

often packed with information about the pure-tone audiogram as well as speech and immittance audiometry. Because it is so comprehensive, it is often difficult to read and interpret and can defy the important requirement of clarity in reporting. The requirement for thoroughness inherent in the medical record makes it even more important that the summary and conclusions are concise and to the point.

An audiogram is also usually sent with a *letter report.* In this case, the report is usually going out of the office or clinic, and a patient record is maintained electronically or in file form in the audiologist's office. In this case, the audiogram form can be designed to be less thorough, but clearer, to the reader. Detailed supporting documentation can be stored in the patient's file. An example of an audiogram that might accompany a letter report is shown in Figure 9–1.

It is not uncommon for an audiogram to include information about speech audiometry, either in tabular form, including speech recognition threshold, word recognition scores, and levels of testing, or in graphic form as a performance-versus-intensity function. The latter probably communicates better, although the former requires less space. Regardless, information about speech thresholds and word recognition scores are often generally understood and should be included with the audiogram form.

Most audiologists also send information on results of immittance audiometry. Again, the form can vary from a tabular summary on an audiogram to a separate sheet of paper showing the tympanogram and acoustic reflex patterns, along with a space for summary information. An example is shown in Figure 9–2. As in all cases, this information will be understood by some who might receive a report and be quite foreign to others. Therefore, care should be taken to provide a clear and concise interpretation on the letter report.

If auditory evoked potentials have been carried out, it is not uncommon for the results to be summarized on an auditory brain stem response latency-intensity summary form. This form shows a graph of wave V latency as a function of stimulus intensity, along with summary information about relevant absolute and interpeak latencies. The form also includes a summary section in case the form is not accompanied by a letter report. An example is shown in Figure 9–3. If the audiologist feels that the referral source will benefit from specific signal and recording parameter information, then actual waveforms with these data may also be included with the summary.

Supplemental Material

Clinical reports are simply not the place to include lengthy descriptions of testing procedures, outcomes, or rehabilitative strategies. Quite frankly, few people read lengthy reports; most just skip to the summary and recommendations. Nevertheless, there

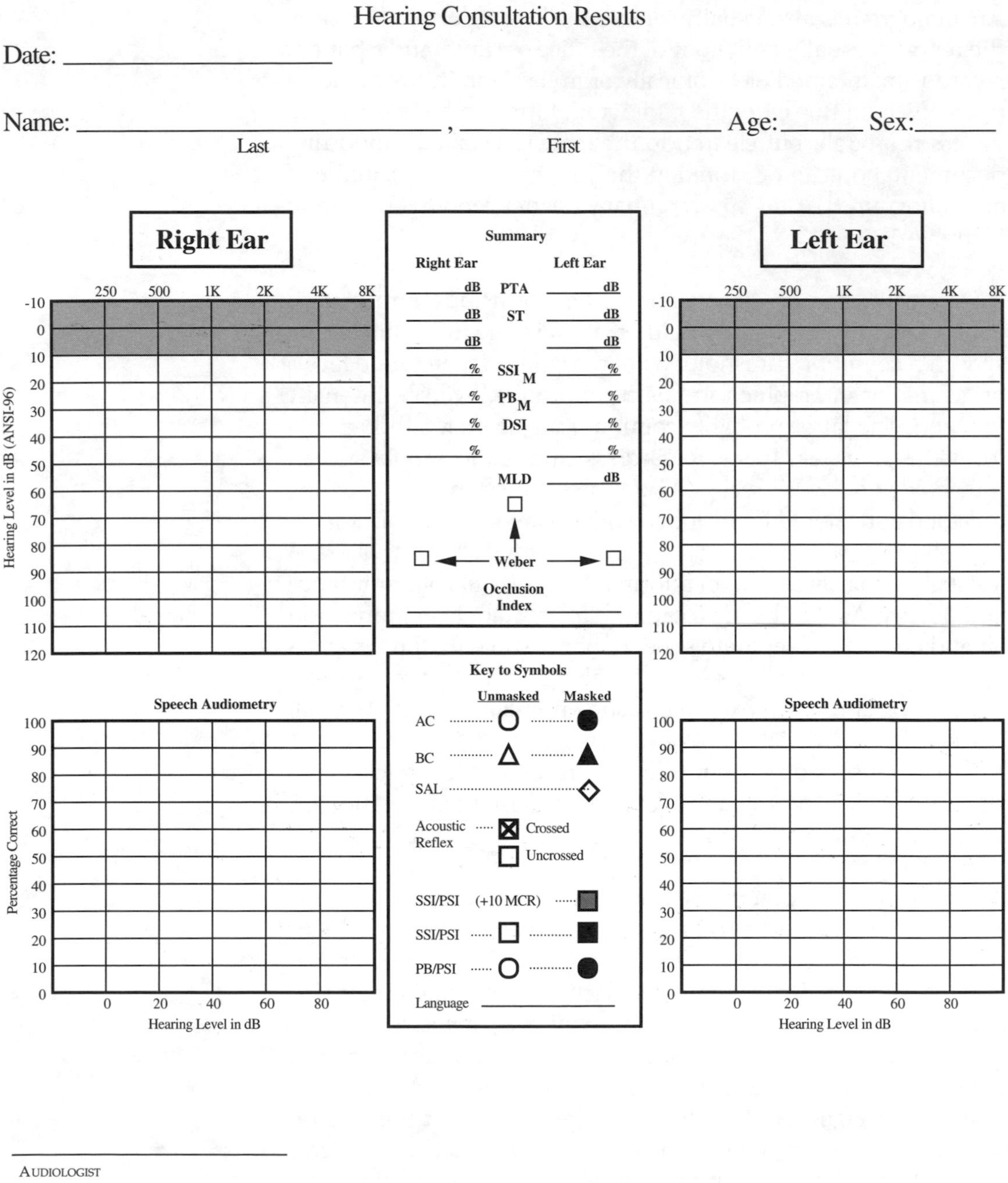

Hearing Consultation Results

Date: _____

Name: _____ , _____ Age: _____ Sex: _____
Last   First

Right Ear		

	250	500	1K	2K	4K	8K

Hearing Level in dB (ANSI-96)

-10, 0, 10, 20, 30, 40, 50, 60, 70, 80, 90, 100, 110, 120

Summary

	Right Ear		Left Ear
dB	PTA	dB
dB	ST	dB
dB		dB
%	SSI M	%
%	PB M	%
%	DSI	%
%		%
	MLD	dB

□

Weber

Occlusion Index

Left Ear		

	250	500	1K	2K	4K	8K

-10, 0, 10, 20, 30, 40, 50, 60, 70, 80, 90, 100, 110, 120

Speech Audiometry

Percentage Correct

100, 90, 80, 70, 60, 50, 40, 30, 20, 10, 0

0   20   40   60   80
Hearing Level in dB

Key to Symbols

	Unmasked	Masked
AC	○	●
BC	△	▲
SAL		◇
Acoustic Reflex	⊠ Crossed	
	□ Uncrossed	
SSI/PSI (+10 MCR)		▣
SSI/PSI	□	■
PB/PSI	○	●
Language		

Speech Audiometry

100, 90, 80, 70, 60, 50, 40, 30, 20, 10, 0

0   20   40   60   80
Hearing Level in dB

_____
AUDIOLOGIST

Figure 9-1. Hearing consultation results form.

420

Acoustic Immittance Results

Name: _____ , _____ Age: _____ Sex: _____
      Last   First

Date: _____ Test Room: _____ Audiologist: _____

Right Ear

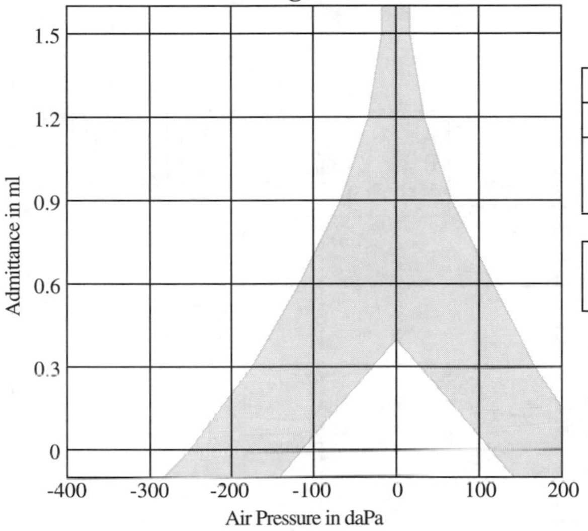

Signal to RE	BBN	500	1K	2K	4K
Crossed					
Uncrossed					

_____ — _____ + _____ = [_____]
  PTA   BBN   Corr   SPAR

RE Volume = [_____]

Impression: _____
_____
_____
_____

Left Ear

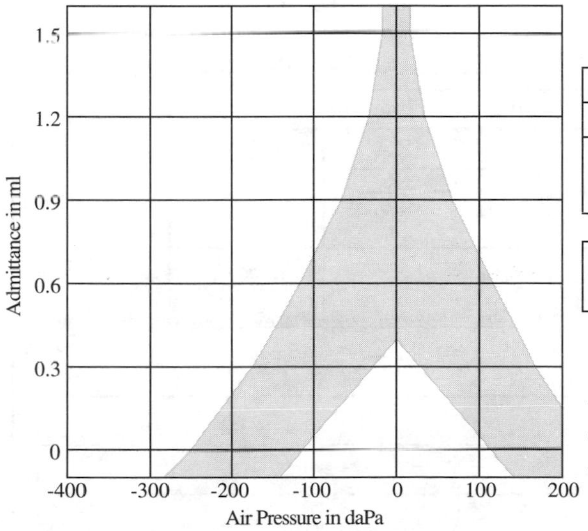

Signal to LE	BBN	500	1K	2K	4K
Crossed					
Uncrossed					

_____ — _____ + _____ = [_____]
  PTA   BBN   Corr   SPAR

LE Volume = [_____]

Impression: _____
_____
_____
_____

Figure 9-2. Immittance results form.

Figure 9–3. ABR report form.

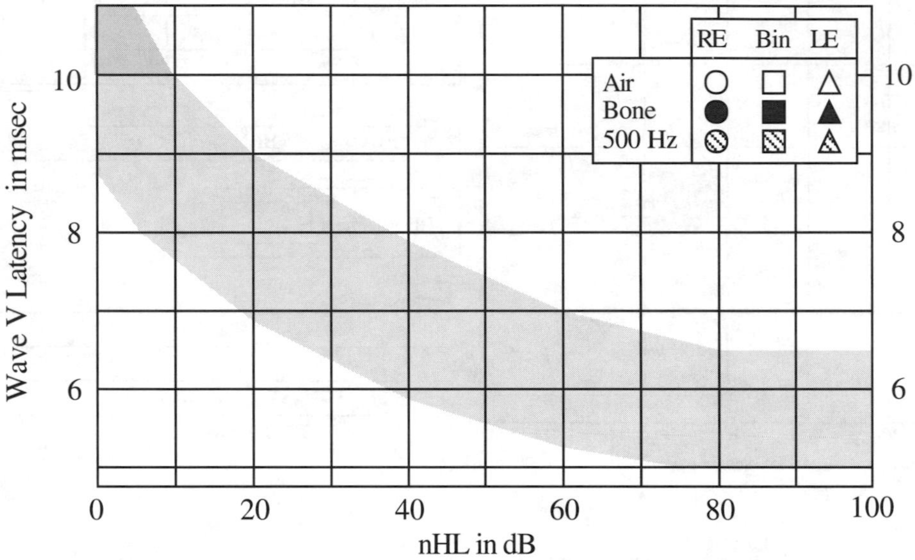

are important times to include descriptive information, and it should be included as supplemental material to the main report and sent only to individuals who might read it.

Information that has proven to be useful as supplemental material includes, for example, pamphlets explaining:

- the nature and consequence of hearing loss;
- the measurement and consequences of auditory processing disorder;
- home and classroom strategies for optimizing listening;
- the nature of tinnitus and its control; and
- the importance of hearing aids and how they can be obtained.

Information such as this is less likely to be read if it is included in a report than if it is presented as supplemental material. It also helps to make reports clearer and more concise.

Sample Reporting Strategy

Computer-based reporting strategies make it possible to generate reports rapidly, with excellent accuracy and consistency. One such strategy is presented here to illustrate the approach.

Experienced audiologists know that there is a finite number of ways they can describe the outcomes of their various audiometric measures. That is, there are only so many ways to describe an audiogram or the results of immittance audiometry. With a little discipline, over 90% of reports written can be generated from "stock" descriptions of testing outcomes. These stock descriptions can be saved in glossaries or other forms in word-processing software and can be called up as appropriate.

An example of this strategy is shown in Figure 9–4. Results of the audiologic evaluation are shown in A and B. These results show a moderate, bilateral, symmetric, sensorineural hearing loss, with maximum word-recognition scores predictable from the degree of hearing loss and no evidence of abnormality. Results of immittance audiometry show normal Type A tympanograms and crossed and uncrossed acoustic reflexes within normal limits, suggesting normal middle ear function. From these audiometric data, descriptors can be chosen that reflect these results in a clear and concise way. A form that might be used to give to the clerical staff is shown in Figure 9–4C. From these descriptors,

Date: __January 1__

Name: _____S_____ , _____B_____ Age: __41__ Sex: __M__
Last   First

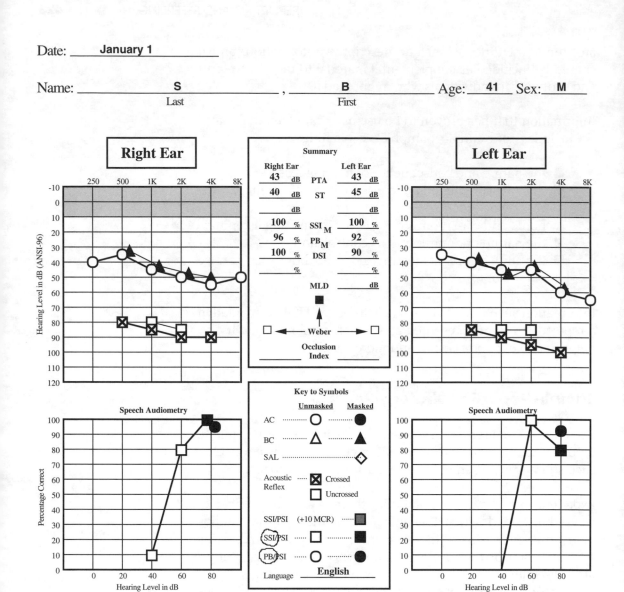

A

Figure 9-4. Example of a reporting strategy, showing (A) hearing consultation results and (B) immittance results, (C) an impression form with computer-based reporting descriptors, and (D) a final report to the referral source.

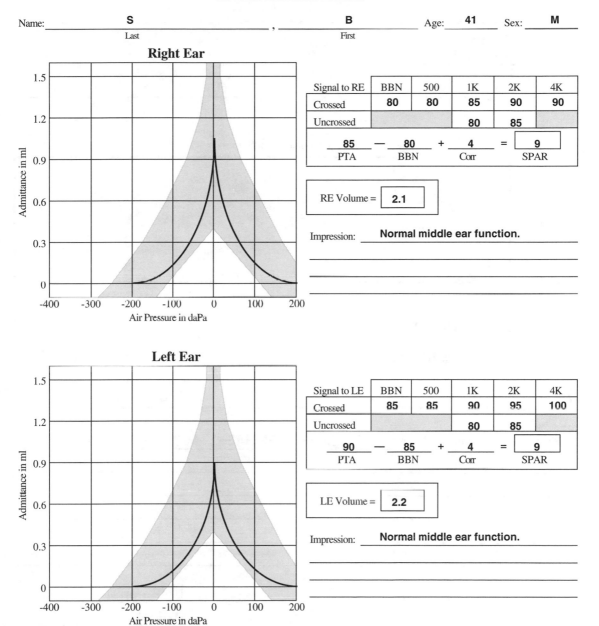

Acoustic Immittance Results

stock paragraphs are generated and placed into a report form template. The final results are shown in Figure 9–4D.

An example of a pediatric report is shown in Figure 9–5. Here, the template needs to be more flexible, but most of the reporting can be done with stock statements of testing outcome.

Impression Form

Date: **January 1**

Name: _____ **S** _____ , _____ **B** _____ Age: **41**

Last   First

Hearing Consultation Summary

Right Ear	**SNMO** **IMPNORM**
Left Ear	**SNMO** **IMPNORM**

Comments and Recommendations: **HAEPOS.   EMHAE.** _____

_____

_____

_____

_____

_____

Report to: **Dr. Referral** _____

Patient _____

_____

_____

C

426

January 2

Hearing Consultation Results

Name: B.S.
Age: 41 years

Dear Dr. Referral

We evaluated your patient, B.S., on January 1. Audiometric
results are as follows:

<u>Right Ear</u>

— Moderate sensorineural hearing loss.
— Acoustic immittance measures are consistent with
normal middle ear function.

<u>Left Ear</u>

— Moderate sensorineural hearing loss.
— Acoustic immittance measures are consistent with
normal middle ear function.

In view of the significant sensitivity loss, we recommend a
hearing aid evaluation to assess the potential for successful use
of amplification. Ear impressions were made, and a hearing aid
consultation has been scheduled.

Sincerely,

Audiologist

D

It is important to remember that not all reports can be written
using this approach. For example, results on a patient who is
exaggerating a hearing loss need to be carefully crafted and do
not lend themselves well to this type of automation. Neither do
some reports of pediatric testing. Nevertheless, the majority of
outcomes and reports can be managed in this way.

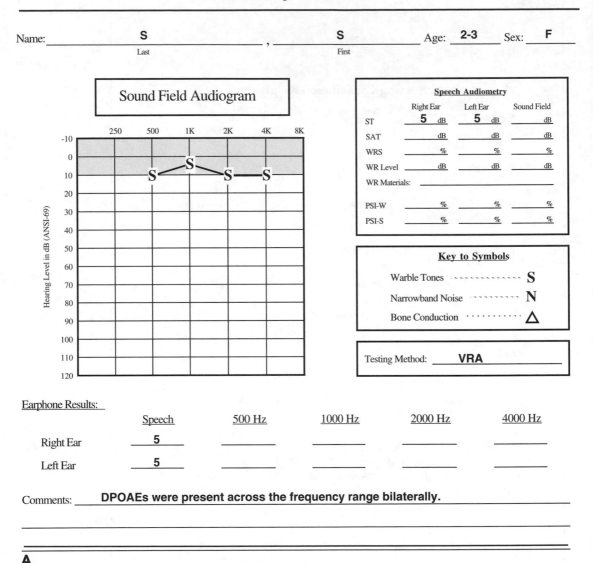

Pediatric Hearing Consultation Results

Name: _____ S _____ , _____ S _____ Age: **2-3** Sex: **F**
　　　　　　　　Last　　　　　　　　　　　　　　First

Sound Field Audiogram

Speech Audiometry

	Right Ear	Left Ear	Sound Field
ST	**5** dB	**5** dB	dB
SAT	dB	dB	dB
WRS	%	%	%
WR Level	dB	dB	dB
WR Materials:			
PSI-W	%	%	%
PSI-S	%	%	%

Key to Symbols

Warble Tones ------------- **S**

Narrowband Noise --------- **N**

Bone Conduction .... **Δ**

Testing Method: **VRA**

Earphone Results:

	Speech	500 Hz	1000 Hz	2000 Hz	4000 Hz
Right Ear	5				
Left Ear	5				

Comments: **DPOAEs were present across the frequency range bilaterally.**

A

Figure 9–5. Example of a pediatric reporting strategy, showing (A) hearing consultation results, (B) immittance results, and (C) a final report to the referral source.

The advantages of using this approach are important. First, it is a very efficient approach to report writing. In most cases the reporting can be completed before the patient leaves the clinic. Second, the accuracy of the report itself is enhanced by simply reducing the opportunity for errors. Third, the approach creates a consistency in reporting test results that will be welcomed by any referral source. Finally, the approach facilitates the creation of a concise report.

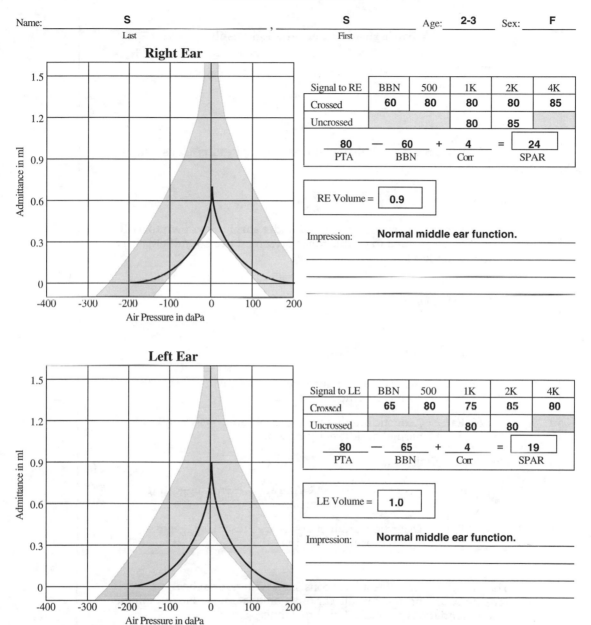

Acoustic Immittance Results

Name: _____ **S** _____ , _____ **S** _____ Age: **2-3** Sex: **F**
Last   First

Right Ear

Signal to RE	BBN	500	1K	2K	4K
Crossed	60	80	80	80	85
Uncrossed			80	85	

$$\underset{\text{PTA}}{80} - \underset{\text{BBN}}{60} + \underset{\text{Corr}}{4} = \underset{\text{SPAR}}{24}$$

RE Volume = **0.9**

Impression: **Normal middle ear function.**

Left Ear

Signal to LE	BBN	500	1K	2K	4K
Crossed	65	80	75	85	80
Uncrossed			80	80	

$$\underset{\text{PTA}}{80} - \underset{\text{BBN}}{65} + \underset{\text{Corr}}{4} = \underset{\text{SPAR}}{19}$$

LE Volume = **1.0**

Impression: **Normal middle ear function.**

A list of descriptors and stock paragraphs were presented in Tables 9–1 through 9–6. These have been modified over the past two decades and have proven to be quite useful in a number of clinical settings. They are easily adaptable to most audiology clinics.

January 2

Pediatric Hearing Consultation Results

Name: S.S.

Age: 2-3 years

Dear Dr. Referral

Your patient, S.S., was evaluated on January 1. Results are as follows:

<u>Behavioral Audiometry</u>

SS responded to speech presented under earphones down to 5 dB HL. SS responded to warble tones presented in a soundfield at the following levels:

        500 Hz: 10 dB
        1000 Hz: 5 dB
        2000 Hz: 10 dB
        4000 Hz: 10 dB

<u>Immittance Audiometry</u>

Right Ear: Acoustic immittance measures are consistent with normal middle ear function.

Left Ear: Acoustic immittance measures are consistent with normal middle ear function.

<u>Otoacoustic Emissions</u>

Right Ear: Distortion-product OAEs are present, suggesting normal cochlear function.

Left Ear: Distortion-product OAEs are present, suggesting normal cochlear function.

The overall pattern of results is consistent with normal hearing sensitivity and normal middle ear function bilaterally. No audiologic recommendations are indicated at this time.

Sincerely,

Audiologist

C

REFERRING

Patients arrive in the audiology clinic for a hearing consultation for many reasons. One reason is that they have a hearing problem, want to have it evaluated, and call to make an appointment. That is, they are self-referred. In other cases, family members and friends encourage someone to have a hearing evaluation and refer him or her to an audiologist. In many other cases, patients are referred for a hearing consultation by another health-care provider, such as an otolaryngologist, pediatrician, oncologist, or general medical practitioner.

The nature of the referral to an audiologist dictates many things. As delineated in earlier chapters, the audiometric testing itself may vary as a function of the referral source, as may the nature of a clinical report. In fact, the audiologist's professional obligation varies depending on who is making the referral. The referral *in* dictates that obligation and influences the referral *out.*

Lines and Ethics of Referral

As a health-care provider, it is important to understand the lines of referral and the boundaries that are dictated by those lines. Audiologists play different roles in hearing health care, and those roles and their boundaries can vary significantly as a function of the reason for a referral. In one case, a patient might be turned over to you to evaluate and manage his or her hearing care. In another case, you might be consulted for an opinion on the nature and degree of hearing loss as part of a patient's medical workup. What you say, to whom you communicate, and how you proceed can be very different in these two cases. Some examples may help to illustrate this concept.

If a patient is self-referred *and* is paying for the evaluation, the audiologist's complete obligation is to the patient. The outcome of testing and the disposition of a report are dictated by the interests of the patient. Therefore, if a patient does not want a report sent out, you are obligated to refrain from sending a report. There is an exception, of course, if the patient is not paying for the evaluation. In that case, the audiologist may also be obligated to report to the third-party. But, in general, the audiologist is free to evaluate and manage the patient and to make whatever other referrals are deemed appropriate for the patient.

If a patient is referred to the audiologist by a physician for a hearing consultation to assist the physician in the medical diagnosis and treatment of the patient, then the audiologist's obligation is to the referral source. If the audiologist feels that the patient needs additional testing, needs to be referred to a medical specialist, needs to have a hearing aid evaluation, and so on, the audiologist is obligated to make that recommendation to the referral source, not to the patient. This is an important concept and cannot be overstated. Under these circumstances, you as an audiologist are being consulted for your opinion, and that opinion should be given to the person who consulted you. You have not been given authority to manage this patient, and you must not assume that authority.

If a patient is referred to the audiologist by a physician to assess the potential benefit from amplification and to provide it if necessary, then the physician is making a referral to you to manage the patient. In this case, your obligation is once again to the patient, with consideration to the referral source in terms of reporting the outcome.

The concept of lines of referral and the ethics related to it are fairly simple to manage if you know the answer to two questions: (a) who referred the patient? and (b) for what reason? The biggest challenge an audiologist faces is either not knowing the answer to one of these two questions or having the answer obscured for some reason. One of the most common sources of trouble for any practitioner is the secondary referral, or the consult within a consult, wherein the audiologist might follow the line of referral, but the referral source may not. The Clinical Note on the facing page provides an example of an instance where this confusion might occur.

Another source of trouble occurs when the audiologist is challenged by the patient or by his or her knowledge to refer the patient for more specialized treatment. An example is given in the Clinical Note on page 434. Here the audiologist is challenged by conflicting ethical issues. One is the critical concept of making referrals back only to the referral source. The other is the important concern of the welfare of the patient. In such instances, the audiologist will do well to remember who is managing the patient and, thus, is ultimately responsible for the patient's care.

When to Refer

As a health-care provider, the audiologist is obligated to understand when it is appropriate to refer a patient for additional as-

Did You Steal that Patient?

One common source of confusion surrounding referral lines comes when there is a secondary referral, or a consult within a consult, and the audiologist is not clearly aware of the sequence that led to the patient sitting in the waiting room.

Let's look at an example. Audiologist 1 is in private practice in a professional building down the street from the medical center in which you work. She evaluates a patient who is interested in pursuing hearing aid use and notes the presence of a middle-ear disorder. The patient has significant sensorineural hearing loss bilaterally and will be a candidate for hearing aid amplification following management of the middle-ear disorder, but first things first. Audiologist 1 refers the patient down the street to an otolaryngologist who works in the same department that you do. The otolaryngologist evaluates the patient and, as a matter of routine, refers to you for an audiologic consultation, and, if indicated, a hearing-aid consultation. You graciously receive the referral, evaluate the patient, and begin the hearing aid process.

The problem here is that you do not know about Audiologist 1. Somewhere in the sequence of referrals, the information about the original referral source is lost, and you assume that this is an otolaryngology referral just like any of the others that you have managed that day. The patient may be equally confused, not always understanding the sometimes obscure relationships among health care providers. Regardless of the source of the confusion, it is difficult to reach any conclusion other than that this hearing-aid patient was stolen from Audiologist 1, who simply made a referral in the patient's best interest for an otology consult.

The lesson and course of action here are simple. The lesson is that you are obligated to understand how this patient made it to your door. The course of action is to refer the patient back to Audiologist 1 once you discover the error.

This type of dilemma becomes more difficult if the patient decides at this point that your services are more desirable than those of Audiologist 1. Your actual obligation is to the source of the referral to you, the otolaryngologist. But you also have a professional obligation to your colleague. These challenges are usually managed best with open dialogue among heath-care providers.

Should You Refer Onward?

A challenging referral dilemma often occurs when a patient who is referred to you by one medical practitioner requests that you provide referral information about more specialized medical care.

Perhaps the most common example of this occurs in the child who has recurrent otitis media with effusion and is being treated by a pediatrician. In this example, the pediatrician refers to you as an audiologist to monitor the child's hearing status and middle ear function.

A typical medical treatment approach for otitis media is the initial use of antibiotics. If the treatment fails to solve the problem, surgical placement of pressure-equalization tubes in the tympanic membrane may be indicated. The decision about how long to follow the antibiotic course and when to intervene with tube placement is often a difficult one for both pediatrician and otolaryngologist. Thrown into the mix is an anxious parent and an audiologist who is concerned about the long-term effects of otitis media.

At some point in the course of care, the parent may want more aggressive treatment of her child's problem. That parent may seek your opinion for a referral to an otolaryngologist, because of an unfounded fear that to ask such a question of the pediatrician would be offensive.

What is your obligation here? You will do well to remember the original line of referral. Did you see this patient initially and refer to the pediatrician? If so, your obligation is to the patient. Did the pediatrician initially refer the patient to you for an audiologic consult? If so, your obligation is to the referral source.

As in all things, dialogue among professionals is usually the best solution to referral issues.

sessment or treatment. Again, it is important to remember that the recommendation for referral out should be made back to the original referral source, whether that be another health-care provider or the patient. For audiologists, the most common referrals are made to otolaryngologists because of identification or suspicion of active otologic disease and to speech-language pathologists because of identification or suspicion of speech and/or language impairment.

Guidelines have been developed to assist health-care providers in identifying signs and symptoms of ear disease that warrant referral for otologic consultation. The American Academy of Oto-laryngology suggest that there are seven signs of serious otologic disease that warrant referral for evaluation to an otolaryngologist. The seven signs are:

ear pain and fullness;
discharge or bleeding from the ear;
sudden or progressive hearing loss, even with recovery;
unequal hearing between ears or noise in the ear;
hearing loss after an injury, loud sound, or air travel;
slow or abnormal speech development in children; and
balance disturbance or dizziness.

Based on the results of the audiologic evaluation, the audiologist should refer for otologic consultation if:

otoscopic examination of the ear canal and tympanic membrane reveals inflammation or other signs of disease;
immittance audiometry indicates middle ear disorder;
■ acoustic reflex thresholds are abnormally elevated;
air- and bone-conduction audiometry reveals a significant air-bone gap;
speech recognition scores are significantly asymmetric or are poorer than would be expected from the degree of hearing loss or patient's age; or
other audiometric results are consistent with retrocochlear disorder.

There are also generally held guidelines for referring to the speech-language pathologist due to suspicion of speech-language delays or disorder. These include:

parental concern about speech and/or language development;
speech-language development that falls below expected milestones, as delineated in the next Clinical Note;
observed deficiency in speech production; or
observed delays in expressive or receptive language ability.

In addition to referrals to otolaryngologists and speech-language pathologists, the audiologist may also make referrals for educational evaluations, neuropsychological assessment, genetic

Hearing, Speech, and Language Expectations

If a child is suspected of having a speech or language problem, a referral should be made to a speech-language pathologist. The following questions reflect milestones in speech and language development that parents can expect from their child. Parents should consider these questions in evaluating their child's speech, language, and hearing development. Failure to reach these milestones, or a "no" answer to any of these questions, is sufficient cause for a speech-language consultation.

Behaviors Expected by 6 Months of Age

■ Does your infant stop moving or crying when you call, make noise, or play music?
■ Does your infant startle when he or she hears a sudden loud sound?
■ Can your infant find the source of a sound?

Behaviors Expected by 12 Months of Age

■ Does your baby make sounds such as *ba, ga,* or *puh*?
■ Does your baby respond to sounds such as footsteps, a ringing telephone, a spoon stirring in a cup?
■ Does your baby use one word in a meaningful way?

Behaviors Expected by 18 Months of Age

■ Does your child follow simple directions without gestures, such as *Go get your shoes; Show me your nose; Where is mommy*?
■ Will your child correctly imitate sounds that you make?
■ Does your child use at least three different words in a meaningful way?

Behaviors Expected by 24 Months of Age

■ When you show your child a picture, can he or she correctly identify five objects that you name?
■ Does your child have a speaking vocabulary of at least 20 words?
■ Does your child combine words to make little sentences, such as *Daddy go bye-bye; Me water;* or *More juice*?

Behaviors Expected by 3 Years of Age

■ Does your child remember and repeat portions of simple rhymes or songs?
■ Can your child tell the difference between words such as *my-your; in-under; big-little*?
■ Can your child answer simple questions such as *What's your name?* or *What flies?*

Behaviors Expected by 4 Years of Age

■ Does your child use three to five words in an average sentence?
■ Does your child ask a lot of questions?
■ Does your child speak fluently without stuttering or stammering?

Behaviors Expected by 5 Years of Age

■ Can your child carry on a conversation about events that have happened?
■ Is your child's voice normal? (is not hoarse; does not talk through his or her nose?)
■ Can other people understand almost everything your child says?

counseling, and so on, depending on the nature of any perceived problems.

SUMMARY

■ One important aspect in the provision of health care is the reporting of results of an evaluation or treatment outcome.
■ The challenge of reporting is to describe what was found or what was done in a clear, concise, and consistent manner.
■ The actual nature of a report can vary greatly depending on the setting and the referral source to whom a report is most likely written.
■ The goal of any report is to communicate the outcome of your evaluation and/or treatment.

■ One of the biggest challenges in report writing is to provide *all* relevant information while *only* reporting relevant information.

■ An audiologic report typically includes a description of the audiometric configuration, type of hearing loss, status of middle ear function, and recommendations.

■ Under certain circumstances, an audiologic report might also include case history information, speech audiometric results, auditory electrophysiologic results, and a statement about site of the auditory disorder.

■ Clinical reports are simply not the place to include lengthy descriptions of testing procedures, outcomes, or rehabilitative strategies. Descriptive information should be included as supplemental material and sent only to individuals who might read it.

■ As a health-care provider, it is important to understand the lines of referral and the boundaries that are dictated by those lines.

■ The concept of lines of referral and the ethics related to it are fairly simple to manage if you know the answer to two questions: who referred the patient? And for what reason?

■ As a health-care provider, the audiologist is obligated to understand when it is appropriate to refer a patient for additional assessment or treatment.

■ Referral challenges are usually managed best with open dialogue among health-care providers.

10

Introduction to Hearing Rehabilitation

A program or therapy designed to help people with hearing impairment redevelop abilities or skills they once had is described as **rehabilitative treatment.**

A program or therapy designed to help people with hearing impairment develop abilities or skills they never had is described as **habilitative treatment.**

As you have learned, the most common consequence of an auditory disorder is a loss of hearing sensitivity. In most cases, the disorder causing the sensitivity loss cannot be managed by medical or surgical intervention. Thus, to ameliorate the impairment caused by hearing sensitivity loss, **habilitative** or **rehabilitative treatment** must be implemented.

The fundamental goal of hearing rehabilitation is to limit the extent of any communication disorder that results from a hearing loss. The first step in reaching that goal is to maximize the use of residual hearing. That is, every effort is made to put the remaining hearing that a patient has to its most effective use. Once this has been done, treatment often proceeds with some form of aural rehabilitation.

The most common first step in the rehabilitation process is the use of hearing aids. More precisely, the most common treatment aimed at maximizing the use of residual hearing is the introduction of hearing-aid amplification. The most common form of amplification is the conventional hearing aid. In some cases, other assistive listening devices may be used to supplement or substitute for hearing aid use. In individuals with a profound loss of hearing, a cochlear implant may be indicated.

When hearing aids were first developed, they were relatively large in size and inflexible in terms of their amplifying characteristics. Hearing aid use was restricted almost exclusively to individuals with substantial conductive hearing loss. Today's hearing aids are much smaller, and their amplification characteristics can be programmed at will. Hearing aids are now used almost exclusively by those with sensorineural hearing loss.

Candidacy for hearing aid amplification is fairly straightforward. If a patient has a sensorineural hearing impairment that is causing a communication disorder, the patient is a candidate for amplification. Thus, even when a hearing impairment is mild, if it is causing difficulty with communication, the patient is likely to benefit from hearing aid amplification. If a patient has a conductive hearing loss, it can usually be treated medically. If all attempts at medical treatment have been exhausted, then the same rule of candidacy applies for conductive hearing loss.

When a hearing loss is the same in both ears, it is considered **symmetric.** When a hearing loss is moderate in one ear and severe in the other, it is considered **asymmetric.**

A person wearing two hearing aids is fitted **binaurally**; a person wearing one is fitted **monaurally.**

If a patient has hearing impairment in both ears that is fairly **symmetric**, it is a good idea to fit that patient with two hearing aids. In fact, up to 95% of individuals with hearing impairment are **binaural** candidates. Benefits from binaural hearing aids include enhancements in:

- audibility of speech originating from different directions,
- localization of sound, and
- hearing speech in noisy environments.

In addition, evidence exists that the use of only one hearing aid in patients with **bilateral** hearing loss may have a long-term detrimental effect on the ear that is not fitted with an aid. Except for cost, there are no good reasons not to wear two hearing aids.

When a hearing loss occurs in both ears, it is **bilateral**; when it occurs in only one ear it is **unilateral.**

The process of obtaining hearing aids begins with a thorough audiological assessment. Following the audiological assessment, prudent hearing health care dictates a medical assessment to rule out any active pathology that might contraindicate hearing aid use. Following medical clearance, impressions of the ears and ear canals are made for customizing earmolds or hearing aid devices. When the devices are received from the manufacturer, they are adjusted and fitted to the patient, and an evaluation is made of the patient's performance with the hearing aids. After successful fitting and dispensing, the patient usually returns for any necessary minor adjustments or to discuss any problems related to hearing aid use. At that time, self-assessed benefit or satisfaction is often measured as a means of assessing treatment outcome.

Although the goal of hearing rehabilitation is relatively constant, the approach can vary significantly depending on patient age, the nature of the hearing impairment, and the extent of communication requirements in daily life. For example, in infants and young children, the extent of sensitivity loss may not be precisely quantified, making hearing aid fitting of children a more protracted challenge than it is in most adults. In addition, extensive habilitative treatment aimed at ensuring oral language development will be implemented in young children, whereas little rehabilitation beyond hearing aid orientation may be required in adults.

Hearing rehabilitation will also vary based on the nature and degree of hearing impairment. For example, patients with profound hearing loss are likely to benefit more from a cochlear implant than from conventional hearing aid amplification. As another example, patients with auditory processing disorders associated with aging may benefit from the use of assistive listening devices as supplements to their conventional hearing aids.

Finally, hearing rehabilitation can vary depending on the communication demands that patients have in their daily lives. For example, an older patient who lives a solitary lifestyle will have different rehabilitative needs than a patient with job-related communication demands and an active lifestyle. The type of amplification system required and the need for aural rehabilitation can vary considerably between these extremes of communication demand.

THE FIRST QUESTIONS

Rehabilitation really begins with assessment—not only assessment of hearing, but also assessment of rehabilitative needs. The hearing evaluation serves as a first step in the rehabilitation process. Toward this end, there are some important questions to be answered from the audiological evaluation. They include:

■ Is there evidence of a hearing disorder?
■ Can medically treatable conditions be ruled out?
■ What is the extent of the patient's hearing sensitivity loss?
■ How well does the patient understand speech and process auditory information?
■ Is the hearing disorder causing impairment?
■ Does the hearing impairment cause a hearing handicap?
■ Are there any auditory factors that contraindicate successful hearing-device use?

Answers to these questions will lead to a decision about the patient's candidacy for hearing aid amplification from an auditory perspective. Equally important, however, are the questions to be answered from an assessment of rehabilitative needs. They include:

■ Why is the patient seeking hearing aid amplification?
■ How motivated is the patient to use amplification successfully?
■ Under what conditions is the hearing loss causing communication difficulty?
■ What are the demands on the patient's communication abilities?
■ What is the patient's physical, psychological, and sociological status?
■ What human resources are available to the patient to support successful amplification use?
■ What financial resources are available to the patient to support audiological rehabilitation?

The answers to these questions help to determine candidacy for hearing aid amplification and begin to provide the audiologist with the insight necessary to determine the type and extent of the hearing rehabilitation process.

The Importance of Asking Why

Why is the patient seeking hearing aid amplification? It sounds like such a simple question. Yet the answer is a very important step in the treatment process because it guides the audiologist to an appropriate rehabilitative strategy. There are usually two main issues related to this *why* question, one pertaining to the patient's motivation and the other pertaining to the need-specific nature of the amplification strategy.

The first reason for asking why a patient is pursuing hearing aid use is to determine, to the extent possible, the factors that motivated the patient to seek your services. Motivation is important because it is highly correlated with prognosis; **prognosis** is important because it is highly correlated with success and tends to dictate the strength and direction of your efforts.

Prognosis is the prediction of the course or outcome of a disease or treatment.

Do you want to see an audiologist wince? Watch as a patient states that the only reason he or she is pursuing hearing aid use is because his or her spouse is forcing the issue. If this truly is the only reason that the patient is seeking hearing aid amplification, the prognosis for successful use is poor.

A patient who is internally motivated to hear better is an excellent candidate for successful hearing aid use. The breadth of amplification options for such a patient is substantial. For example, patients with a moderate sensorineural hearing loss will benefit from conventional hearing aids in many of their daily activities. They might also find a telephone amplifier to be of benefit at home and work and are likely to avail themselves of the assistive listening devices available in many public theaters, churches, or other meeting facilities. Such a patient will use two hearing aids, permitting better hearing in noise and better localization ability, and will probably want digitally programmable hearing aids to ensure better adaptation to changing acoustic environments.

In contrast, a patient who seeks audiologic care as a result of external factors will find any of a number of reasons why hearing aid amplification is not satisfactory. The patient will find the sound of a hearing aid to be unnatural and noisy, the battery replacement costs to be excessive, and the gadgetry associated with assistive devices to be a nuisance. Such a patient will insist on wearing one hearing aid and will complain about the difficulty hearing in noise when the aid is on. The patient will probably want a nonprogrammable hearing aid and be dissatisfied when it cannot be adjusted limitlessly to address the patient's hearing needs.

The contrast in motivation can be striking, as can the contrast in your ability as an audiologist to meet the patient's needs and expectations. Knowing *why* from a motivation viewpoint is an important first question.

Another reason that the *why* question is so important is that it can lead to successful yet unconventional solutions to the patient's hearing needs. Twenty years ago, this did not really matter. Hearing aids varied little, and there was no need to distinguish between conventional and **need-specific amplification**, because need-specific amplification was not readily available. Today, amplification options are numerous and growing. You will learn more in subsequent chapters about the burgeoning technology available to those with hearing impairment. The growing advantage is that amplification can be tailored to a patient's communication needs rather than used generically for all hearing losses and all individuals. The result is that patients can be treated more effectively by adapting the technology to the patient's needs rather than asking the patient to adapt to the technology.

Need-specific amplification includes such devices as FM systems, TV amplifiers, doorbell and telephone amplifiers, and other assistive listening devices designed to meet a specific need.

A simple example of need-specific amplification may serve to make the point. Suppose that a patient's only hearing concern is that she cannot hear the television when it is set to a volume that is comfortable for her spouse. In the past, there was a tendency on the part of hearing care providers to ignore this information, assuming that they knew what was best for this patient and insisting on a general solution (i.e., conventional hearing aids) to this specific problem. The general solution was helpful, of course, but it could have been much better if it had been tailored to the patient's need to hear the television. Today's technology is making need-specific amplification so much of a reality that the question *why* is becoming ever more important.

Assessment of need can be carried out informally, or it can be carried out formally with a questionnaire. An example of a questionnaire that addresses the situational-specific needs of individuals with hearing impairment is shown in Figure 10–1. Either the formal or informal approach can lead the audiologist to an impression of whether the individual's amplification needs are

Sample Questions from the Abbreviated Profile of HearingAid Benefit	A Always (99%) B Almost Always (87%) C Generally (75%) D Half-the-time (50%) E Occasionally (25%) F Seldom (12%) G Never (1%)

When I am in a crowded grocery store, talking
with the cashier, I can follow the conversation .... A B C D E F G

Unexpected sounds, like a smoke detector or
alarm bell are uncomfortable .... A B C D E F G

I have trouble understanding dialogue in a
movie or at the theater.................................... A B C D E F G

When I am listening to the news on the car
radio, and family members are talking, I have
trouble hearing the news .... A B C D E F G

Traffic noises are too loud .... A B C D E F G

When I am in a small office, interviewing or
answering questions, I have difficulty
following the conversation................................ A B C D E F G

When I am having a quiet conversation with a
friend, I have difficulty understanding .... A B C D E F G

When a speaker is addressing a small group,
and everyone is listening quietly, I have to
strain to understand .... A B C D E F G

I can understand conversation even when
several people are talking................................. A B C D E F G

It's hard for me to understand what is being
said at lectures or church services .... A B C D E F G

**Answers are divided into subscales. Results are expressed as
percentage of benefit for each subscale.**

Figure 10-1. Sample questions from a self-assessment questionnaire, the Abbreviated Profile of Hearing Aid Benefit. (From The Abbreviated Profile of Hearing Aid Benefit (APHAB), by R. M. Cox and G. C. Alexander, 1995, *Ear and Hearing, 16,* 176–186.)

general, requiring the use of conventional amplification solutions, or more specific, requiring a more tailored solution.

Once patients' motivation and needs are known, the rehabilitative assessment proceeds to using the available audiometric and self-assessment data to determine candidacy for rehabilitation and to help determine an effective amplification approach.

Assessment of Rehabilitative Candidacy

The goal of the rehabilitative assessment is to determine candidacy for auditory rehabilitation. The process for doing so includes several important steps. The first step is often the audiological evaluation, which will determine the type and extent of hearing loss. Following the audiological evaluation, the patient is counseled about the nature of the results and recommendations to assist in the decision about whether to pursue amplification. Once the decision is made to go forward, the rehabilitation assessment continues with an evaluation of the patient's communication needs, self-assessment of handicap, psychosocial status, physical capacity, and financial status.

If the decision is made to pursue hearing aid use, medical clearance will need to be procured from a physician. This typically involves otoscopic inspection of the external auditory meatus and tympanic membrane, in an effort to ensure that no medical conditions exist that would contraindicate use of a hearing aid.

Audiological Assessment

The audiologic assessment for rehabilitative purposes is the same as that described in detail in Chapters 5 and 6. For the most part the strategies and techniques used for diagnostic assessment and rehabilitative assessment are identical. The reasons for the assessment are different, however, and that tends to change the manner in which the outcomes are viewed. For example, air-conduction and bone-conduction audiometry are used to determine the extent of any conductive component to the hearing loss. Diagnostically that information might be used to confirm the influence of middle ear disorder and for pre- and postassessment of surgical success. From the nonmedical rehabilitation perspective, a conductive component to the hearing loss has a significant impact on how much amplification a hearing aid will need to deliver to the ear. Although the clinical strategy, instrumentation, and techniques are the same, the outcome has different meaning diagnostically and rehabilitatively.

As always, assessment begins with the case history. The audiologist will begin here to pursue information about and develop impressions of the patient's motivation for hearing aid amplification, should it prove to be indicated by the audiometric results.

The next step in the evaluation is the otoscopic inspection of the auricle, external auditory canal, and tympanic membrane. The fundamental reasons for doing this are to inspect for any obvious signs of ear disease and to ensure an unimpeded canal for insert earphones or immittance probe placement. However, if the patient appears to be a candidate for amplification, the audiologist also uses this opportunity to begin to form an impression of the fitting challenges that will be presented by the size and shape of the patient's ear canal.

Immittance audiometry is used to assess middle-ear function in an effort to rule out middle-ear disorder as a contributing factor to the hearing loss. This is no different for rehabilitative than for diagnostic assessment.

Air-conduction pure-tone audiometry is used to quantify hearing sensitivity across the audiometric frequency range. If immittance measures show middle ear disorder, then bone-conduction audiometry is used to quantify the extent of any conductive component to the hearing loss. The air-conduction thresholds and the size of the conductive component are both crucial pieces of information for determination of the appropriate hearing aid amplification characteristics.

Speech audiometry is at least as important to the rehabilitative assessment as it is to the diagnostic assessment. Speech recognition ability is an important indicator of how the ear functions at suprathreshold levels. If speech perception is significantly degraded or if it is unusually affected by the presence of background noise, the prognosis for successful conventional hearing aid use may be reduced. Conventional speech audiometric measures of word recognition ability in quiet may be useful in this context, but more sophisticated assessment of speech recognition in competition is probably a better prognostic indicator of satisfaction with hearing aid use.

Determination of frequency-specific thresholds of discomfort is a very important component of the rehabilitation assessment but is seldom carried out as part of a diagnostic assessment. A *threshold of discomfort* (TD) is just as it sounds, the level at which a sound becomes uncomfortable to the listener. Many terms are used to describe this level, the most generic and perhaps useful of which is the threshold of discomfort. Some of the other terms and a technique for determining TDs are described in the following Clinical Note. Determination of the TD across the frequency range is important because it provides guidance about the maximum output levels of a hearing aid that will be tolerable to the patient. More will be said about all of that in Chapters 11 and 12.

All of the information gleaned from the case history and audiologic evaluation is taken together to determine the potential candidacy of the patient for hearing aid amplification. Once the determination is made, a rehabilitation assessment is completed.

Rehabilitation Assessment

The rehabilitation assessment is carried out using a patient-centered approach and is designed to determine the self-perception and family-perception of handicap; the patient's physical, psychological, and sociological status; and the sufficiency of human and financial resources to support hearing rehabilitation. Specifically, the following areas are assessed in one manner or another:

- communication needs
- self- and family-assessment of handicap or disability
- motoric and other physical abilities
- psychosocial status
- financial status

Assessment of communication needs was discussed earlier. Its importance is paramount in the provision of properly focused hearing rehabilitation services. Communication needs should be thoroughly examined prior to determination of an amplification strategy.

Self-assessment of handicap or disability is an important component of the rehabilitation process. Many examples of self-assessment scales are available, one of which is described in the Clinical Note on page 451. There are several important reasons for measuring the extent to which a hearing impairment is disabling or handicapping to a patient. One is that it provides the audiologist with additional information about the patient's communication needs and motivation. Another is that it serves as a

How to Determine a TD

Determination of a threshold of discomfort (TD) is an important early step in the hearing aid fitting process. The goal of determining discomfort levels is to set the maximum output of a hearing aid at a level that permits the widest dynamic range of hearing possible without letting loud sounds be amplified to uncomfortable levels. This is critical to the patient's satisfaction.

Numerous terms have been used to describe the threshold of discomfort, including uncomfortable loudness (UCL), uncomfortable level (UL), upper limits of comfortable loudness (ULCL), uncomfortable loudness level (ULL), and loudness discomfort level (LDL). The term *threshold of discomfort* is a reasonable alternative to these because discomfort can be related to quality of a signal as well as its loudness.

Many factors need to be considered in determining a discomfort level. Instructions to patients, type of signals used, and response strategies can all influence the measurement of TDs.

Following is a protocol for determining threshold of discomfort (after Mueller & Bright, 1994):

1. Provide concise instructions to the patient about the purpose of the test and the desired response. You are trying to find a level that is somewhere between "initial discomfort" and "extreme discomfort." That level is usually described as "definite discomfort" or "uncomfortably loud."
2. Provide patients with a list of descriptions, such as those in the following figure, relating to the loudness of sounds that will be presented.
3. Use pure-tone signals of 500, 1000, 1500, 2000, and 3000 Hz.
4. Use an ascending method, in 2 or 5 dB steps. Present the pure-tone signal to the patient and increase it until the listener indicates uncomfortable loudness. Reduce the intensity to a comfortable level and then increase again until it is uncomfortable. The TD is taken as the level that gives the perception of loudness between "loud but O.K." and "uncomfortably loud" on two out of three trials.

Mueller, H. G., & Bright, K. E. (1994). Selection and verification of maximum output. In M. Valente (Ed.), *Strategies for selecting and verifying hearing aid fittings* (pp. 38–63). New York: Thieme Medical Publishers, Inc.

continued

Loudness Levels

- Painfully loud
- Extremely uncomfortable
- Uncomfortably loud
- Loud, but O.K.
- Comfortable, but slightly loud
- Comfortable
- Comfortable, but slightly soft
- Soft
- Very soft

Response card containing a list of descriptions relating to the loudness of sounds that can be used to determine threshold of discomfort.

baseline assessment against which to compare the eventual benefits gained from hearing aid amplification.

Some audiologists will ask a patient to have a spouse or significant other complete an assessment scale along with the patient. By doing so, the audiologist can gain insight into communication needs that the patient may overlook or underestimate. The process has an added benefit of providing the family with a forum for communicating about the communication disorder.

Physical ability, particularly fine motor ability, can be an important factor in successful use of hearing aid amplification. Particularly in the aging population, reduced fine motor control can make manipulation of conventional hearing aids and hearing aid batteries a challenging endeavor. Assessment should occur prior to the time of fitting a particular hearing device.

Self-Assessment Scales

Self-assessment scales are an important part of the rehabilitation process. They provide quantifiable information about communication needs and motivation and serve as a baseline assessment against which to compare hearing-aid benefit.

Many good self-assessment scales are available. Some are designed for specific populations, such as the elderly; others are designed to be generally applicable. One example of the self-assessment scale that enjoys widespread use is the APHAB, or Abbreviated Profile of Hearing Aid Benefit (Cox & Alexander, 1995). The APHAB consists of 24 items that describe various listening situations. A sample of these items is shown in Figure 10–1. The patient's task is to judge how often a particular situation is experienced, ranging from *never* to *always*. Answers are assigned a percentage, and the scale is scored in terms of those percentages.

Results of the assessment scale can be analyzed into four subscales:

- ease of communication, describing communication effort in easy listening environments;
- reverberation, describing speech recognition ability in reverberant conditions;
- background noise, describing speech recognition ability in the presence of competing sound; and
- aversiveness to sound, describing negative reactions to sound.

The APHAB is often administered at the time of the initial hearing aid consultation. If hearing aids are fitted, the scale can be readministered at a follow-up appointment to quantify self-perceived benefit from the devices.

Cox, R. M., & Alexander, G. C. (1995). The abbreviated profile of hearing aid benefit. *Ear and Hearing, 16,* 176–186.

Visual ability is also an important component of the communication process and can have an impact on hearing rehabilitation. Most people benefit to some extent from the compensation afforded high-frequency hearing loss through the use of speechreading of the lips and face. A reduction in visual acuity can reduce the prognosis for successful hearing rehabilitation.

Mental status, psychological well-being, and social environment can all have an impact on the success of a hearing rehabilitation program. Memory constraints or other affected cognitive functioning can limit the usefulness of certain types of amplification approaches. Attitude, motivation, and readiness are all psychological factors that can impact hearing rehabilitation. In addition, the availability of human resources, such as family and friends, can have a significant positive impact on the prognosis for successful hearing aid use. Although most audiologists do not assess these factors directly, most do use directed dialogue techniques during the preliminary rehabilitative counseling to assess these various areas for obvious problems.

Hearing aid amplification is expensive. A frank discussion of the expenses related to hearing aids is an important component of any rehabilitation evaluation.

Once the rehabilitative assessment is completed, the rehabilitation challenge begins. Prepared with a knowledge of the patient's hearing ability, communication needs, and overall resources, the audiologist can begin the challenge of implementing hearing aid rehabilitation.

THE AUDIOLOGIST'S CHALLENGE

The audiologist faces a number of clinical challenges during the rehabilitative process. One of the first challenges is to determine whether the patient is an appropriate candidate for amplification or whether the prognosis is such that hearing aids should not be considered. Certain types of disorders and audiometric configurations pose daunting hearing aid challenges. Thus, the first step in the rehabilitative process is to determine whether the patient is likely to benefit from amplification. Once a decision has been made that the patient is a candidate, the rehabilitation process includes a determination of type of amplification system, implementation of the actual fitting of the devices, validation of the fit, and specification of additional treatment needs.

Amplification—Yes or No?

As a general rule, most patients who seek hearing aids can benefit from their use. Thus, in most cases the answer to the question of whether a patient should pursue amplification is an easy *yes,* and the challenges are related to getting the type and fitting correct.

Even in cases in which the prognosis for successful hearing aid use is poor, most audiologists will make an effort to find an amplification solution if the patient is sufficiently motivated. In the extreme case, however, the potential for benefit is sufficiently marginal that pursuit of hearing aid use is not even recommended. Some of the factors that negatively impact prognosis for success include:

- patient does not perceive a problem
- not enough hearing loss
- too much hearing loss
- a "difficult" hearing loss configuration
- very poor speech recognition ability
- central auditory processing disorder
- active disease process in the ear canal

Although none of these factors preclude hearing aid use, they can limit the potential that might otherwise be achieved by well fitted amplification.

A patient who does not perceive the hearing loss to be a significant problem is usually one with a slowly progressive, high-frequency hearing loss. This tends to be the patient who can "hear a (low-frequency) dog bark three blocks away" or could understand his spouse "if she would just speak more clearly." Some of this denial is understandable because the loss has grown gradually, and the patient has adjusted to it. Many people with a hearing loss of this nature will not view it as sufficiently handicapping to require the assistance of hearing aids. As an audiologist you might be able to show the patient that he will obtain significant benefit from hearing aid use, and you probably should try. But the prognosis for successful use is limited by the patient's lack of motivation and recognition of the nature of the problem. In this case, greatest success will probably come with patience. It would be a wise clinical decision to simply educate the patient about hearing loss and the potential benefit of hearing aid use. Then, when the patient's hearing loss progresses and becomes a handicap, he will be aware of his amplification options.

Some patients have a hearing loss, but it is not sufficient in magnitude for hearing aid use. The definition of "sufficient" has changed dramatically over the years. Currently, even patients with minimal hearing losses can wear mild gain hearing aids with success. As a general rule, if the hearing impairment is enough to cause a problem in communication, the patient is a candidate for hearing aids. Nevertheless, a certain minimum degree and configuration of loss must occur before hearing aid use is warranted.

Some patients have too much hearing loss for hearing aid use. Profound hearing loss can limit the usefulness of even the most powerful hearing aids. You will learn in the next chapter that the amount of amplification boost or gain that a hearing aid can provide has its limits. In many cases of profound hearing loss, a hearing aid can provide only environmental awareness or some rudimentary perception of speech. Many patients will not consider this to be valuable enough to warrant the use of hearing aids. In these cases, cochlear implantation is often the rehabilitation strategy that is most beneficial.

For some audiometric configurations, it is very challenging to provide appropriate amplification. Two examples are shown in Figure 10–2. One difficult configuration is the high-frequency precipitous loss. In this case, hearing sensitivity is normal through 2000 Hz, and drops off dramatically at higher frequencies. Trying to amplify the higher frequency sounds exclusively presents a whole series of challenges, not the least of which is that the sound quality is usually not very pleasing to the patient. Depending on the frequency at which the loss begins and the slope of the loss, these types of hearing loss can be very difficult to fit effectively. The other extreme is the so-called *reverse slope* hearing loss, a relatively unusual audiometric configuration in which a hearing loss occurs at the low frequencies, but not the high frequencies. The first problem with respect to amplification is that this type of loss seldom causes enough of a communication problem to warrant hearing aid use. When it does, certain aspects of the fitting can be troublesome, and the prognosis for successful fitting is somewhat limited.

Some types of cochlear hearing loss, such as that due to endolymphatic hydrops, can cause substantial distortion of the incoming sound, resulting in very poor speech recognition ability. If it is poor enough, hearing aid amplification simply will not be effective in overcoming the hearing loss. Regardless of how much or what type of amplification is used to deliver signals to the ear, the cochlea distorts the signal to an extent that hearing aid benefit may be limited. Fortunately, this type of disorder is seldom bilateral, but when it is, hearing aid use will benefit audibility but may not be satisfactory overall.

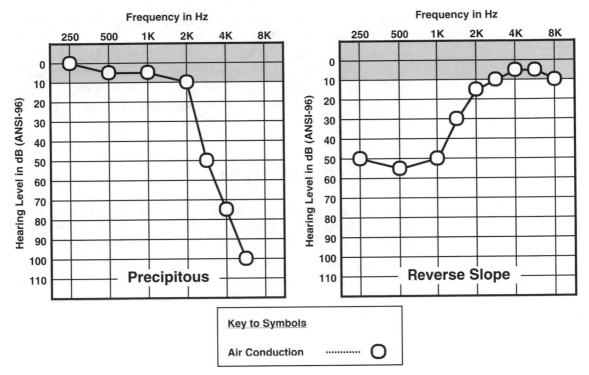

Figure 10-2. Two challenging audiometric configurations for the appropriate fitting of amplification.

Central auditory processing disorders in young children and in aging adults can reduce the benefit from conventional hearing aid amplification. In fact, it is not unusual for geriatric patients who were once successful hearing aid users to experience increasingly less success as their central auditory nervous system changes with age. The problem is seldom extreme enough to preclude hearing aid use, but these patients may benefit more from assistive listening devices to complement conventional hearing aid use.

There are some physical and medical limitations that can make conventional hearing aid use difficult. Occasionally a patient with hearing loss will have external otitis or ear drainage that cannot be controlled medically. Even if the patient has medical clearance for hearing aid use, placing a hearing aid in such an ear can be a constant source of problems. Other problems that limit access to the ear canal include canal stenosis and certain rare pain disorders. In such cases, amplification strategies other than conventional hearing aids must be employed if hearing rehabilitation is to be successful.

These are some of the factors that make hearing aid fitting difficult. It should be emphasized again, however, that if a person is having a communication disorder from a hearing loss, there is a very high likelihood that the person can benefit from some form of hearing aid amplification. That is, the answer to the question of amplification is usually *yes*, although the question of how to do it successfully is sometimes challenging.

Amplification Strategies

Once the decision has been made to pursue the use of hearing aid amplification, the challenge has just begun. At the very beginning of the hearing aid fitting process, the audiologist must formulate an amplification strategy based on the outcome of the rehabilitation assessment. Various patient factors will have an impact on the decisions made about amplification alternatives. These include:

- hearing loss factors
    - type of loss
    - degree of loss
    - audiometric configuration
    - speech perception

- medical factors
    - progressive loss
    - fluctuating loss
    - auricular limitations

- physical factors

- cognitive factors

With these patient-related considerations in mind, the audiologist must make decisions about amplification strategies, approaches, and options, including:

- type of amplification system
    - conventional hearing aids
    - assistive listening device
    - cochlear implant

- which ear

    monaural versus binaural

    better ear or poorer ear

    contralateral routing of signals

- conventional hearing aid options

    signal processing strategy

    device style

The type of amplification strategy is dictated by various patient factors. Clearly though, the vast majority of patients with hearing impairment can benefit from conventional hearing aid amplification. It is only the exceptional patient that will go on to exclusive use of an assistive device or to a cochlear implant. And even in these cases, conventional hearing aids are likely to be tried as the initial amplification strategy. In general then, except in the rare circumstances described in the previous section, the decision is made to pursue hearing aid use.

The second group of options tends to be an easy decision as well. In most cases, the best answer to the question of which ear to fit is *both*. There are several important reasons for having two ears. The ability to localize the source of a sound in the environment relies heavily on hearing with both ears. The brain evaluates signals delivered to both ears for differences that provide important clues as to the location of the source of a sound. This binaural processing enhances the audibility of speech originating from different directions. The use of two ears is also important in the ability to suppress background noise. This ability is of great importance to the listener in focusing on speech or other sounds of interest in the foreground. Hearing is also more sensitive with two ears than with one. All of these factors create a **binaural advantage** for the listener with two ears. Thus, if a patient has symmetric hearing loss or asymmetry that is not too extensive, the patient will benefit more from two hearing aids than from one hearing aid. There is one other compelling reason to fit two hearing aids. Evidence suggests that fitting a hearing aid to only one ear places the unaided ear at a relative disadvantage. This asymmetry may have a long-term detrimental effect on the processing ability of the unaided ear. Thus, in general, it is a good idea to fit binaural hearing aids whenever possible.

Sometimes it is not possible to fit binaural hearing aids effectively. This usually occurs when the difference in hearing between

Enhanced hearing with two ears is called a **binaural advantage**.

the two ears is substantial. In cases where both ears have hearing loss, but there is significant asymmetry between ears, it is generally more appropriate to fit a hearing aid on the better hearing ear than on the poorer hearing ear. The logic is that the better hearing ear will perform better with amplification than the poorer hearing ear. Thus, fitting of the better ear will provide the best aided ability of either monaural fitting. There are exceptions, of course, but they relate mostly to difficult configurations on the better hearing ear.

The extreme case of asymmetry is in the case of unilateral hearing loss, with the other ear being normal. If the poorer ear can be effectively fitted with a hearing aid, then obviously a monaural fitting is indicated. If the poorer ear cannot be effectively fitted, then another option is to use an approach termed *contralateral routing of signals* (CROS). This approach uses a microphone and hearing aid on the poorer or nonhearing ear and delivers signals to the other ear either through bone conduction or via a receiving device worn on the normal hearing ear. Although this type of fitting is rare, it is often used effectively on patients with profound unilateral hearing loss due, for example, to a viral infection or secondary to surgery to remove an VIIIth nerve tumor.

Once the ear or ears have been determined, a decision must be made about the type of signal processing that will be used in the hearing aids. This decision relates to the acoustic characteristics of the response of the hearing aids and includes:

- how much amplification gain to provide in each frequency range;
- whether the amount of amplification varies with the input level of the sound;
- what the maximum intensity level that the hearing aids can generate will be;
- how the maximum level will be limited;
- whether the hearing aids will have analog, digital, or digitally-controlled analog processing; and
- whether the hearing aids will have one setting or multiple settings.

Once the signal processing strategy has been determined, a decision must be made about the style of hearing aids to be fitted. In reality, the decisions might not be made in that order. Some patients will insist on a particular style of hearing aid, which may limit some of the features that can be included. In the best of all worlds, however, the audiologist would decide on processing strategy first and let that dictate the potential styles. There are two general styles of conventional hearing aids. One type is the *behind-the-ear* (BTE) hearing aid. It hangs over the auricle and delivers sound to the ear through a custom-made earmold. The other type is the *in-the-ear* (ITE) hearing aid. An ITE hearing aid has all of its components encased in a customized shell that fits into the ear. Subgroups of ITE hearing aids include *in-the-canal* (ITC) hearing aids and *completely-in-the-canal* (CIC) hearing aids. The decision about whether to choose an ITE or BTE hearing aid is related to several factors, including degree and configuration of hearing loss and the physical size and limitations of the ear canal and auricle. You will learn more about these devices and the challenges of fitting them in Chapter 11.

As you can see, the audiologist has a number of decisions to make about the amplification strategy and a number of patient factors to keep in mind while making those decisions. The experienced audiologist will approach all of these options in a very direct way. The audiologist will want to fit the patient with two hearing aids with superior signal processing capability and maximum programmable flexibility, in a style that is acceptable to the patient at a price that the patient can afford. That is the audiologist's goal and serves as the starting point in the fitting process. The ultimate goal may then be altered by various patient factors until the best set of compromises can be reached.

Approaches to Fitting Hearing Instruments

Preselection of an amplification strategy, signal processing options, and hearing aid style is followed by the actual fitting of a device. There are a number of approaches to fitting hearing instruments, but most share some factors in common. Fitting of hearing instruments usually includes the following:

- estimating an amplification target for soft, moderate, and loud sounds;
- adjusting the hearing aid parameters to meet the targets;
- ensuring that soft sounds are audible;
- ensuring that discomfort levels are not exceeded;
- asking the patient to judge the quality or intelligibility of amplified speech; and
- readjusting gain as indicated.

The first general step in the fitting process is to determine target gain. *Gain* is the amount of amplification provided by the hearing aid and is specified in decibels. *Target gain* is an estimate of how much amplification will be needed at a given frequency for a given patient. The target is generated based on pure-tone audiometric thresholds and is calculated based on any number of gain rules that have been developed over the years. A simple example is a gain rule that has been used since 1944, known as the half-gain rule. It stated that the target gain should be one-half of the number of decibels of hearing loss at a given frequency, so that a hearing loss of 40 dB at 1000 Hz would require 20 dB of hearing aid gain at that frequency. A number of such gain rules have been developed to assist in the preliminary setting of hearing aid gain.

Current hearing aid technology permits the setting and achieving of targets in much more sophisticated ways. The audiologist can now specify targets for soft sounds to ensure that they are audible, for moderate sounds to assure that they are comfortable, and for loud sounds to ensure that they are loud, but not uncomfortable. Many of these types of targets can be calculated from pure-tone air-conduction thresholds and patient discomfort levels.

Once a target or targets have been determined by the audiologist, the hearing aids are adjusted in an attempt to match those targets. Typically, this is done by measuring the output of the hearing aids in a hearing aid analyzer or in the patient's ear canal. The gain of the hearing aids is then adjusted until the target is reached or approximated across the frequency range.

One important goal of fitting hearing aids is to make soft sounds audible. Often in the fitting process this will be assessed by delivering soft sounds to the hearing aids and measuring the amount of amplification at the tympanic membrane or, more directly, by measuring the patient's thresholds in the sound field.

Another important goal of fitting hearing aids is to keep loud sounds from being uncomfortable. Again, this can be assessed indirectly by measuring the output of the hearing aids at the tympanic membrane to high-intensity sound. Or it can be assessed directly by delivering loud sounds to the patient and having the patient judge whether the sound is uncomfortably loud.

Once the parameters of the hearing aids have been adjusted to meet target gains, the patient's response to speech targets is assessed. This can be accomplished in a number of ways, some of which are formal and some informal. The general idea, however, is the same: to determine whether the quality of amplified speech is judged to be acceptable and/or whether the extent to which speech is judged to be intelligible is acceptable. Should either be judged to be unacceptable, modifications are made in the hearing aid response.

Challenges in the fitting of hearing aids are numerous. Specific approaches, gain targets, instrumentation used, and verification techniques can vary from clinic to clinic or from audiologist to audiologist within a clinic. The goal, however, is usually the same: to deliver good sound quality and maximize speech intelligibility.

Approaches to Defining Success

With so many hearing aid options and so many different fitting strategies, one of the audiologists' biggest challenges is knowing when they got it right. That is, how does the audiologist know that the fitting was successful, and against what standards is it judged to be good enough?

Defining hearing aid success has been a challenging and elusive target for many years. In the early years, when type of hearing aid and circuit selection were limited to a very few choices, the question was often simply of a yes or no variety—yes, it helps, or no, it doesn't. Today, there are so many options that validation of the one chosen is much more difficult. In general, there are two approaches to validating the hearing aid selection and fitting procedures:

- aided speech recognition measures, and
- self-assessment scales.

Aided speech recognition measures are designed to assess the patient's ability to recognize speech targets with and without hearing aids. They are typically presented in the presence of background competition in an attempt to mimic real-life listening situations. The goal of carrying out aided speech recognition testing is to ensure that the patient is provided with some expected level of performance. These measures can also be used if there is an issue about the potential benefits of monaural versus binaural amplification fitting.

Another method for defining amplification success is the use of self-assessment scales. An example of one scale was described earlier in this chapter in the Clinical Note on page 451. This measure is often given to the patient prior to hearing aid fitting and then again at some later date after the patient has had time to adjust to using the hearing aids. The goal again is to ensure that the patient is provided with some expected level of benefit from the devices. Self-assessments scales are now used extensively as a means for judging clinical outcomes of hearing aid fitting.

Treatment Planning

The fitting of hearing aids is the first component of the treatment plan. The process attempts to address the first goal, that of maximizing the use of residual hearing. From that point, the audiologist is challenged to determine the benefit of the amplification and, if it is inadequate, to plan additional intervention strategies. In all cases, the audiologist must convey to patients and families the importance of understanding the nature of hearing impairment and the benefits and limitations of hearing aids.

The need for and the nature of additional intervention strategies are usually not a reflection of the adequacy of the initial amplification fitting. Rather, needs vary considerably, depending on patient factors, such as age, communication demands, and degree of loss.

Many patients do not require additional treatment. Theirs is a sensory loss, the hearing aids ameliorated the effects of that loss, and their only ongoing needs are related to periodic re-evaluations.

For other patients, the fitting of hearing aids simply constitutes the beginning of a long process of habilitation or rehabilitation. Children may need intensive language stimulation programs, classroom assistive devices, and speech therapy. Adults may need speechreading classes, telephone amplifiers, and personal FM systems.

SUMMARY

- ■ The fundamental goal of hearing rehabilitation is to limit the extent of any communication disorder that results from a hearing loss.
- ■ The first step in reaching that goal is to maximize the use of residual hearing, usually by the introduction of hearing-aid amplification.

- If a patient has a sensorineural hearing impairment that is causing a communication disorder, the patient is a candidate for amplification.
- The goal of the rehabilitative assessment is to determine candidacy for auditory rehabilitation.
- The rehabilitation assessment determines the self-perception and family-perception of handicap; the patient's physical, psychological, and sociological status; and the sufficiency of human and financial resources to support hearing rehabilitation.
- The first step in the rehabilitative process is to determine whether the patient is likely to benefit from amplification.
- Patient factors, including hearing impairment, medical condition, physical ability, and cognitive capacity, impact the decisions made about amplification alternatives.
- Preselection of amplification includes decisions about type of amplification system, signal processing strategy, and device style.
- Fitting of hearing instruments usually includes estimation of amplification targets, adjustment of hearing aid parameters to meet those targets, and verification of hearing aid performance and benefit.
- Many patients do not require additional treatment; for others, hearing aid fitting is only the beginning of the rehabilitative process.

SUGGESTED READINGS

Alpiner, J. G., & McCarthy, P. A. (1993). *Rehabilitative audiology: Children and adults* (2nd ed.). Baltimore: Williams & Wilkins.

Hull R. H. (1996). *Aural rehabilitation: Serving children and adults* (3rd ed.). San Diego: Singular Publishing Group.

Ripich, D. (Ed.). (1991). *Handbook of geriatric communication disorders.* Austin, TX: Pro-Ed.

Valente, M. (Ed.). (1994). *Strategies for selecting and verifying hearing aid fittings.* New York: Thieme Medical Publishing.

The Audiologist's Rehabilitative Tools: Hearing Instruments

Hearing-instrument technology advances at a rapid pace. Today's hearing instruments use digital signal processing, provide high fidelity sound reproduction, are small enough to fit into the ear canal, have low battery drain, and are computer programmable, providing tremendous flexibility for precise fitting.

Some aspects of hearing aids have not changed over the years. There is still a microphone to convert acoustical energy to electrical energy, an amplifier to boost the energy, and a receiver or loudspeaker to turn the signal back from electrical to acoustical energy. We still discuss the output of a hearing aid in terms of the amplification or gain that is provided across the frequency range and the maximum level of sound that is delivered to the ear. Similarities to past technology end there, however, as many of the old rules have changed or are changing.

A **body-worn hearing aid** has its components encased in a small box worn on the chest with a cord connected to a receiver worn on the ear. **Eye-glass hearing aids** were an early style of hearing aid, in which the microphone and amplifier were built into one or both sides of the eyeglass frames with earmolds attached.

BTE = behind-the ear
ITE = in-the-ear
ITC = in-the-canal
CIC = completely-in-the-canal

Cy Libby, a master hearing aid dispenser and writer, introduced the concept of the hearing aid **pyramid**.

If you were a student in the not-so-distant past, you would probably learn about antiquities such as **body-worn hearing aids** and **eye-glass hearing aids**. Now you might see these instruments in a hearing-aid museum. Today when you look at a picture of a behind-the-ear **(BTE)** hearing aid, you may be looking at the next addition to that museum.

The burgeoning technological advances can make it difficult for beginning students to appreciate some of the challenges audiologists have faced over the years in the fitting of hearing aids. When you look at a picture of a BTE hearing aid today, it does not look much different than it did 5 years ago, although its capacity has advanced remarkably in even that short a period of time.

One of the best ways to view the progress of advances in amplification may be to think of it in terms of a **technology pyramid**. The concept is shown in Figure 11–1. At the bottom of the pyramid is standard technology with something called linear amplification and simple output limiting. Linear amplification means that soft, medium, and loud sounds are all amplified to the same extent. Output limiting is the way that the maximum output is capped. The next step up the pyramid is advanced technologies, which include more sophisticated nonlinear amplification and output limiting. Nonlinear amplification usually means that soft sounds are amplified more than loud sounds. Next up is miniaturization. This has allowed even the most sophisticated signal processing circuits to be fitted into a completely-in-the-canal **(CIC)** style of hearing aid. Its advantages are numerous. Above that is programmable technology, which provides extremely flex-

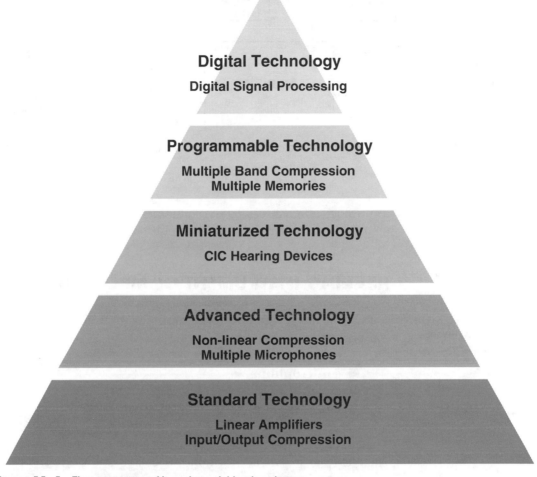

Figure 11-1. The progress of hearing aid technology.

ible control of hearing aid characteristics and multiple memories for programming different response parameters for different listening situations. At the top of the pyramid is digital technology. Digital signal processing provides the opportunity to use almost any of the technologies in the pyramid in a flexible manner to meet the needs of patients and put them all in a small package.

In this chapter, you will learn about the fundamental characteristics of hearing aids and about some of the current signal processing strategies. You will also learn about assistive listening devices, which are often used as supplements to conventional amplification, and cochlear implants, which are the devices of choice for many patients with profound hearing loss. Armed with a basic understanding, you should be able to appreciate the

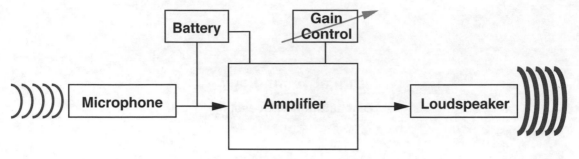

Figure 11–2. Schematic representation of the components of a hearing aid.

technological advances as they emerge into the reality of commercially available hearing instruments.

HEARING INSTRUMENT COMPONENTS

A hearing aid is an electronic amplifier that has three main components:

A hearing aid contains a **microphone**, an **amplifier**, and a **loudspeaker**.

■ a **microphone**,
■ an **amplifier**, and
■ a **loudspeaker**.

A schematic of the basic components is shown in Figure 11–2. The *microphone* is a vibrator that moves in response to the pressure waves of sound. As it moves, it converts the acoustical signal into an electrical signal. The electrical signal is boosted by the *amplifier* and then delivered to the loudspeaker. The *loudspeaker* then converts the electrical signal back into an acoustical signal to be delivered to the ear. A battery is used to provide power to the amplifier. Most hearing aids have some forms of external control as well, including a volume control and certain adjustments for shaping the amplifier's frequency response. Hearing aids may also contain a *telecoil* or t-coil. A telecoil allows the hearing aid to pick up electromagnetic signals directly, bypassing the hearing aid microphone. This allows for direct input from devices such as telephone receivers.

Microphone

A microphone is a transducer that changes acoustical energy into electrical energy. A microphone is essentially a thin membrane

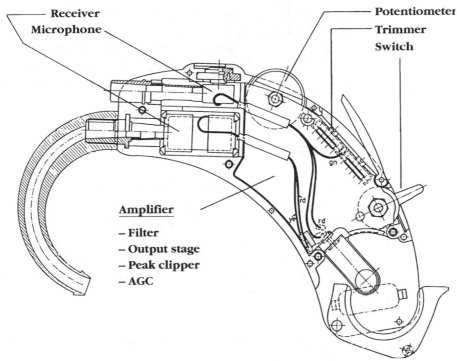

Figure 11-3. Drawing of a BTE hearing aid. (From *Hearing Instrument Technology*, by A. Vonlanthen, 1995, p. 9. Switzerland: Phonak AG. Reprinted with permission.)

that vibrates in response to the wave of compression and expansion of air molecules emanating from a sound source. As the membrane of the microphone vibrates, it creates electrical energy flow that corresponds to the amplitude, frequency, and phase of the acoustic signal. This energy is then pre-amplified before it is filtered. A microphone and its port are shown on the diagram of a behind-the-ear hearing aid in Figure 11–3.

Most conventional hearing devices use an **omnidirectional microphone**. An omnidirectional microphone provides wide-angle reception of acoustic signals. That is, it is sensitive to sound coming from many directions. A **directional microphone**, which has a more focused field, is sometimes substituted for the omnidirectional microphone. The purpose of using a directional microphone is to focus its sensitivity toward the front of the listener, thereby attenuating or reducing unwanted "noise" or competition emanating from behind the listener.

An **omnidirectional microphone** is sensitive to sounds from all directions; a **directional microphone** focuses on sounds in front of a person.

Microphone technology has also been designed that provides the capability of both directional and omnidirectional microphone reception in the same hearing device. This is sometimes accomplished by using two microphones in the same hearing aid. The directional microphone in some devices can be switched from omnidirectional to directional setting via remote control. Others have been designed so that switching is done manually with a push button.

Amplifier

The heart of a hearing aid is its power amplifier. The amplifier boosts the level of the electrical signal that is delivered to the hearing aid's loudspeaker. The amplifier contains a filtering component that controls how much amplification occurs at certain frequencies. The amplifier can also be designed to differentially boost higher or lower intensity sounds. It also contains some type of limiting devices so that it does not deliver too much sound to the ear.

Most patients have more hearing loss at some frequencies than at others. As you might imagine, it is important to provide more amplification at frequencies with more hearing loss and less amplification at frequencies with less loss. Thus, hearing aids contain a filtering system, which is usually adjustable, that permits the "shaping" of frequency response to match the configuration of hearing loss.

An example of the effects of filtering is shown in Figure 11–4. Here, the response of the hearing aid varies as a function of the filter settings on the hearing aid. When little filtering is used, the response of the device is relatively flat across the frequency range. When high-pass filtering is used (to pass the highs and cut the lows), the response of the hearing aid shows little amplification in the low frequencies and relatively greater amplification in the high frequencies.

An amplifier can be designed to provide linear amplification or nonlinear amplification. *Linear* amplification means that the same amount of amplification, or gain, is applied to an input signal regardless of the intensity level of that signal. That is, if the gain of the amplifier is, say, 20 dB, then a linear amplifier will increase an input signal of 40 dB to 60 dB, an input of 50 dB to 70 dB, an input of 60 dB to 80 dB, and so on. This relationship is shown in Figure 11–5. *Nonlinear* amplification means that the amount of gain is different for different input levels. For example, a nonlinear amplifier might boost a 30 dB signal to 65 dB,

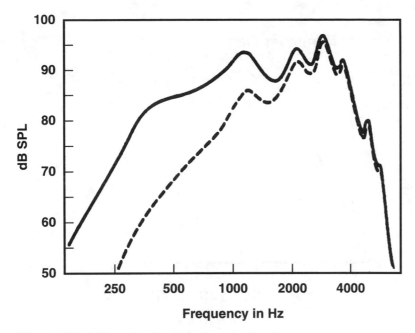

Figure 11-4. The effects of filtering on the frequency response of a hearing aid.

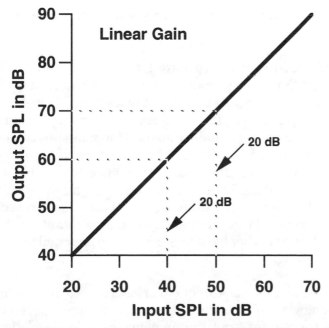

Figure 11-5. The relationship of sound input to output in a linear hearing aid circuit. Gain remains at a constant 20 dB, regardless of input level.

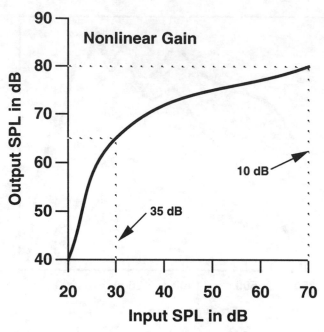

Figure 11–6. The relationship of sound input to output in a nonlinear hearing aid circuit. Amount of gain changes as a function of input level.

but a 70 dB signal to only 80 dB. This relationship is shown in Figure 11–6.

An amplifier also contains circuitry that limits its output. The output can be limited by simply putting a lid on it and not letting peaks of the signal exceed a certain predetermined level. This output limiting technique, known as *peak clipping,* is shown schematically in Figure 11–7. Another method for doing this is called *compression limiting.* Here, the amplifier is designed to become nonlinear as input signals reach a certain level, so that the amount of gain is diminished significantly at the maximum output level. This compression limiting technique is shown schematically in Figure 11–8. Compression limiting introduces less distortion than peak clipping and is usually the preferred method of output limiting.

Hearing aid amplifiers have frequency responses with a wide and smooth bandwidth. That is, the upper frequency limit is extended into high frequencies, and the amplifier provides a relatively smooth or constant output across the frequency range. The wider and smoother the aid's frequency response is, the better the fi-

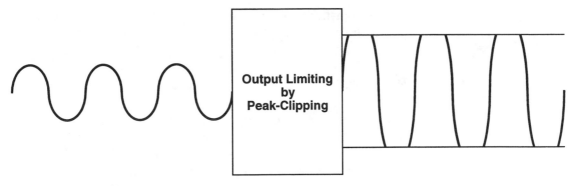

Figure 11-7. Schematic representation of output limiting by peak clipping.

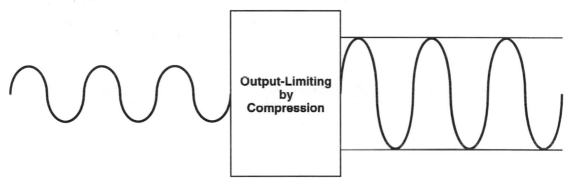

Figure 11-8. Schematic representation of output limiting by compression.

delity of signal reproduction and the better a person wearing the device will understand speech. In most patients, sensorineural hearing loss is greater in the higher frequencies. It is in these higher frequencies that consonant sounds, which carry so much of the meaning of speech, have most of their acoustic energy. In the early days of hearing aids, amplifiers had limited capacity for boosting the higher frequencies of speech that are so critical for its perception. Problems arose due to an inability to reduce distortion in the amplification of the high frequencies. This distortion made it difficult for hearing-device wearers to tolerate high-level speech or music, and there was a tendency to limit high-frequency amplification, thereby sacrificing fidelity for tolerability. Much of the difficulty in extending amplification to the high frequencies without distortion related not to amplifier limitations, but to the need to drive the amplifiers with low power batteries. To obtain reasonable battery life, amplifiers were altered in ways that also exaggerated distortion. Enhancements in amplifier technology now permit high-fidelity signal reproduction of the high-frequency range of amplification without excessive power drain.

Receiver

The amplifier of a hearing aid delivers its electrical signal to a receiver, or loudspeaker. The loudspeaker is a transducer that changes electrical energy back into acoustical energy. That is, it acts in the opposite direction of a microphone.

The loudspeaker is also an important component of a hearing aid. Think for a moment what a good, high-fidelity stereo system sounds like when you are playing your favorite CD through very good headphones or speakers. Now imagine what it would be like if you were to replace your good speakers with cheap ones. What a waste of a good amplifier.

The receiver, or loudspeaker, of a hearing aid must have a broad, flat frequency response in order to accurately reproduce the signals being processed by the hearing aid amplifier.

Controls

A **potentiometer** is a resistor connected across a voltage that permits variable change of a current or circuit. On a hearing aid, it is a small dial that can be rotated to change some parameter of the response.

A **matrix** is a group of electroacoustic frequency gain curves that describes the range of the output characteristics of a hearing aid.

The various output parameters of a hearing aid amplifier can be manipulated by hardware controls, such as dials, switches, and **potentiometers**, or by software control.

A hearing aid amplifier has a general response curve that characterizes the circuit. Most response curves can be manipulated to a certain extent, usually to reduce or enhance the low- and/or high-frequency range. Thus, a given hearing aid amplifier is capable of producing several response curves within a generalized range. These curves, taken together, form a **matrix** of responses that a given hearing aid is capable of producing. A hearing aid matrix is shown in Figure 11–9. Any hearing aid has a matrix of potential responses that can be adjusted by the audiologist or the patient with certain controls.

Newer hearing aid circuits use digital signal processing or conventional analog processing that is under digital control. These newer devices tend to have a more generic frequency response that can be manipulated to a far greater extent under computer or programmer control. Thus, fewer matrices are available, but the response within a matrix can be adjusted to vary significantly.

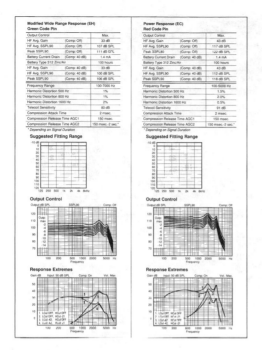

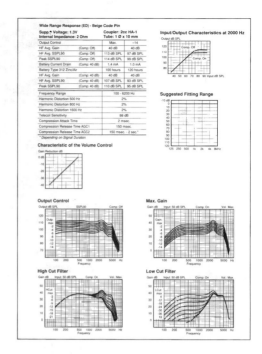

Figure 11-9. An example of a hearing aid matrix. (Courtesy of Widex Hearing Aid Company, Inc.)

This creates sort of a "one-size-fits-all" concept for hearing aid circuitry.

The issue of how much control to give and to whom is ongoing and tends to vary as a function of technology. For example, linear amplifiers require a volume control that the patient uses to turn the volume or output of the hearing aid up or down depending on the listening situation. Newer nonlinear amplifiers provide different levels of gain for different inputs, thus reducing the need for a volume control.

The nature of controls has also changed with technological advances. Older hearing aids used switches and pots (potentiometers), requiring audiologists to own a good set of tiny screwdrivers. Newer devices are controlled by plugging them into a programmer or computer interface. Patient controls have changed as well, moving in some cases to remote control of various signal parameters.

Manual Control

A conventional hearing aid will usually have one or two controls that the patient can manipulate and one or two others that the

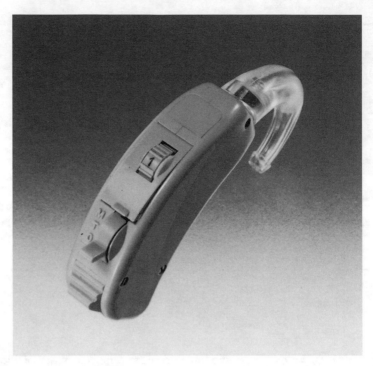

Figure 11-10. Photograph of a BTE hearing aid, with a MTO switch and rotating volume control. (Courtesy of Siemens Hearing Instruments, Inc.)

audiologist manipulates. Controls include an on-off switch, volume or gain control, frequency response potentiometer, and maximum output limiter.

On-off switches and volume controls can take many forms on a hearing aid. The classic on-off switch is the **MTO** switch, and the classic volume control is a rotating wheel, as shown in Figure 11–10. The MTO switch stands for **M**icrophone, **T**elecoil, **O**ff. *Microphone* means on; *telecoil* means that the microphone is turned off and that the telecoil of a hearing aid is activated to pick up signals from a telephone or other electromagnetic transducer; *off* means off. If a hearing aid does not have a telecoil, then the control is an M-O switch. In some hearing aids, the on-off switch is contained as part of the volume control wheel.

M = microphone
T = telephone
O = off

Other controls are usually less obvious, hidden as small potentiometers within the hearing aid case or at some location on the hearing aid faceplate. An example of a hidden potentiometer is shown in Figure 11–11. This dial can be rotated to change an

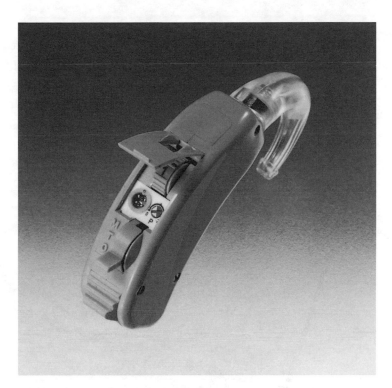

Figure 11-11. Photograph of a potentiometer on a BTE hearing aid. (Courtesy of Siemens Hearing Instruments, Inc.)

acoustic characteristic of the hearing aid, such as the frequency response or maximum output.

Other controls are used for various other amplifier manipulations related to certain signal processing strategies. For example, you will learn more later about compression circuits, which essentially change a linear hearing instrument into a nonlinear one. Often, certain parameters of the compression circuitry can be controlled by the audiologist, usually through a potentiometer.

Programmable Control

Many hearing aids are either completely digital in their control paths or have analog processing that is under digital control. Adding digital capabilities to hearing aids has made them *programmable*, or manipulable under computer control. Under such computer control, the response parameters of a hearing device can be manipulated with flexibility and relative ease. In some cases, the programming unit is a **proprietary**, stand-alone instrument (Figure 11–12), and in other cases, it is one that can be

Proprietary means belonging to a proprietor, in this case a hearing instrument manufacturer.

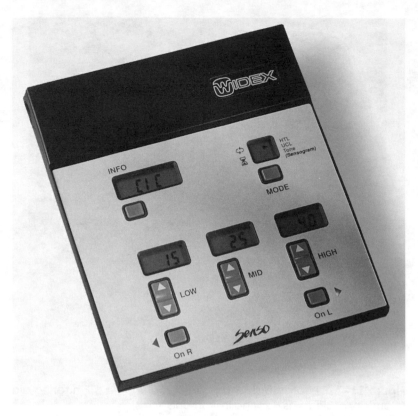

Figure 11–12. Photograph of a proprietary, stand-alone hearing-aid programming instrument. (Courtesy of Widex Hearing Aid Company, Inc.)

used for various makes of hearing devices and is controlled by proprietary computer software (Figure 11–13).

Sophistication of programmable hearing devices varies substantially. In its simplest form, a programmable hearing device is little more than a conventional linear hearing aid that allows computer control over variables that were formerly controlled by potentiometers and screwdrivers. The most sophisticated programmable device has two or more frequency **channels** with nonlinear compression circuitry that can be adjusted in all or some of the channels, as well as several memories for storing responses programmed for different listening situations.

A **channel** is a frequency region that is processed independently of other regions.

Programmability of hearing instruments provides several benefits that have led to improved fitting capability. Because the electroacoustic parameters of a programmable device can be manipulated over a fairly broad range at the time of fitting, manufactur-

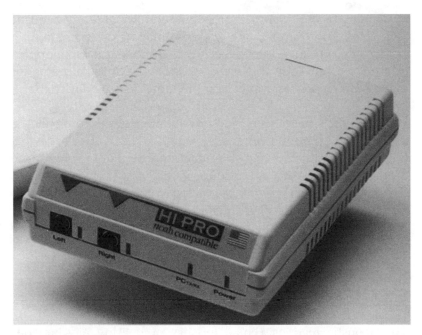

Figure 11-13. Photograph of a programmer designed as an interface for hearing aids from different manufacturers. (Courtesy of Madsen Electronics, Inc.)

ers can produce programmable instruments in a one-size-fits-all manner. A typical programmable device contains four to six parameter adjustments, an impossibility in a nonprogrammable device the size of an in-the-ear or in-the-canal aid. The main advantages of programmability are enhanced efficiency, flexibility, and precision of electroacoustic adjustments that can be made to fit an individual's particular hearing loss configuration. All of these adjustments can be made at the time of the fitting or during follow-up appointments in a manner that provides more appropriate amplification for a patient.

Most programmable instruments have acoustic parameters that can be manipulated over a wide range, permitting gain and output modifications as hearing loss progresses or fluctuates. This feature is particularly useful in fitting young children whose hearing ability may not be precisely quantified at the time of the initial evaluation.

Another advantage of programmability is that it provides access to automatic signal processing algorithms not available to nonprogrammable devices. Still another aspect of programmable hearing aids that has proven to be useful for some wearers is the availability of multiple memories that contain different acoustic responses. For example, one response may be appropriate for a certain acoustic environment such as telephone use, but inappropriate for listening in a noisy environment. Multiple memories make both responses available in the same hearing device.

Various efforts have been made by manufacturers to develop a uniform programming interface. When programmable devices first became available, each manufacturer had a unique hardware module and software interface for its devices. Early attempts to develop a universal programmer failed to gain widespread acceptance. Now, software platforms are available so that proprietary software from various hearing-instrument manufacturers can be integrated onto a single computer.

ELECTROACOUSTIC CHARACTERISTICS

The acoustic response characteristics of hearing aids are described in terms of frequency gain, input-output, and output limiting. Gain of the hearing aid is the amount of sound that is added to the input signal. If a speech signal enters the hearing aid at 50 dB and is amplified to 90 dB, the amount of gain is 40 dB. The frequency gain response of a hearing aid is the amount of gain as a function of frequency. Because most hearing losses are greater at some frequencies than at others, the ability to manipulate gain selectively in different frequency regions is important. *Input-output characteristic* of a hearing aid is the amount of gain as a function of the input intensity level. The input-output function can be linear or nonlinear. *Output limiting* refers to the maximum intensity of the amplified signal. If a signal of 100 dB were delivered to a hearing aid that had 40 dB of gain, without a limiting circuit, the output would be 140 dB. Such a high-intensity signal would not only be intolerable, but would be damaging to the cochlea, so it is necessary to limit the maximum intensity level the aid can generate.

Frequency Gain Characteristics

The most recognizable "signature" of a hearing aid is its frequency response. A frequency response curve is a graphic representation of the amplification characteristics of a hearing aid in decibels as a function of frequency. It is determined by delivering to the hearing aid a signal at a fixed-intensity level across the frequency range. Figure 11–14 illustrates the frequency response

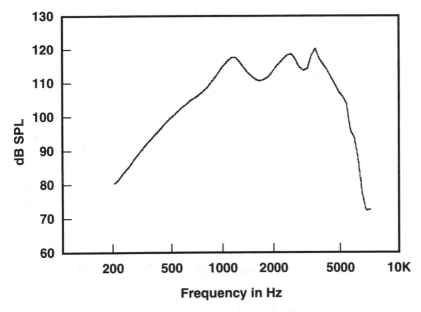

Figure 11-14. Frequency response of a hearing aid.

of a hearing aid. This curve represents how much acoustical energy the hearing aid generates for a given level of input signal.

The frequency response of a hearing aid is a standard that is used to describe its amplification characteristics. Often, the first step taken by an audiologist after receiving a hearing aid from the manufacturer is to evaluate the frequency response of the device on a hearing aid analyzer to ensure that it meets specifications.

The frequency response curve provides information about the *absolute* response of a hearing aid. Although important in describing the performance of an aid, we are usually more interested in the *relative* response of a hearing aid, or how much amplification was added at each frequency by the hearing aid. The most common way of describing this relative response is by a frequency gain curve. The term **gain** refers to the magnitude of amplification of sound by a hearing aid. In other words, gain represents how much the sound is boosted by the hearing aid amplifier. A frequency gain response is a graph of the gain produced by a hearing aid to a specified intensity level of a signal presented across the frequency range. Thus, it is a picture of the difference between the intensity level of the output of the hearing aid and the intensity level of the input. An example of a frequency gain response is shown in Figure 11–15.

Gain is the amount, expressed in dB, by which the output level exceeds the input level.

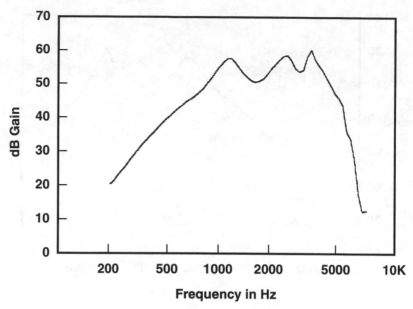

Figure 11–15. Frequency gain response of a hearing aid.

The frequency gain characteristics are important to the audiologist in the hearing-aid fitting process. Most of the methods used for prescribing a hearing aid are based on providing a specified amount of gain at a given frequency, based on a patient's puretone audiogram. Thus, the audiologist is usually more interested in knowing the amount of gain provided to a given input level than the decibel level of the device's output.

Input-Output Characteristics

A frequency gain response provides information about the amount of gain produced for a given input intensity level. Now suppose you were interested in knowing the response at various input intensity levels. Figure 11–16 shows frequency response curves to signals presented at several intensity levels. If you were to take a single frequency and plot the output intensity level as a function of the input intensity level, you would have an **input-output function** of the hearing aid at a specified frequency.

An **input-output function** is used to describe the gain characteristics of a hearing aid.

The input-output characteristics of a hearing aid are important because they describe how a hearing aid functions at different intensity levels. That is, they tell us how many decibels the amplification increases with an increase in the input signal. For some

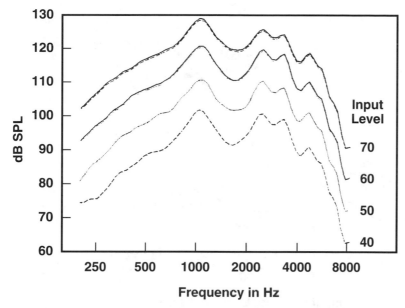

Figure 11-16. Frequency responses of a hearing aid to different input levels.

hearing aids, this input-output relationship is a simple matter of a 1 dB increase in output for every 1 dB increase in input until the hearing aid's maximum level is reached. This is called a linear input-output relationship. For other hearing aids the input-output relationship may change throughout the intensity range in a nonlinear manner.

Linear Amplification

Linear amplification means that the relationship between input and output is proportional, so that low-intensity sounds are amplified to the same extent as high-intensity sounds. An example of a linear input-output function was shown previously in Figure 11–5. Here, for every dB increase in the input, there is a corresponding dB increase in the output.

Fitting of linear amplification was a fairly standard approach over the years and remains applicable for conductive hearing loss and mild sensorineural hearing loss.

A problem with this type of linear amplification is that it does not address the nonlinearity of loudness growth that occurs with sensorineural hearing impairment. You will recall from Chapter 3 that many patients with sensorineural hearing loss do not hear

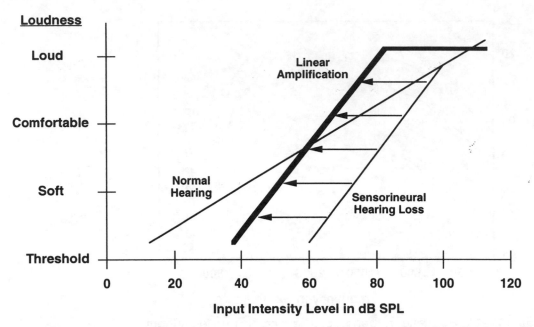

Figure 11-17. Schematic representation of loudness as a function of intensity level for normal hearing and for sensorineural hearing loss. A linear hearing aid amplifies both soft and loud sounds identically, making moderate intensity sound comfortable, but high intensity sound too loud.

soft sounds, but can hear loud sounds normally. A linear device amplifies both soft and loud sounds identically. As a result, if a low-intensity sound is made loud enough to be audible, a high-intensity sound is likely to be made too loud for the listener. This idea is shown schematically in Figure 11–17.

Nonlinear Amplification

Nonlinear amplification means that the relationship between input and output is not proportional, so that, for example, low-intensity sounds are amplified to a greater extent than high-intensity sounds. An example of a nonlinear input-output function was shown previously in Figure 11–6.

Nonlinear amplification is achieved with something called compression circuitry. *Compression* is a term that is used to describe how the amplification of a signal is reduced as a function of its intensity. Compression techniques are used both to limit the maximum output of a hearing aid and to provide nonlinear amplification across a wide range of inputs.

Wide-range nonlinear amplification is designed to "package" speech into a listener's residual dynamic range. Dynamic range, in this case, is a term used to describe the decibel difference between the level of a person's threshold of hearing sensitivity and the level that causes discomfort. In a normal-hearing person, that range is from 0 dB HL to about 100 dB HL. In a patient with a sensorineural hearing loss, that range is reduced. For example, a patient with a 50 dB hearing loss and a discomfort level of 100 dB has a dynamic range of only 50 dB. Compression circuitry used in nonlinear amplification is designed to fit speech signals into this reduced dynamic range. The idea is to boost the gain of low-intensity sounds so that they are audible but to limit the gain of high-intensity sounds so that they are not uncomfortable. The term *dynamic range compression* has been used to describe this nonlinear amplification process because it is meant to provide compression throughout a patient's range of useable hearing.

The need for nonlinear amplification is based on the knowledge that sensorineural hearing loss results in a reduced dynamic range and also on the knowledge that the loudness growth function in that ear is different from a normal ear. Again, the loudness growth of an ear with sensorineural hearing loss can be nonlinear, and the linearity may differ as a function of frequency. For example, our patient with the 50 dB hearing loss hears moderate-intensity sounds at reduced loudness but hears high-intensity sounds at normal loudness. A linear hearing aid amplifies all sounds to the same extent, so that low-intensity sounds become audible, moderate sounds become louder than desired, and high intensity sounds become intolerable. Nonlinear, dynamic-range-compression devices, in contrast, are designed in various ways to account for the nonlinear nature of loudness growth resulting from hearing impairment. Figure 11–18 illustrates the difference between linear compression and dynamic-range compression as it relates to an ear with sensorineural hearing loss and nonlinear loudness growth.

A number of nonlinear compression strategies have been developed to address the dynamic-range issue, and they vary in their approach and complexity. Some strategies are designed to provide compression over part of the dynamic range. Partial dynamic-range compression typically provides linear amplification for low input signals and some level of compression once the input reaches a certain level. Other strategies are designed to provide compression over a wider portion of the dynamic range. Wide dynamic-range compression has as its basis the enhanced amplification of quiet sounds and relatively reduced amplification

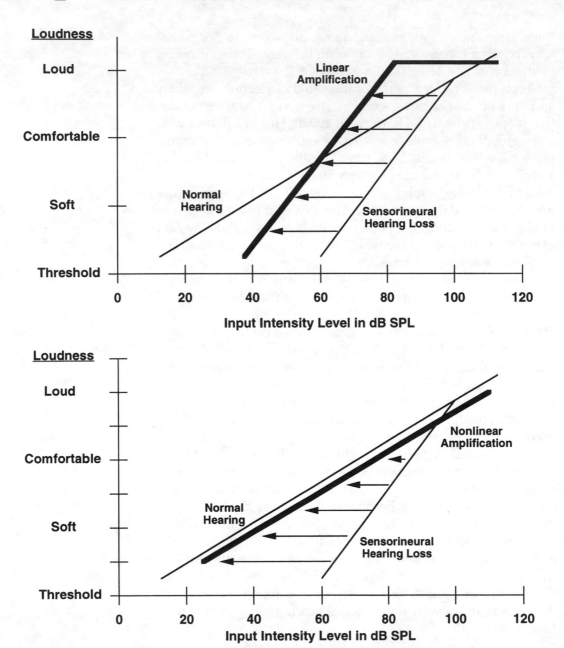

Figure 11–18. Schematic representation of the difference between linear and nonlinear amplification in an ear with sensorineural hearing loss and nonlinear loudness growth.

of loud sounds. A person with a sensorineural hearing loss cannot hear soft sounds; therefore, these sounds need to be amplified. In contrast, at high levels, hearing may be essentially normal, and no amplification is needed. Thus, gain is high for low-level sounds and low for high-level sounds. These changes in gain are gradual enough throughout the dynamic range that they cannot be perceived by the listener. The overall effect is to make soft sounds audible, moderate sounds comfortable, and loud sounds loud, but not too loud.

For some systems, wide dynamic-range compression can be altered in multiple frequency bands; in others compression is limited to a single band. For the multiband systems, if a patient's dynamic range is reduced in one frequency range and nearly normal in another, then the compression can be tailored to the frequency band where it is needed, and the other band can act as more of a linear amplifier.

Output Limiting

It is important that the output level of a hearing aid be limited to some maximum because high-intensity sounds can be both damaging to the ear and uncomfortable to the listener. Output limiting strategies are of two general types, peak clipping and compression limiting.

Peak Clipping

Peak clipping is a common technique used to limit output. Peak clipping removes the extremes of alternating current amplitude peaks at some predetermined level. A schematic representation of this output limiting technique was shown previously in Figure 11–7.

Although peak clipping is effective in limiting hearing aid output, it can produce substantial distortion when **saturation** is reached at high input levels. An alternative method is the use of some type of compression to approach output limiting in a more gradual manner.

Saturation is the level in an amplifier circuit at which an increase in the input signal no longer produces additional output.

Compression Limiting

Compression circuitry was developed in response to limitations inherent in peak clipping. A schematic representation of this output limiting technique was shown previously in Figure 11–8.

Many terms are used to describe compression, and it is not always easy to sort them out. One of the older terms used is *automatic gain control,* or AGC. AGC is used to describe both partial dynamic range compression and output limiting compression.

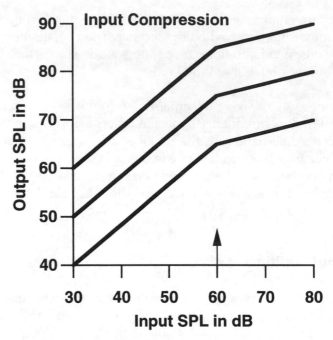

Figure 11-19. Schematic representation of the effect of input compression at three gain settings. Compression activation occurs when input reaches 60 dB.

Attack time is the amount of time it takes for compression to engage.
Release time is the amount of time it takes for compression to disengage.

The difference in these two types of compression strategies is in the threshold of activation, range over which compression occurs, ratio of input to output, and **attack** and **release time**.

One other aspect of compression circuitry that is important is whether the limiting compression is input or output compression. With *input compression,* the hearing aid microphone and preamplifier detect that a certain intensity, or activation threshold, is reached and goes into its compression mode. This occurs regardless of where the gain control of the hearing aid is set. A schematic of the effect of input compression is shown in Figure 11–19.

Impulse noises, such as a door slamming or a dish breaking are considered **transient signals.**

Output compression is activated at a high output level or threshold, such as 100 or 110 dB SPL. It has a fast reaction time so that it can reduce **transient signals**. Output-limiting compression also has a high input-output ratio, so that as input grows above the threshold, output is reduced substantially. Output compression limits the output of the hearing aid at the same intensity levels for all gain control settings. A schematic of the effect of output compression is shown in Figure 11–20.

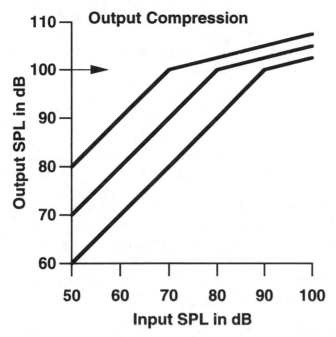

Figure 11-20. Schematic representation of the effect of output compression at three gain settings. Compression activation occurs when output reaches 100 dB.

A number of compression parameters have become adjustable, and some have become automatically adjustable. The result is that compression limiting, and compression in general, can be implemented in a flexible manner that allows patients to benefit from its effects without perception of its activation and functioning.

SIGNAL PROCESSING

Sophisticated, high-fidelity electronic processing of acoustic signals is commonplace in modern hearing aids. Three main processing strategies are used:

- analog,
- digitally controlled analog, and
- digital.

In analog hearing aids, acoustic signals follow an analog path that is under analog control. In digitally controlled analog (DCA) hearing aids, acoustic signals follow an analog path that is under digital control. In digital signal processing (DSP) hearing aids, acoustic signals are converted from analog to digital and back again, with digital control over various amplification parameters.

Analog

Analog has been the predominant signal processing strategy used in hearing aids since their inception. The term *analog* means that a signal is processed in a manner that is continuously varying over time. It is used in contrast to the term *digital,* in which a signal is represented as discrete numeric values at discrete moments in time. A waveform represented in analog and digital form is shown in Figure 11–21. The term *analog hearing aid* is a **neologism** that was created to describe conventional hearing aids when digital processing was introduced.

Neologism means a new word or a new meaning for an established word.

A schematic of an analog hearing aid is shown in Figure 11–22. Here, an acoustical signal is converted by a microphone into electrical energy in a continuously variable manner. The energy is filtered, amplified, and delivered to the hearing aid loudspeaker. Controls are mostly analog as well; for example, the volume or gain control provides adjustment along an uninterrupted continuum.

Analog signal processing has been refined to deliver amplified signals with high fidelity and low distortion and to incorporate sophisticated compression-limiting and nonlinear dynamic-range compression circuitry.

Digitally Controlled Analog

A digitally controlled analog hearing aid uses analog signal processing along its amplification path, with digital control over the amplification parameters. A schematic of a DCA hearing aid is shown in Figure 11–23. Here, the acoustical-to-electrical-to-acoustical flow of energy is identical to the analog hearing aid. The difference is that adjustments to the frequency gain response, compression parameters, and other electroacoustic parameters are made under digital control.

The main advantage of DCA hearing aids is the flexibility that results from the ability to program the devices. Digital control

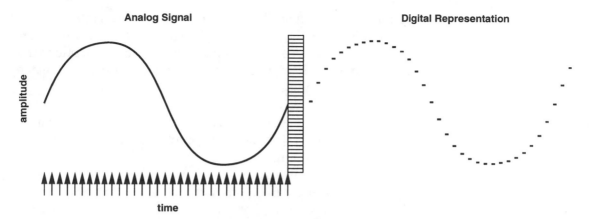

Figure 11–21. Schematic representation of a waveform converted from analog to digital form.

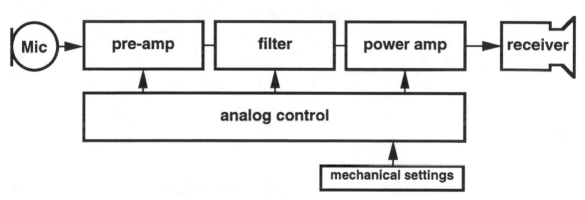

Figure 11–22. Schematic representation of an analog hearing aid.

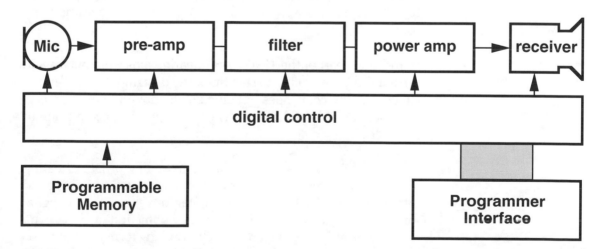

Figure 11–23. Schematic representation of a digitally controlled analog hearing aid.

permits fine tuning of a hearing aid remotely via an interface that communicates with a personal computer or dedicated hearing-aid programmer. As a result, fine adjustments can be made to the electroacoustic parameters of the hearing aid in real time while the patient is wearing the device.

Another advantage of DCA technology is that a given hearing aid can have a greater range of output. That is, instead of a hearing aid containing a single amplifier matrix that can only be varied minimally, a DCA device often contains a variety of matrices, any of which can be programmed to be used by the hearing aid.

In addition to a greater *range* of control, DCA hearing aids include a greater *number* of controls than their analog predecessors. This is related simply to the physical size of hearing devices. DCA hearing aids have separate controls for on-off, gain control, frequency response, compression parameters, output limiting, and other characteristics. Analog instruments are limited by size as to how many of these controls can be included in a single device.

Digital

The first commercially available DSP hearing aid was marketed in the late 1980s. However, due to size of the device, battery consumption, and other technological constraints of the time, the device did not gain widespread acceptance. During the same period, DCA devices were introduced, and their use became fairly routine.

In the latter part of the 1990s, DSP hearing aids were once again introduced to the market. This time, the design of the integrated circuit met the challenges of being small enough to fit in an ear-level hearing aid and having low enough power consumption to be practical.

A DSP hearing aid is different from an analog or DCA hearing aid in that the analog signals from the microphone are converted into digital form by an analog-to-digital converter. Once in digital form, the signals are manipulated by sophisticated processing algorithms and then converted back to analog form by digital-to-analog conversion. A schematic of a DSP hearing aid is shown in Figure 11–24.

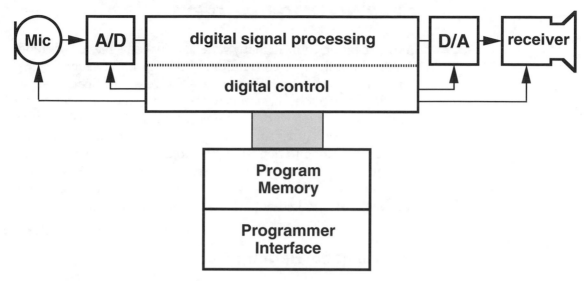

Figure 11–24. Schematic representation of a digital signal processing hearing aid.

Digital signal processing eliminates many of the barriers faced in trying to design analog circuits to fit in a small hearing aid and run on low-powered batteries. Indeed, the degree of sophistication of signal processing that is used in a DSP hearing aid is limited only by our conceptual framework of how hearing aid amplification should work. Some DSP hearing aids are designed as hardware DSP devices under software control. The limitations of such devices relate to the limitations of our knowledge about the processing algorithms that will best overcome the consequences of sensorineural hearing loss. Thus, the hardware DSP devices are designed to accomplish specific processing tasks. Other DSP hearing aids are designed as general purpose hardware platforms with an array of general purpose software algorithms that simultaneously performs multiple signal processing functions, not unlike a very small PC on which multiple operating systems or computer programs can run.

The clinical value of real-time digital processing for achieving appropriate sound reproduction through a hearing aid is clear. Along with the flexibility inherent in enhanced programmability, DSP provides more precise and flexible frequency shaping, better acoustic feedback reduction, more sophisticated compression algorithms, and enhanced noise reduction.

HEARING INSTRUMENT SYSTEMS

Aids to hearing come in many varieties. For convenience, we tend to talk about them as conventional hearing aids, assistive listening devices, and cochlear implants. A conventional hearing aid is any device with the basic microphone-amplifier-receiver components contained within a single package that is worn in or around the ear. An assistive listening device generally uses a remote microphone to deliver signals to an amplifier worn by the patient. A cochlear implant consists of an external microphone-amplifier-transmitter package that sends electrical signals to a receiver or electrode that has been implanted into the cochlea.

Conventional Hearing Aids

Conventional hearing aids come in several styles and with a range of functionality. The most common styles of hearing aids are known as

- behind-the-ear (BTE),
- in-the-ear (ITE),
- in-the-canal (ITC), and
- completely-in-the-canal (CIC)

hearing aids. All are shown in Figure 11–25. A BTE hearing aid consists of the microphone, amplifier, and loudspeaker housed in a case that is worn behind the ear. The aid is held in place by a plastic hook that fits over the top of the ear. Amplified sound is delivered to the ear canal through a tube that leads to a custom-fitted earmold. An ITE hearing aid has all of the components contained in a custom-fitted case that fits into the outer ear. A canal hearing aid is a smaller version of an ITE, which fits mostly into the ear canal. A CIC hearing aid is an even smaller version of an ITE that fits completely in the canal.

Behind-the-Ear

Figure 11–10 shows a picture of a BTE hearing aid. The aid itself contains the microphone-amplifier-receiver in a package that hangs behind a patient's ear. The microphone is usually located on the top or on the back side of the device. External controls for patient manipulation, including an MTO switch and volume control, are also located on the back side. Other controls are usually hidden under a removable plate on the underside of the hearing aid case.

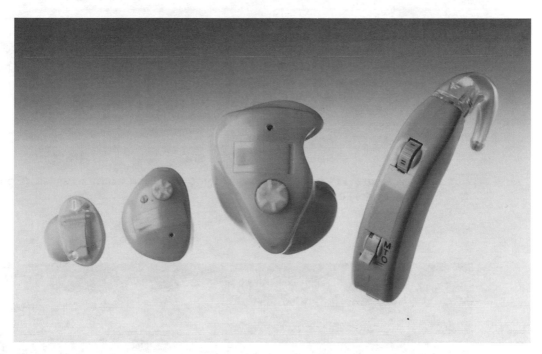

Figure 11-25. Photograph of CIC, ITC, ITE, and BTE hearing aids. (Courtesy of Siemens Hearing Instruments, Inc.)

Sound emanating from the hearing aid receiver leaves through an earhook that extends over the top of the auricle and holds the hearing aid in place. From here, sound is directed through hollow tubing to an earmold.

An earmold is a customized coupler formed to fit into the auricle. It is designed to channel sound from the earhook and tubing into the external auditory meatus. Earmolds come in a variety of shapes and sizes. Illustrations of some of the available earmold styles are shown in Figure 11–26. The acoustical properties of the sound that leaves the hearing aid are altered significantly by the tubing and earmold. Earmold and tubing modifications are often used to alter the frequency gain characteristics of the hearing aid in a controlled manner. The earmold may or may not be **vented**, depending on gain needs and requirements for ear canal ventilation.

A **vent** is a bore made in an earmold that permits the passage of sound and air into and out of the otherwise blocked external auditory meatus.

In-the-Ear

An ITE hearing aid is shown in Figure 11–27. Here, the micro-phone-amplifier-receiver are all contained in a custom-fitted case that fits into the concha of the auricle.

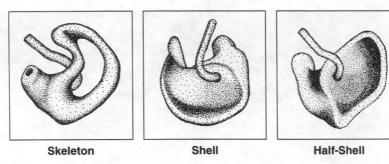

| Skeleton | Shell | Half-Shell |

Figure 11-26. Illustrations of three common earmold styles. (Courtesy of Earmold Design, Inc.)

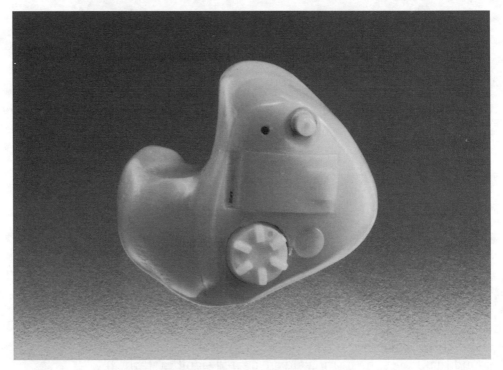

Figure 11-27. Photograph of an ITE hearing aid. (Courtesy of Siemens Hearing Instruments, Inc.)

The microphone port is located on the hearing aid faceplate. This provides an advantage over BTE hearing aids in that the microphone is located in a more natural position on an ITE. This advantage increases with ITC and CIC devices.

External controls for patient manipulation, including an MTO switch and volume control are also located on the faceplate. If

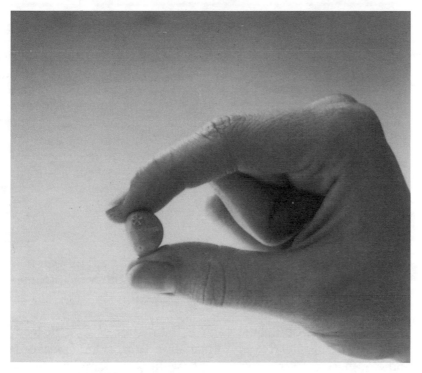

Figure 11-28. Photograph of an ITC hearing aid. (Courtesy of Siemens Hearing Instruments, Inc.)

the hearing aid is DCA or DSP, the interface connection is there as well. Other controls are usually located in the battery compartment or on the inside surface of the case.

In-the-Canal

An ITC or canal hearing aid is a smaller version of an ITE that tends to be fitted more deeply in the canal and extends outward into the concha to a lesser extent than an ITE. A canal hearing aid is shown in Figure 11–28.

Not unlike the ITE, the microphone port, external controls, and programmable interface controls are located on the hearing aid faceplate. Other controls are usually located in the battery compartment or on the inside surface of the case.

Completely-in-the-Canal

A CIC hearing aid is a small canal device that has its lateral end 1 to 2 mm inside the opening of the ear canal and terminates close to the tympanic membrane. Because it does not protrude beyond the meatal opening, it is barely visible.

A CIC hearing aid is shown in Figure 11–29. Here, the microphone-amplifier-receiver are all contained in a custom-fitted case that fits deeply into the ear canal. The microphone port is located on the faceplate. There is also a thin filament protruding from the faceplate which serves primarily as an extraction device for the aid. Some hearing aids have attached this to a volume control for patient manipulation. Any controls that can fit on a CIC are located on the faceplate as well.

Style Considerations

Although the decision on which type of hearing aid to wear may be based on cosmetic considerations, several other factors must be considered.

Acoustic Feedback. First, there is the matter of acoustic feedback. If the amplified sound emanating from a loudspeaker is directed back into the microphone of the same amplifying system, the result is *acoustic feedback* or whistling of the hearing aid. Most students are familiar with this concept from their experiences listening to public address systems. If the amplified sound of a public address system gets routed back into the microphone, a rather loud and annoying feedback occurs. One way to control feedback on hearing aids is to separate the microphone and loudspeaker by as much distance as possible. This solution favors the BTE hearing aid, in which the output of the loudspeaker is in the ear canal, and the microphone is behind the ear. Another solution is to attempt to seal off the ear canal so that the amplified sound cannot escape and be re-amplified. The tradeoff here is usually between isolation of the microphone from the sound port and amount of output intensity that is desired. The higher the intensity of output, the more likely it is that feedback will occur. Thus, if a person has a severe hearing loss, greater output intensity is required, and greater separation of the microphone and loudspeaker will be necessary. Thus, canal hearing aids are generally used for milder hearing losses and BTE hearing aids for more severe hearing losses.

Venting. Placement of an earmold or hearing aid into an ear canal creates two potentially detrimental effects. One is that it seals off the ear canal, reducing natural aeration of the external auditory meatus. In some patients, this can lead to problems associated with **external otitis**. The other problem is that plugging

External otitis is inflammation of the outer ear.

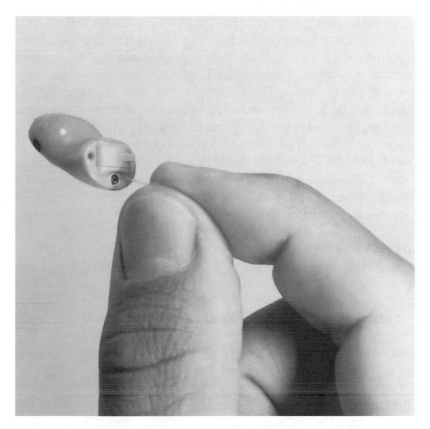

Figure 11-29. Photograph of a CIC hearing aid. (Courtesy of Siemens Hearing Instruments, Inc.)

the ear canal creates an additional hearing loss, often referred to as **insertion loss**. This is particularly problematic in patients with normal hearing sensitivity in the low frequencies.

The solution to these problems is called venting. *Venting* refers to the creation of a passageway for air and sound around or through a hearing device by the addition of a vent. A vent is a bore made in an earmold or in-the-ear hearing aid that permits the passage of sound and air into the otherwise blocked ear canal.

Venting creates both an opportunity and a challenge. The opportunity is that the electroacoustic characteristics of the hearing aid can be manipulated by the size and type of venting. Low-frequency amplification can be eliminated and natural sound

The difference in SPL at the tympanic membrane with the ear canal open and the ear canal occluded by an earmold or hearing aid is called **insertion loss**.

allowed to pass through the hearing aid for patients with normal low-frequency hearing and high-frequency hearing loss. Thus, venting can be used to shape the frequency gain response in very beneficial ways. Generally, the larger the vent, the more pronounced is the effect. The challenge associated with this opportunity is related to **feedback**. The larger the vent, the more likely it is that amplified sound will find its way out of the ear canal and back into the microphone port. Various venting strategies can be used to reduce feedback problems, but there always remains some tradeoff between the amount of gain that can be delivered by the hearing aid and the amount of venting necessary to achieve a proper frequency gain response.

Device Size. Another factor in style selection relates to size of the device. Because the BTE is larger in size, the number and size of electronic components that can be included are greater. More controls and more circuitry provide enhanced flexibility of fitting, which cannot be included in smaller ITE instruments. DSP technology makes this a non-issue, because sophisticated processing in a small package, low battery drain, and programmable control permit more functionality in a smaller case.

Durability. Another consideration is related to durability of the instruments. In ITC and CIC instruments, all of the electronic components are placed within the ear canal and subject to the detrimental effects of perspiration and cerumen.

Deep Insertion. CIC hearing aids have some unique advantages over the other styles of hearing aid that are worth noting. The external ear and ear canal provide acoustic enhancements that are eliminated when an earmold or ITE hearing aid is placed in the ear. To make matters worse, these natural acoustic enhancements are in the higher frequencies that play such a crucial role in speech perception. Therefore, the placement of a hearing aid into the ear adds an additional hearing loss that the device must overcome.

CIC devices provide an acoustic advantage over larger devices by preserving the natural influences of the auricle and concha and by terminating close to the tympanic membrane. These two factors result in an increase in sound pressure level delivered to the eardrum for the same amount of amplifier gain, with particular emphasis of the high frequencies. The auricle and concha effectively increase high-frequency input to the microphone. Their collection and resonance properties enhance sounds above 2000 Hz. The concha causes resonance of 6 to 8 dB in the 4000 to

When a hearing aid whistles, it is called **feedback**.

5000 Hz region. This extra boost in the high frequencies can be very helpful for understanding speech in background noise. The reduced residual volume of the ear canal between the earmold bore and the tympanic membrane additionally increases the sound pressure level by approximately 9 to 13 dB across the frequency range. Thus, a CIC device requires less amplifier gain than a larger device to produce the same amount of amplification. Because less amplifier gain is required, feedback and saturation-induced distortion are reduced. The requirement of less gain also permits increased battery life. This, in turn, provides the additional capacity necessary for advanced signal processing.

Other advantages of CICs include reduced wind noise, ease of telephone use, and enhanced listening with headsets and stethoscopes. In addition, it is likely that because the microphone is in the ear canal, the advantage of using two ears for both sound localization and for listening in noise will be realized to an extent not possible with conventional devices.

Assistive Listening Devices

Amplification systems other than conventional hearing aids have been designed for more specific listening situations. These devices are collectively known as assistive listening devices or ALDs. ALDs are usually not used as general purpose amplification devices; rather, they are used as need-specific amplification in a particular environment or listening situation.

Among the devices considered to be ALDs are personal amplifiers, FM systems, telephone amplifiers, and television listeners. In general, these devices are designed to enhance an acoustic signal over background noise by the use of a remote microphone. That is, rather than the microphone being built into the same case as the amplifier and receiver, it is separated in some way to close the gap between the signal source and the listener.

At least three categories of patients benefit from the use ALDs. One category includes patients who simply do not receive sufficient benefit from their conventional hearing aids. As a general rule, individuals who have more severe hearing losses often find that supplementing hearing aid use with ALDs is necessary under certain circumstances. Other individuals, because of communication demands in their workplace or social life, welcome the additional use of ALDs. A second category includes patients who have amplification needs that are so specific that the general use of a hearing aid is not indicated. For example, some individuals feel as if their only communication problems occur when viewing television or attending church. For those individuals, an ALD tailored to that particular need is often an appropriate alternative to a conventional hearing aid. A final category includes patients who have hearing disorders due to changes in central nervous system function. The resulting central auditory processing disorder is not necessarily accompanied by a loss in hearing sensitivity, but rather is characterized by difficulty understanding speech in background noise. For these patients, use of a remote microphone for enhancement of signal-to-noise ratio is more appropriate than amplification from a conventional hearing aid.

Hearing in the presence of background noise remains a problem for individuals with hearing loss and particularly for those who wear conventional hearing devices. Strides have been made over the past few years to address this issue. In conventional ear-level hearing aids, the introduction of sophisticated compression strategies has enhanced listening in noise, as has the use of deep-canal devices, and, most recently, the use of dual-microphone systems. Despite this progress, some patients need additional assistance with hearing in unfavorable listening situations. In these patients, use of remote-microphone technology can provide substantial assistance.

Personal FM Systems

One type of ALD is a personal FM system. A photograph of a personal FM system is shown in Figure 11–30. The system consists of two parts, a microphone-transmitter and an amplifier-receiver. The microphone is connected to, or is a part of, the case that contains the FM transmitter. The person who is talking wears the microphone and transmitter. Signals from the transmitter are sent to a receiver via FM radio waves. The listener wears the amplifier-receiver, which acts like a FM radio and "picks up" the transmitted signal. The receiver is usually coupled to the listener's ear via earphones or to hearing aid t-coils via a neck loop that transmits the signal.

The obvious advantage of this type of remote-microphone, personal FM system is that the listener's ear is no farther from the speaker than the microphone is from the speaker's mouth. Thus, the gap from the speaker to the listener is bridged, thereby eliminating the influence of all the intervening noise. This idea of signal-to-noise ratio enhancement is shown in Figure 11–31.

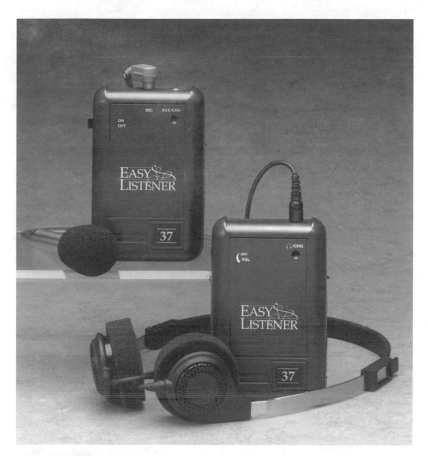

Figure 11–30. Photograph of a personal FM system. (Courtesy of Phonic Ear, Inc.)

By detaching the microphone from the remainder of the amplification device, certain listening situations that can be very difficult for a patient using a conventional hearing aid are made much easier. These situations include listening in a classroom, restaurant, car, church, theater, or in a party situation.

Advances in both transmitter and receiver technology have placed remote-microphone technology into the mainstream. Some transmitters have sophisticated **array microphones**, which are designed for directionality. The transmitter can be enclosed in a small hand-held case that can be directed at a sound source or handed to speaker during communication in a noisy environment (Figure 11–32). FM transmitters can also be included in hearing instrument remote controls. Similar advances have been made on the receiver portion of the FM system. Entire FM receiver systems can be integrated into a conventional BTE or ITE

An **array** is an orderly grouping. An **array microphone** system contains multiple microphones aligned in a row, designed for directionality.

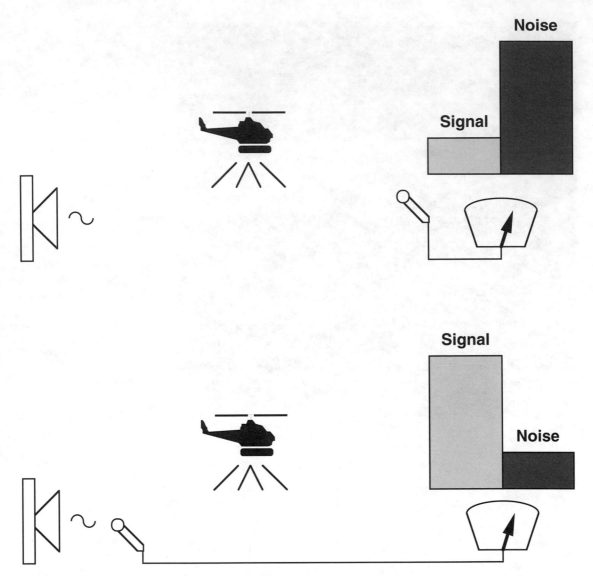

Figure 11-31. Schematic representation of the enhancement of signal-to-noise ratio by placing the microphone closer to the signal source.

hearing device or other coupler. An example of an FM "boot" for a BTE is shown in Figure 11–33. As these transmitters and receivers have become more practical and advanced, the use of remote-microphone technology has become a more common option.

Other Remote Microphone Systems

Personal FM systems are considered general purpose remote-microphone systems. Other systems are designed as instruments

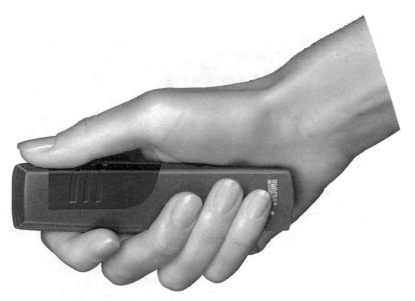

Figure 11–32. Photograph of a hand-held array microphone and FM transmitter. (Courtesy of Phonak AG)

dedicated to a single purpose, such as television viewing. Television listeners are similar in concept to the FM system, except that the transmitter is connected directly to the television. Audio signals from the television are transmitted, either by FM or by infrared light waves, to a dedicated receiver that is worn by the patient.

These types of dedicated systems are installed in many theaters. The transmitter is interfaced to the sound system of the theater, and patrons can request the use of a receiver during a performance. Again, some of the systems use FM waves as the carrier of the signal, and others use infrared light waves. Regardless, the effect is to bring the sound source closer to the listener's ear.

Personal Amplifiers

Another type of assistive listening device is called a personal amplifier. A photograph is shown in Figure 11–34.

A personal amplifier consists of a microphone that is connected to an amplifier box, usually by a cord. The microphone is held by the person who is talking. The signal is then routed to a small case, which is often about the size of a deck of cards. The box contains the battery, amplifier electronics, and volume control.

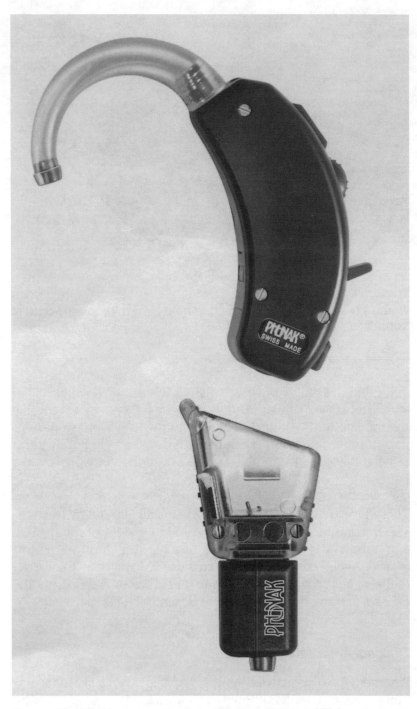

Figure 11-33. Photograph of an FM "boot" for a BTE hearing aid. (Courtesy of Phonak AG)

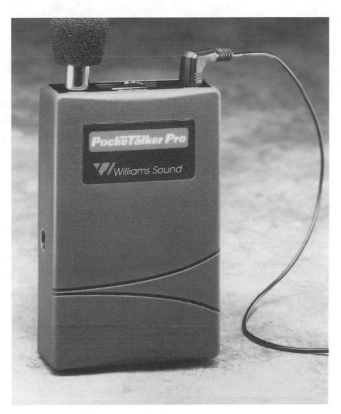

Figure 11-34. Photograph of a personal amplifier. (Courtesy of Williams Sound®)

The loudspeaker is typically a set of lightweight headphones or an ear-bud transducer. By separating the microphone from the amplifier, it can be moved closely to the signal of interest. In doing so, the signal-to-noise ratio is enhanced.

Personal amplifiers are often used as generic replacements for conventional hearing aids in acute listening situations. A common example of personal amplifier use is in a hospital. Patients who are in the hospital without their hearing aids or who have developed hearing loss while in the hospital may need amplification during their stay. The personal amplifier provides a good temporary solution. A physician who specializes in geriatric treatment will often carry a personal amplifier while making rounds in case it is needed to communicate with a patient. Another common use for a personal amplifier is the patient receiving **palliative care** who needs amplification only on a temporary basis.

Palliate means to lessen the severity of without curing; **Palliative care** is that which is provided to patients with terminal illnesses.

Other Assistive Technologies

Assistive devices come in other forms as well. Telephone amplifiers are popular assistive listening devices and are available in several forms. Some handsets have built-in amplifiers with a volume control. There are also portable telephone amplifiers that can be attached to any phone. The telephone receiver can also be adapted to transmit over FM waves to a personal FM system.

Other assistive devices that are available for individuals with hearing impairment have been designed to replace what is typically an acoustic signal with a different signal that can be perceived by one of the other senses. One of the most commonly used assistive device is a text telephone, whereby communication over the telephone lines is achieved by typing messages. Another type of assistive device is closed captioning of television shows. Closed captioning presents the dialogue of a television show as text along the bottom of the television screen. Other assistive devices include alerting devices, such as alarm clocks, fire alarms, and doorbells, which are designed to flash a light or vibrate a bed when activated.

Cochlear Implants

Individuals who have severe or profound deafness and do not benefit from conventional amplification are candidates for cochlear implants. Profound deafness results from a loss of hair cell function in the cochlea. As a result, neural impulses are not generated, and electrical activity in the auditory nerve is not initiated. A cochlear implant is designed to stimulate the auditory nerve directly. An electrode array is surgically implanted into the cochlea. The electrode array is attached to a magnet which is implanted into the temporal bone. Acoustic signals are received via a microphone attached to a sophisticated amplifier. The amplifier then sends signals to the electrode via the implanted magnet/receiver. When the electrode receives a signal, it applies an electrical current to the cochlea, thereby stimulating the auditory nerve.

Cochlear implants are different from conventional hearing aids in that hearing aids simply amplify sound, whereas cochlear implants bypass the cochlear damage and stimulate the auditory nervous tissue directly. The potential advantages are numerous and include better high-frequency hearing, enhanced dynamic range, better speech recognition, and no feedback-related problems.

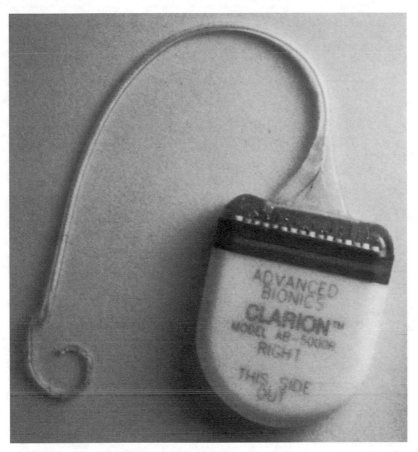

Figure 11–35. Photograph of a cochlear implant receiver and electrode array. (Courtesy of Advanced Bionics® Corporation)

Cochlear implants have been shown to be valuable in two groups of patients. Adults who have lost their hearing **adventitiously** can derive substantial benefit from a cochlear implant, especially as an aid to lipreading. Young children with adventitious hearing loss or with congenital hearing loss that is identified early can also benefit substantially from a cochlear implant, especially when implanted at an early age.

A person who has lost his or her hearing **adventitiously** did so after acquiring speech and language.

Internal Components

The surgically implanted portion of a cochlear implant has two components, a receiver and an electrode array. A photograph of the implant is shown in Figure 11–35. The receiver is surgically embedded into the temporal bone. The electrode array is inserted into the round window of the cochlea and passed through the

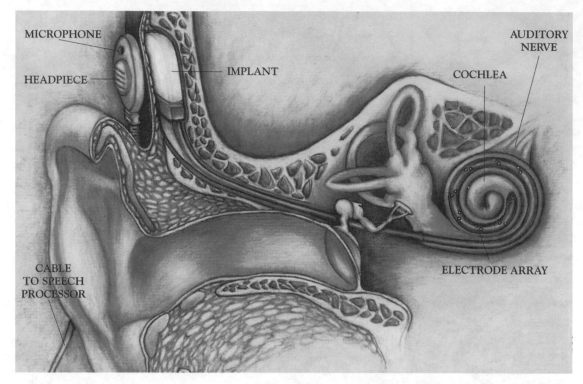

Figure 11–36. Schematic representation of an electrode array in the cochlea. (Courtesy of Advanced Bionics® Corporation)

cochlear labyrinth in the scala tympani, curving around the modiolus as it moves toward the apex. A schematic drawing of the electrode array in the cochlea is shown in Figure 11–36.

The receiver is essentially a magnet that receives signals electromagnetically from the external processor. The receiver then transmits these signals to the proper electrodes in the array. The electrode array is a series of wires attached to electrode stimulators that are arranged along the end of a flexible tube. The electrodes are arranged in a series, with those at the end of the array nearer the apex of the cochlear and those at the beginning of the array nearer the cochlea's base.

External Components

The external components of a cochlear implant are similar to those of a conventional hearing aid. The microphone is located in an ear-level device. Output from the microphone is routed to an amplifier that uses digital signal processing. The amplified

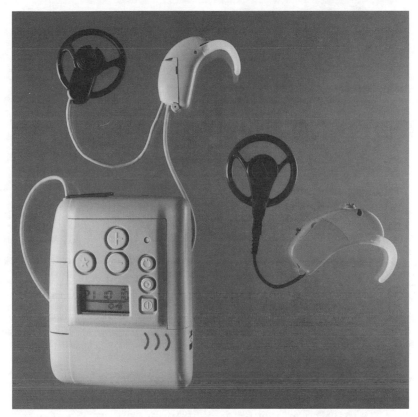

Figure 11-37. Photograph of the external components of a cochlear implant. (Courtesy of Cochlear Corporation)

signal is delivered to a receiver, which, in this case, delivers signals to a transmitter coil. The transmitter coil has a magnet which holds it against the skin opposite to the internal receiver. The signal is then transmitted electromagnetically across the skin.

A photograph of the external components of a cochlear implant is shown in Figure 11–37. Because of the sophisticated nature of signal processing and the power needed to drive the electromagnetic coupling, these external components are often contained in a body-worn case. Ear level processors are also used, subject to processing and power consumption constraints.

Signal Processing

Signal processing strategies used in cochlear implants are sophisticated algorithms designed to analyze speech, extract salient features, and deliver the relevant parameters to the electrode array.

The strategies are numerous and complex, but all are based on extracting frequency, intensity, and temporal cues from the speech signals and translating them to the electrode array in a manner that can be effectively processed by the residual neurons of the auditory nerve.

A simple example of the processing that can be done may be helpful in understanding the potential of cochlear implant signal processing. The spatial characteristics of the electrode array permit some degree of frequency translation to the ear. High-frequency information can be delivered to the basal electrodes, and low-frequency information can be delivered to the apical electrodes. The amount of stimulation of each electrode can be used to translate intensity information to the ear. In this way, the speech processor can detect and extract frequency and intensity information and deliver it at a specified magnitude to an electrode corresponding to the frequency range of the signal.

SUMMARY

■ A hearing aid is an electronic amplifier that has three main components: a microphone, an amplifier, and a loudspeaker.
■ A microphone is a transducer that changes acoustical energy into electrical energy.
■ The heart of a hearing aid is its power amplifier, which boosts the level of the electrical signal that is delivered to the hearing aid's loudspeaker. The amplifier contains a filtering component that controls how much amplification occurs at certain frequencies.
■ The loudspeaker is a transducer that changes electrical energy back into acoustical energy.
■ The various output parameters of a hearing aid amplifier can be manipulated by hardware controls, such as dials, switches, and potentiometers, or by software control.
■ The acoustic response characteristics of hearing aids are described in terms of frequency gain, input-output, and output limiting.
■ The frequency gain response of a hearing aid is the amount of gain as a function of frequency.
■ The input-output characteristic of a hearing aid is the amount of gain as a function of the input intensity level. The input-output function can be linear or nonlinear.

- Linear amplification means that the relationship between input and output is proportional, so that low-intensity sounds are amplified to the same extent as high-intensity sounds.
- Nonlinear amplification means that the relationship between input and output is not proportional, so that, for example, low-intensity sounds are amplified to a greater extent than high-intensity sounds.
- Output limiting refers to the maximum intensity of the amplified signal. Output limiting strategies are of two general types, peak clipping and compression limiting.
- Peak clipping removes the extremes of alternating current amplitude peaks at some predetermined level.
- Compression limiting reduces output gradually as a function of its intensity.
- In analog hearing aids, acoustic signals follow an analog path that is under analog control.
- In digitally controlled analog hearing aids, acoustic signals follow an analog path that is under digital control.
- In digital signal processing hearing aids, acoustic signals are converted from analog to digital and back again, with digital control over various amplification parameters.
- A conventional hearing aid is any device with the basic microphone-amplifier-receiver components contained within a single package that is worn in or around the ear. The most common styles of conventional hearing aids are known as behind-the-ear, in-the-ear, in-the-canal, and completely in the canal.
- An assistive listening device generally uses a remote microphone to deliver signals to an amplifier worn by the patient. Among the devices considered to be ALDs are personal amplifiers, FM systems, telephone amplifiers, and television listeners.
- A cochlear implant consists of an external microphone-amplifier-transmitter package that sends electrical signals to a receiver or electrode that has been implanted into the cochlea.

SUGGESTED READINGS

Chasin, M. (Ed.). (1997). *CIC handbook.* San Diego: Singular Publishing Group.

Clark, G., Cowan, R., & Dowell, R. (1997). *Advances in cochlear implants for infants and children.* San Diego: Singular Publishing Group.

Crandell, C. C., Smaldino, J. J., & Flexer, C. (1995). *Sound-field FM amplification.* San Diego: Singular Publishing Group.

Sandlin, R. E. (Ed.). (1992). *Handbook of hearing aid amplification. Volume I: Theoretical and technical considerations.* San Diego: Singular Publishing Group.

Studebaker, G. A., & Hochberg, I. (1993). *Acoustical factors affecting hearing aid performance* (2nd ed.). Needham Heights, MA: Allyn and Bacon.

Valente, M. (Ed.). (1994). *Hearing aids: standards, options, and limitations.* New York: Thieme Medical Publishing.

12

The Audiologist's Rehabilitative Strategies

Hearing aids are selected and fitted based on an individual's degree of hearing loss, the audiometric configuration of the loss, and estimates of the intensity levels at which sound is perceived to be uncomfortably loud. The first step in the selection process is to determine the targets for approximating the shape of the hearing aids' frequency gain responses. The targets are based on any of a number of rules. The frequency gain responses of the hearing aids are then adjusted to the targets. Output limiting is set in relation to the patient's threshold of discomfort. Verification of the frequency response is often made by **probe-microphone measurement**. A small microphone is placed near the tympanic membrane, and the responses of the hearing aids to sounds of various frequencies and intensities is determined. Following orientation of the patient to the devices, the hearing aid fitting is usually validated with speech audiometry. The patient is tested wearing the hearing aids, listening to speech signals through loudspeakers. The hearing aids are then adjusted for performance on the speech audiometric measures and for comfort of listening. Thus, the process of fitting hearing aids usually follows this course:

Probe-microphone measurement is an electroacoustic assessment of the characteristics of a hearing aid at or near the tympanic membrane using a probe microphone.

- selection of gain and characteristics
- selection of style and other options
- fitting
- verification
- orientation
- validation

HEARING INSTRUMENT SELECTION

The process of hearing instrument selection is one of systematically narrowing choices until a reasonable approximation of the patient's hearing and rehabilitation needs are met. Once the decision has been made to pursue conventional hearing aid amplification, the process begins by determining the appropriate output characteristics of the hearing aids, including frequency gain, maximum output, and input-output characteristics. The process continues with determination of a style and processing type that can achieve those characteristics.

Frequency Gain Characteristics

The first step in the selection process is to determine the target frequency gain responses that must be approximated by the chosen hearing aids. These targets are determined based on any of a number of rules. Examples of some of those rules are provided in the Clinical Note on the following page.

Once the target gains for various inputs have been determined, the approach varies depending on whether the hearing aids are programmable or not. Programmable hearing aids tend to have quite a bit of range in terms of the gain characteristics, so the audiologist's job is to ensure that the target gains fit within that range, preferably at the lower end. If so, then the task of matching the target can be accomplished in the fitting stage. If the hearing aids are not programmable, then their frequency response ranges are relatively more limited, and more care must be taken in determining the appropriate targets when the hearing aids are ordered.

That may not sound very difficult to do: take the pure tone audiometric results, plug them into a formula, determine the desired target gain, and browse through a hearing aid specifications book until you find the gain characteristics that approximate the target. However, the challenge is complicated somewhat by the way in which the electroacoustic characteristics of hearing aids are measured.

A hearing aid is typically measured in a **2-cc coupler** and the hearing aid specifications are expressed in terms of 2-cc coupler measurements. The coupler is much larger than the volume of someone's ear canal. Therefore, the response of the hearing aid in the ear canal will be different than the response of the aid in the coupler. It is ideal for custom corrections to be incorporated in the prescription of the target gain. These corrections are usually based on average correction factors designed to predict insertion gain from coupler responses. Correction factors are available for making this conversion.

A **2-cc coupler** is used to connect a hearing aid receiver to a microphone in order to measure its electroacoustic characteristics.

In a linear hearing instrument, the typical frequency gain target is calculated for average speech, ranging from 60 to 70 dB SPL. If nonlinear signal processing is used, it is common and useful to calculate frequency-specific gain targets for higher and lower input levels as well, because the frequency gain characteristics will be different for different levels of input.

There are other considerations for determining targets, including the type of hearing loss and whether one or both ears are being fitted. When there is a conductive component to the hearing loss, target gain should be increased by approximately 25% of the

The Prescription of Gain

One simple and common way of determining the frequency gain requirements of a hearing aid is the use of pure-tone threshold information to prescribe the gain at each frequency. The goal is to prescribe frequency gain characteristics that will amplify average conversational speech to a comfortable or preferred listening level. The underlying assumption of threshold-based prescriptive gain procedures is that this comfortable level can be predicted from the audiogram.

A number of prescriptive rules have been developed over the years in an effort to predict the appropriate frequency-gain characteristics. As an example, the half-gain rule prescribes gain equal to one half of the amount of hearing loss. A third-gain rule prescribes gain equal to one third of the loss. Most prescriptive rules start with this type of approach and then alter individual frequencies based on some empirically determined correction rules.

The table below shows the rules for three well-known prescriptive procedures, the Berger method, the POGO method, and the NAL–R method. Figure B on the next page shows the amount of gain that would be provided, based on each formula, for the hearing loss shown in the top figure. As you can see, the amount of prescribed gain is different for each rule.

The rules for three well-known prescriptive procedures, the Berger method, the POGO method, and the NAL–R method.

Frequency	Berger	POGO	NAL–R
500	0.30	0.5 (−5)	0.31 (−8)
1000	0.63	0.5	0.31 (+1)
2000	0.67	0.5	0.31 (−1)
3000	0.59	0.5	0.31 (−2)
4000	0.53	0.5	0.31 (−2)
6000	0.50	0.5	0.31 (−2)

Sources: Berger: Berger, K. W., Hagberg, E. N., & Rane, R. L. (1979). Determining hearing aid gain. *Hearing Instruments, 30,* 26–28, 44. POGO: McCandless, G. A., & Lyregaard, P. E. (1983). Prescription of gain and output (POGO) for hearing aids. *Hearing Instruments, 37,* 16–21. NAL–R: Byrne, D., & Dillon, H. (1986). The national acoustic laboratories' (NAL) new procedure for selecting the gain and frequency response of a hearing aid. *Ear and Hearing, 7,* 257–265.

Most clinicians and hearing-aid manufacturers use some prescriptive formula as a basis for circuit selection. Fortunately, most modern hearing aid circuits provide sufficient flexibility to adjust the prescription to individual needs.

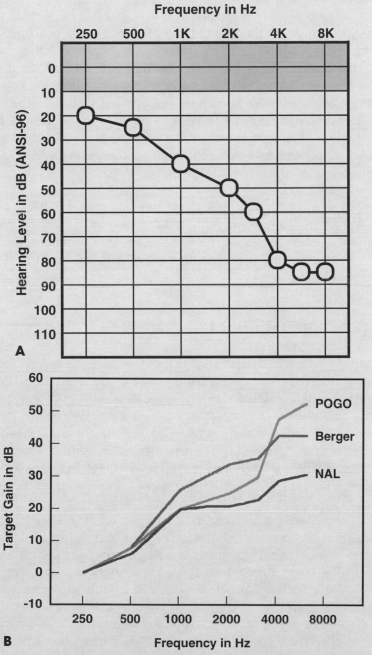

Pure-tone audiometric results (**A**), and the corresponding gain targets (**B**) as prescribed on the basis of the Berger method, the POGO method, and the NAL–R method.

air-bone gap at a given frequency. When the hearing aid fitting is binaural, the target gain for each ear should be reduced by 3 to 6 dB to account for binaural summation.

Maximum Output

It is very important that the maximum output of the hearing aids does not exceed the patient's threshold of discomfort. If it does, the patient will likely reject the hearing aids or turn the gain down to a level at which the hearing aids are no longer effective. Once again, this determination is confounded slightly by the difference between TDs that were determined with earphones, expressed in dB HL and the desired level of hearing aid output in a patient's real ear or the dB SPL in a 2-cc coupler. However, corrections are available for making this conversion.

Sometimes unaided discomfort levels are not available. This often occurs when fitting young children who cannot convey discomfort information reliably. In these cases, the maximum output can be calculated using a prescriptive method based on pure-tone thresholds.

Input-Output Characteristics

A **nonlinear hearing aid** is one that incorporates compression circuitry, so that soft sounds are amplified more than loud sounds.

Specifying target parameters for input-output characteristics is important when the decision has been made to fit **nonlinear hearing aids**. As stated previously, the frequency gain characteristics of a nonlinear hearing aid vary as a function of the input level of the signal. Recall as an example that nonlinear hearing aids are often designed to provide substantial gain for low level inputs and little, if any, gain for high level inputs. In this case, the specification of gain at several input intensity levels is important.

Also important for nonlinear hearing aids is the specification of certain compression characteristics, including threshold and input-output ratio. Fortunately, most newer hearing aids provide a suitable range over which these parameters can be manipulated. Nevertheless, knowledge of these compression characteristics may lead the audiologist to choose one form of circuitry over another, and it is important that a decision be made during the selection process. Several prescriptive fitting methods provide assistance in making decisions about these input-output characteristics. An example of how these might be used is described in the following Clinical Note.

How to Determine I-O?

In the days of linear hearing aid amplification, prescriptive procedures were used to estimate frequency-gain characteristics that would amplify average conversational speech to a comfortable or preferred listening level. The problems with this type of approach were numerous. One important problem was that the linear nature of the amplifiers did not account for the nonlinear nature of loudness growth in patients with sensorineural hearing loss.

As understanding grew, it became apparent that different frequency-gain rules were needed, depending on the intensity of the input signal. That is, soft sounds needed to be amplified differently than loud sounds. Soon, technology caught up with this knowledge, and dynamic range compression became commonly available. As the technology became available, the need arose to develop prescriptive strategies that would address the issue of dynamic range.

Prescriptive rules for I-O vary considerably in approach. For example, one approach is to bisect the dynamic range, so that amplified speech is placed midway between a patient's threshold and discomfort level. Another approach is to simply use pure-tone threshold data to predict the dynamic range and then amplify average speech to a level, say 15 to 20 dB above threshold at each frequency.

Loudness-based approaches have also been developed. For example, one approach uses pure-tone threshold data to calculate gain targets for low-level sounds (40 dB SPL), moderate level sounds (65 dB SPL), and high-level sounds (95 dB SPL). These targets are based on average loudness data. Other approaches are available that use individual loudness data to determine frequency gain targets.

Other Characteristics

As you learned in Chapters 10 and 11, there are a number of other challenges and options that need to be addressed during the hearing aid selection process. These include:

- **binaural** versus **monaural** fitting
- hearing aid style
- number and size of user controls

Binaural means both ears; **monaural** means one ear.

- signal processing options
- volume control considerations
- **telecoil** and telecoil sensitivity
- compatibility with **ALDs**
- programmable options

A **telecoil** is a coiled wire included in hearing aids to receive electromagnetic signals from a telephone.
ALDs = assistive listening devices

Once all of these decisions have been made, the audiologist will have narrowed the selection process down to a tractable set of device options. The audiologist will then compare these options against the knowledge of devices available from several manufacturers and make a decision about exactly which hearing aids to order for the patient.

HEARING INSTRUMENT FITTING AND VERIFICATION

Hearing aid fitting has two important components, getting the actual physical fit of the device right and getting the electroacoustic characteristics of the device right. Both require significant technical knowledge and skill, and both require a bit of artistic talent. The general process of fitting and verification includes:

- making earmold impressions
- inspection of quality control
- assessment of physical fit
- assessment of performance

Ear Impressions

The fitting process begins with the making of impressions of the outer ear and external auditory meatus. These impressions are used by the manufacturer to create custom-fitted earmolds or in-the-ear hearing aids. The quality of the impression dictates the quality of the physical fit of the hearing instruments.

The impression-making process is simple and systematic. The first step is inspection of the ears and ear canals to ensure that they are clear for the introduction of impression material. The inspection process includes an evaluation of:

- the skin of the canals to ensure that no inflammation exists,

- the amount of cerumen in the canals to ensure that it is not impacted or excessive enough to interfere with the task, and
- the tympanic membranes to ensure that they can be visualized and do not have obvious perforations or disease process.

If any concern exists about the condition of the outer-ear structures, it is prudent to seek medical opinion before making the impression or even medical assistance while making the impression.

The next step in the process is to place foam or cotton blocks deep into the ear canals to protect the tympanic membranes from impression material. These blocks should have a string attached for easy removal. Once the blocks are in place, the ear canals are filled with impression material. This is soft material that is mixed just before it is placed into the ear canals and sets shortly after it is in place. After a period of time sufficient for the material to set, the ear impressions are removed from the ears, inspected for quality, and shipped to the manufacturer.

The nature of ear impressions is similar for both earmolds and custom hearing aids. An important exception is the CIC hearing aid and earmolds for profound hearing loss, where care must be taken to make very deep impressions of the ear canals.

If ear impressions are being made into earmolds for use with behind-the-ear hearing aids, decisions will need to be made about the style of earmolds, the material to be used, and the style and size of venting. Earmold materials vary in softness and flexibility. Some materials are nonallergenic. The decision of which material to use is usually based on concerns relating to comfort and feedback.

Quality Control

When hearing aids are received from the manufacturer, they should be inspected immediately for the quality of appearance and function.

The first step is to look at the hearing aids and assess their appearance. Custom hearing aids or earmolds should be inspected to ensure that style, color, and venting are correct. The switches and controls should be checked to ensure that the proper ones were included and that they function.

Electroacoustic analyses of the hearing aids should be conducted to ensure that their output meets design parameters in terms of frequency gain, maximum output, and input-output characteristics. In addition, hearing aids are required to meet specified standards of performance, including minimum hearing aid circuit noise and signal distortion. Measurement of these aspects of performance should be included in any electroacoustic analysis.

Following the electroacoustic analysis, a listening check should be performed to rule out excessive circuit noise, intermittency, and negative impressions of sound quality. Any controls should also be manipulated to ensure that they work and do not add noise to the amplified signal as they are changed.

Assessment of Physical Fit

The first step in the fitting process with the patient is to assess the physical qualities of the devices, including their fit in the ears, the patient's perception of their appearance, and the patient's ease in manipulating the devices. This should include an assessment of:

VC = volume control

- security of fit
- absence of feedback
- appropriate microphone location
- physical comfort
- ease of insertion and removal
- ease of **VC** rotation
- overall patient manipulation
- cosmetic appeal

The **auricular** structures are the external or outer ear.

Assessment of the physical fit of the devices is important. They should fit securely without excessive patient discomfort, the gain should exceed the usable level before feedback occurs, and the microphones should not be obstructed by any **auricular** structures. If the fit is not adequate, the hearing aids or earmolds can be modified to a certain extent.

Patient comfort with using the devices is equally important. The patient should be able to insert and remove the devices without excessive difficulty and should be able to operate the controls easily.

Assessment of Performance

The general strategy of fitting and verification is one of

- assessing the gain and frequency parameters,
- making adjustments,
- verifying that the responses meet targets, and
- verifying that the aids meet some defined perceptual expectations.

Audiologists use a number of techniques to fit hearing aids and verify their suitability. In general, the process includes placing the hearing aids in the patient's ears, measuring their gain and frequency response in the ear canal, adjusting the parameters to meet targets, and then asking the patient to make a perceptual assessment of the quality of the hearing experience with the aids.

Verification Techniques

The methods used to verify the electroacoustic output of the hearing aids are generally designed to assess whether or not the targeted gains are achieved across the frequency range for a given input to the hearing aids. The procedures used to achieve this involve some form of real-ear testing, either probe-microphone or functional gain measurements. Once the electroacoustic output is verified, loudness judgments are performed to ensure that certain criteria for loudness growth are met. Finally, the speech quality of the amplified sound is assessed with some form of quality or intelligibility judgment procedure.

Probe-Microphone Measurement. For most patients, the method of choice for assessing **real-ear gain** characteristics is probe-microphone measurement. In fact, many audiologists think that it should always be used unless it is contraindicated by physical limitations. Using probe-microphone equipment, the real-ear gain is measured with a hearing aid in place and set to an estimated output configuration. The real-ear gain values are then compared to target gain values for different inputs. If the targets are not reached, the hearing aid is adjusted, and the real-ear gain is measured again. This process is repeated until all targets are approximated within some acceptable tolerance. Targets for low, medium, and high intensity sounds can be assessed in this manner.

Real-ear gain is the amount of gain delivered to the ear as opposed to a coupler; it is measured with a probe microphone or by functional gain assessment.

Functional Gain. If probe-microphone measurements cannot be made, an alternative solution is to measure functional gain.

This is done by presenting frequency-specific signals via loud-speaker to the patient. The patient is tested in both unaided and aided conditions in the sound field. The difference between aided and unaided thresholds is functional gain. These gain values are then compared to target values determined from a prescriptive fitting protocol. The hearing aid controls are adjusted until the functional gain approximates the prescriptive gain target.

Loudness Judgment Ratings. The goal of loudness judgment ratings is to ensure that low-intensity sounds are audible and that high-intensity sounds are not uncomfortable. Typically, the patient is asked to judge loudness for speech or narrow bands of noise. The signals are presented at various intensity levels, and the patient is asked to rate the loudness at each level. For example, a speech signal presented at 45 dB SPL should be judged as "soft," a speech signal presented at 65 dB SPL should be judged as comfortable, and a speech signal presented at 85 dB SPL should be judged as loud, but not uncomfortable. The hearing aid controls are then adjusted until appropriate aided loudness judgments are obtained for all three presentation levels of the speech signal.

Speech Perceptual Judgments. Once the parameters of the hearing aids have been set to meet gain and loudness targets, the patient is often asked to make perceptual judgments about the nature of the amplified speech sound. Judgments are usually made along the perceptual dimensions of quality or intelligibility. For quality judgments, the patient is presented different speech signals and makes judgments about whether the speech sounds natural, clear, harsh, and so on. The hearing aid controls are then adjusted until the quality of speech is judged to be maximal. For intelligibility judgments, the patient is presented different speech signals, often in quiet and in noise, and makes judgments about the intelligibility of speech. The hearing aid controls are then adjusted until the intelligibility of speech is judged to be acceptable.

Speech Recognition Measurements. Another technique that has been used for verification over the years is speech recognition measurement. Here, the patient is presented with one of several types of speech materials, such as sentences or monosyllabic words, and performance scores are obtained. Testing is usually done in the presence of one or multiple levels of noise or competition. The patient's score is compared to some predetermined performance level.

One benefit of speech recognition measurement is that performance of monaural hearing fitting can be compared to binaural fitting, and the ears can be compared to each other. This is important, especially in older patients who can show marked asymmetry in their ability to use hearing aids. Verification with other strategies will not permit this evaluation.

Tournament Strategies. Hearing aid output characteristics can also be determined by subjecting some aspect of them to competition. Programmable hearing aids permit modification of response parameters by computer control. In a tournament strategy, the patient is asked to decide between competing responses which is better along some perceptual parameter. The computer then determines the next challenger, and the circuit characteristics are evaluated until a winner is found.

Verification of Outcomes

One of the more compelling verification strategies is the determination of loudness judgments as a means for assuring that speech is packaged appropriately within a patient's dynamic range. The presumption of achieving this goal is that speech will be audible and tolerable to the listener and that maximal perception will follow naturally.

Audibility of Soft Sounds. One of the goals of hearing aid fitting is to make soft sounds audible. The audibility of soft sounds can be verified in one of three ways:

- real-ear gain response for a soft input of approximately 50 dB SPL should achieve its prescriptive target;
- functional gain in the soundfield should be between 20 and 30 dB; or
- a low-intensity speech signal of approximately 45 to 50 dB should be judged as very soft, soft, or comfortable but slightly soft.

Average-Speech Comfort. Another goal of hearing aid fitting is to make average speech comfortable. The comfort of average speech can be verified in one of two ways.

- real-ear gain response for an average input of 65 dB SPL should achieve its prescriptive target for average speech; or

■ an average speech signal of approximately 60 to 65 dB SPL should be judged as comfortable but slightly soft, comfortable, or comfortable but slightly loud.

Comfort for Loud Sounds. A third goal of hearing aid fitting is to make loud sounds loud, but not uncomfortable. The comfort of loud sounds can be verified in one of two ways:

■ real-ear gain response for an input of 90 dB SPL should achieve its prescriptive target based on a patient's unaided discomfort level; or
■ a loud speech signal of approximately 80 to 85 dB SPL should be judged as comfortable but slightly loud or loud but okay.

HEARING INSTRUMENT ORIENTATION

Following the completion of hearing aid fitting and verification, a hearing aid orientation program is implemented. An orientation program consists of informational counseling for both the patient and the patient's family. Topic areas include of the nature of hearing and hearing impairment, the components and function of the hearing aids, and care and maintenance of the hearing aids. One of the most critical aspects of the hearing aid orientation is a discussion of reasonable expectations of hearing aid use and strategies for adapting to different listening environments. The hearing aid orientation program also provides an opportunity to discuss and demonstrate other assistive devices that might be of benefit to the patient.

In some programs, groups of patients with hearing impairment are brought together for orientation. Such groups serve at least two important functions. First, they provide a forum for expanded dissemination of information to patients and their families. Second, they provide a support group that can be very important for sharing experiences and solutions to problems.

Topics

The orientation process involves the dissemination of information on a number of topics and details about the hearing aid, its function, and its use. Topics that should be covered during the orientation period include:

- instrument features and landmarks
- working knowledge of the components
- ■ usage patterns
- use and routine maintenance
- storage
- battery management
- telephone use
- ALD coupling

It is important for the audiologist to recognize the likely novelty of this information and provide the patient with as much in the way of handout material as possible. In addition to the manufacturer's manual for the hearing aids, the audiologists should provide written instructions on use and routine maintenance, including troubleshooting guidelines.

The orientation also provides an excellent opportunity to educate the patient and family about successful communication strategies for those with hearing impairment. Information about manipulation of the acoustic environment for favorable listening and information about how to speak clearly and effectively to those with hearing impairment will be invaluable to both patient and family.

During the orientation, the patient should also be familiarized with other assistive devices that might be valuable for his or her communication needs. Familiarity with the availability of telephone amplifiers and remote microphone systems will provide patients with a perspective on the options that are available to them beyond the hearing aids. It is also a good opportunity to inform patients about the public facilities that are available to them in terms of group amplification for theaters and the like.

Performance Expectations

If a patient expects hearing aids to restore hearing to normal similar to the way that eyeglasses restore vision to normal, then that patient may be disappointed with the hearing aids that you have worked so hard to get just right. Hearing aids amplify sound. Some hearing aids amplify sounds extremely well. Regardless, the sound is being delivered to an ear that is impaired, and amplified sound cannot correct the impairment. If a patient has a reasonable understanding of that, and his or her expectations are in line with that understanding, then the prognosis for successful hearing aid use is good. Conversely, if patient expectations are unreasonable, the prognosis is guarded at best.

Patients should expect certain things from hearing aid amplification. They should expect:

- acceptable hearing in most listening environments
- communication to improve, but not be perfect
- environmental sounds to not be uncomfortably loud
- feedback-free amplification
- that hearing aids are visible to some degree
- reasonable physical comfort, but not tactile transparency
- more benefit in quiet than in noise
- that background noise will be amplified

These expectations should be reviewed at the time of follow-up. If they are not being met, the hearing aids probably need to be adjusted. If they are being met, and the patient accepts them as reasonable, the likelihood is that the patient will be a satisfied hearing aid wearer.

HEARING INSTRUMENT VALIDATION

Outcome validation is important in the provision of any aspect of health care. Hearing aid rehabilitation is no exception. It is common practice to evaluate the success of hearing aid fitting at some point after the patient has had an opportunity to wear and adjust to the use of his or her hearing devices.

Validating the outcome of hearing aid fitting means asking if the treatment, in this case hearing aid use, is doing what it is supposed to do. The goal of the hearing rehabilitation process is to reduce the communication disorder imposed by a hearing loss. We have a tendency to define success at reaching this goal in terms of whether the patient understands speech better with the hearing aids and whether the hearing aids helps to reduce the handicapping influences of hearing impairment.

Aided Speech Recognition Measures

The goal of evaluating speech recognition for validation purposes is to ensure that the patient is hearing and understanding speech in a manner that meets expectations of performance. Performance in absolute terms is usually measured against expectations

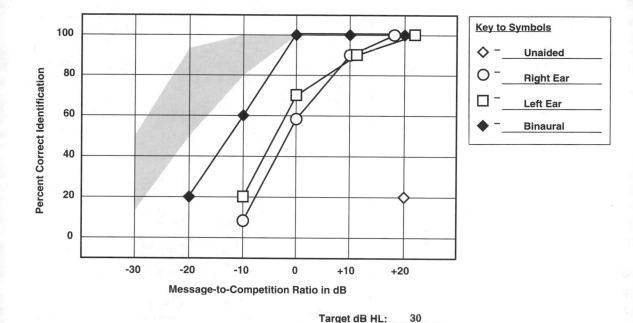

Figure 12-1. Results of aided speech recognition testing. Speech targets are presented at a fixed intensity level from a loudspeaker placed in front of a patient, with background competition presented from a loudspeaker located above or behind. Percent correct identification of target sentences is plotted as a function of message-to-competition ratio for three aided conditions: right, left, and binaural.

related to a patient's degree and configuration of hearing loss. Performance in relative terms is usually measured against unaided ability or as a comparison of monaural to binaural ability.

A number of strategies are used to assess aided speech recognition performance. A common approach is to present speech signals at a fixed intensity level from a loudspeaker placed in front of a patient, with background competition of some kind delivered from a speaker above or behind. Performance in recognizing the speech targets is then measured, and the intensity level of the competition is varied to assess ability at various target-to-competition ratios.

Figure 12–1 provides an example of results from this type of speech recognition testing. Performance in the monaural aided condition is compared to the binaural aided condition, and all are compared to normal performance. If speech recognition performance meets expectations, then the fitting is considered to be successful. If not, then the hearing aids can be adjusted or alternative amplification methods pursued.

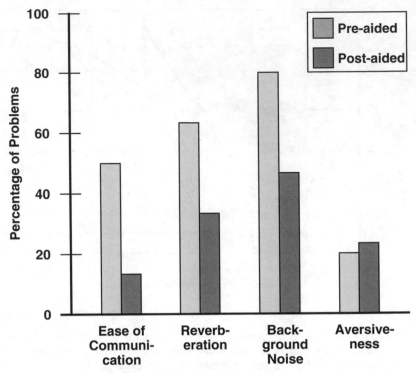

Figure 12–2. Results on the APHAB self-assessment scale in a patient before and after hearing aid use.

Self-Assessment Scales

Another way of validating outcome related to hearing aid fitting is to assess its impact on self-perception of communication handicap. Results from self-assessment scales administered after amplification use can be compared to pretreatment results to assess whether the hearing aids have had an impact on communication ability or handicap. Similarly, assessment can be done by spouses or others to verify the success of the rehabilitation approach.

A number of self-assessment scales are available for this purpose. Results from one that enjoys widespread use are shown in Figure 12–2. These results show pre- and postaided assessment of communication ability and indicate significant improvement.

Self-assessment validation is useful in identifying success or failure and may be useful in differentiating between major types of hearing aids or approaches to hearing aid fitting. It is probably not sensitive enough to differentiate between minor changes in electroacoustic output characteristics.

POSTFITTING REHABILITATION

For many adult patients, the proper fitting of appropriate hearing aid amplification, accompanied by extensive orientation and follow-up, constitutes enough rehabilitation to sufficiently ameliorate their communication disorders. For others, however, hearing aid fitting represents only the beginning of the process.

Postfitting rehabilitation for adults may involve auditory training to maximize the use of residual hearing and speechreading training to maximize use of the visual channel to assist in the communication process. Postfitting rehabilitation for children is usually much more protracted. It often involves language stimulation, speech therapy, auditory training, and extensive educational programming.

Auditory Training and Speechreading

Auditory training and speechreading are treatment methods that are sometimes used following the dispensing of hearing aids. Auditory training programs are designed to bring awareness to the hearing task and to improve listening skills. Extensive focus is placed on maximizing the use of residual auditory function. Auditory training programs typically include structured exercises in speech detection, discrimination, identification, and comprehension.

Speechreading programs are designed to enhance the skills of patients in supplementing auditory input with information that can be gained from lip movements and facial expressions.

Educational Programming

The goal of any treatment program for children is to ensure optimal acquisition of speech and language. In children with mild hearing sensitivity losses, such a goal can be accomplished with careful fitting of hearing aids, good orientation of parents to hearing loss and hearing aids, and very careful attention to speech and language stimulation during the formative years. For more severe hearing losses the task is more difficult, and the decisions are more challenging.

For many years there has been controversy about the best method of communication development training for children

The **oral approach** is a method of communication that involves the use of verbal communication and residual hearing.

The **manual approach** is a method of communication that involves the use of fingerspelling and sign language.

The **total communication** approach is a method of communication that incorporates both the oral and manual approaches.

with severe and profound hearing losses. One school of thought champions the **oral approach**, in which the child is fitted with hearing aids, or a cochlear implant, and undergoes very intensive training in oral/aural communication. The goal is to help the child to develop oral skills that will allow for a mainstreamed education and lifestyle. Another school of thought champions the **manual approach**. The manual approach teaches the child sign language as the method of communication. The goal is to help the child develop language through a sensory system that is not impaired. Yet another school of thought champions the idea of combining oral and manual communication in a **total approach**. The total approach emphasizes language development without regard to the sensory system. This approach seeks to maximize both language learning and oral communication.

Although the topic of education of the children with deafness has always been controversial, the acrimony has grown in recent years with the advent of cochlear implantation. Implants are proving to be a successful alternative to conventional hearing aid use, particularly in terms of ease of learning language. Many individuals who ascribe to the manual school of thought consider such an approach to be near heresy, however, because of their contention that deafness is an attribute not a disorder.

Regardless of the habilitation strategy, the most important component of a rehabilitation program is early identification and early intervention. The sooner a child is identified, the sooner the channels of communication required for language development can be opened.

SUMMARY

- Hearing aids are selected and fitted based on an individual's degree of hearing loss, the audiometric configuration of the loss, and estimates of the intensity levels at which sound is perceived to be uncomfortably loud.
- The first step in the selection process is to determine the target frequency gain responses that must be approximated by the chosen hearing aids. These targets are determined based on any of a number of rules.
- It is very important that the maximum output of the hearing aids does not exceed levels that are greater than the patient's threshold of discomfort.
- Specifying target parameters for input-output characteristics is important when the decision has been made to fit nonlinear hearing aids.

- The fitting process begins with the making of impressions of the outer ear and external auditory meatus. These impressions are used by the manufacturer to create custom-fitted earmolds or in-the-ear hearing aids.
- When hearing aids are received from the manufacturer, they should be inspected immediately for the quality of appearance and tested for function.
- The first step in the fitting process with the patient is to assess the physical qualities of the devices, including their fit in the ears, the patient's perception of their appearance, and the patient's ease in manipulating the devices.
- The general strategy of fitting and verification is one of assessing the gain and frequency parameters, making adjustments, verifying that the responses meet targets, and verifying that the aids meet some defined perceptual expectations.
- Verification of the frequency response is usually made by probe-microphone measurement. A small microphone is placed near the tympanic membrane, and the responses of the hearing aids to sounds of various frequencies and intensities are determined.
- One of the more compelling verification strategies is the determination of loudness judgments as a means of ensuring that speech is packaged appropriately within a patient's dynamic range.
- Following verification, a hearing aid orientation program is implemented, which consists of informational counseling about the nature of hearing and hearing impairment, the components and function of the hearing aids, and care and maintenance of the hearing aids.
- One of the most critical aspects of the hearing aid orientation is a discussion of reasonable expectations of hearing aid use and strategies for adapting to different listening environments.
- It is common practice to evaluate the success of hearing aid fitting after the patient has had an opportunity to wear and adjust to the use of the devices.
- Success is usually defined in terms of whether the patient understands speech better with the hearing aids and whether the hearing aids help to reduce the handicapping influences of hearing impairment.
- Postfitting rehabilitation for adults involves auditory training and speechreading training.
- Postfitting rehabilitation for children involves language stimulation, speech therapy, auditory training, and extensive educational programming.

SUGGESTED READINGS

Alpiner, J. G., & McCarthy, P. A. (1993). *Rehabilitative audiology: Children and adults* (2nd ed.). Baltimore: Williams & Wilkins.

Mueller, H. G., Hawkins, D. B., & Northern, J. L. (1992). *Probe microphone measurements. Hearing aid selection and assessment.* San Diego: Singular Publishing Group.

Sandlin, R. E. (Ed.). (1992). *Handbook of hearing aid amplification. Volume II: Clinical considerations and fitting practices.* San Diego: Singular Publishing Group.

Valente, M. (Ed.). (1994). *Strategies for selecting and verifying hearing aid fittings.* New York: Thieme Medical Publishing.

13

Different Rehabilitative Approaches For Different Populations

Although the overall goal of any hearing rehabilitation strategy is to reduce hearing handicap by maximizing the use of residual hearing, the approach used to reach that goal can vary across patients. The approach chosen to evaluate and fit hearing aids is sometimes related to patient factors such as age, sometimes related to type of hearing disorder, and other times related to patient need. For example, the strategy used for an adult patient with a sensorineural hearing impairment is considerably different from that used for a child with central auditory processing disorder. In the former, emphasis is placed on matching gain targets and approximating loudness growth; in the latter, emphasis is placed on classroom amplification strategies. Within these broad categories, the approach may also vary depending on a patient's age. For example, achieving hearing aid success in a geriatric patient may require a different approach than that used in a 20-year-old. Finally, there are patients with severe and profound deafness who might benefit from cochlear implantation, which requires an altogether different approach to fitting.

Although hearing rehabilitation must be adapted to the needs and expectations of individual patients, several broad categories of patients present common challenges that can be approached in a similar clinical manner. These categories include adults with sensorineural impairment, aging patients, children with sensorineural hearing impairment, children with CAPD, patients with conductive hearing loss, and patients with severe to profound hearing impairment.

ADULT POPULATIONS

Adult Sensorineural Hearing Impairment

Rehabilitative Goals

The challenges of fitting hearing aids to adults with sensorineural hearing impairment are, of course, related to the difficulties that sensorineural hearing losses cause. To review, sensorineural hearing loss results in the following problems, to a greater or lesser extent:

- loss of hearing sensitivity, so that soft sounds need to be amplified to become audible;
- sensitivity loss that varies with frequency and is generally greater in the higher frequencies;

- reduced dynamic range from the threshold of sensitivity to the threshold of discomfort;
- nonlinearity of loudness growth;
- diminished speech recognition ability, proportionate to the degree and configuration of the sensitivity loss; and
- reduced ability to hear speech in background noise.

Hearing aid amplification, then, is targeted at these manifestations of sensorineural hearing impairment. A hearing aid must amplify soft sounds to a level of audibility, must "package" the range of sound so that soft sounds are audible and loud sounds are not uncomfortable; must limit the maximum output to avoid discomfort; must reproduce sound faithfully, without distortion, to ensure adequate speech perception; and must do so in a manner that maintains or enhances the relation of the signal to the background noise.

Rehabilitative Strategies

Adult patients with sensorineural hearing impairment tend to be both easy and challenging in terms of hearing aid selection and fitting—easy because they are cooperative and can provide insightful feedback throughout the fitting process and challenging because there is not much to limit the audiologist's options. Following are general guidelines for fitting adults. The most important variables in this population are the degree and configuration of hearing loss.

Hearing Aid Selection. The adult patient should be fitted with binaural hearing aids, unless contraindicated clinically or because of some substantial ear asymmetries. Most adults will prefer custom hearing aids, and most can be accommodated in one way or another. Some hearing losses that formerly required the use of **BTE** hearing aids can now be fitted with **CIC** devices. Programmable hearing aids, with either **DCA** processing or **DSP**, should be the first choice because of their flexibility in matching the response gains to target. Dynamic range compression is usually indicated in patients with sensorineural hearing loss, especially those in the mild to moderate hearing loss categories.

BTE = behind-the-ear
CIC = completely-in-the-canal
DCA = digitally controlled analog
DSP = digital signal processing

Hearing Aid Fitting and Verification. Gain targets should be matched and verified with probe-microphone measurements. Loudness judgments can be obtained reliably in adults and should be used to verify that soft sounds are audible and loud sounds not uncomfortable. Finally, verification can be confirmed in adult patients with sensorineural hearing impairment with speech quality or speech intelligibility judgments.

Hearing Aid Validation. Aided speech recognition testing can quantify any binaural advantage or difference between ears and may be useful in helping the patient to develop reasonable performance expectations. A self-assessment scale should prove useful in pre- and postfitting assessment of communication abilities and needs.

Rehabilitation Treatment Plan. The treatment plan is usually uncomplicated in adult patients and consists of thorough orientation and follow-up to fine tune the hearing aid's functioning. Some patients, especially those with significant hearing loss and communication demands, will benefit from assistive listening devices, including the use of telephone amplifiers and personal FM systems.

Illustrative Case

Illustrative Case 13–1 is a patient with a long-standing sensorineural hearing impairment. The patient is a 54-year-old man with bilateral sensorineural hearing loss that has progressed slowly over the past 20 years. He has a positive history of noise exposure, first during military service, and then at his workplace. The patient reports that he has used hearing protection on occasion in the past, but has not done so on a consistent basis. In addition, there is a family history of hearing loss occurring in middle age. He was having his hearing tested at the urging of family members who were having increasing difficulty communicating with him.

An audiological assessment revealed normal middle ear function, a bilateral, fairly symmetric, high-frequency sensorineural hearing loss, and speech-recognition ability consistent with the degree of hearing loss.

A rehabilitation assessment showed that the patient has significant communication needs at work. Results of a hearing handicap assessment showed that he has communication problems a significant proportion of the time that he spends in certain listening environments, especially those involving background noise. He has no motoric and other physical disabilities and is financially able to pursue hearing aid use. The patient expressed a preference for the "computerized hearing aids that are invisible in the ear."

Target gains were calculated based on the patient's hearing thresholds with a commonly used prescriptive gain formula. Programmable CIC DSP hearing devices were chosen based on the patient's stated preference. Thus, the general prescriptive gain was all that was specified because of the flexibility of the device for controlling other electroacoustic characteristics. The particular devices chosen use wide dynamic range compression for the input-output characteristics and compression limiting of maximum output. Ear impressions were made, and the hearing aids were ordered.

Real-ear assessment of the output of the hearing aid was made with probe-microphone measurements. Figure 13–1A shows the responses of the right-ear hearing aid to three levels of input signals and how they compare to a targeted frequency gain. Verification of the fitting was made by asking the patient to judge the loudness of speech presented at 45, 65, and 85 dB SPL. Adjustments were made to ensure that the patient heard the speech as soft, moderate, and loud, but not too loud.

Validation was assessed after 1 month of hearing aid use. The patient's speech-recognition performance with the hearing aids is shown in Figure 13–1B. Here, performance is plotted as a function of message-to-competition ratio. In addition, the self-assessment scale that was given at the time of the initial rehabilitation assessment was readministered. Results were compared to the earlier evaluation and showed that communication problems were reduced for him in most listening environments with the hearing aids.

Geriatric Sensorineural Hearing Impairment

Rehabilitative Goals

Hearing loss that occurs with aging is not necessarily different than that which occurs in younger adults. In some older patients, however, the sensitivity loss is confounded by changes in central auditory nervous system function. As a consequence, in addition to the problems described above, hearing impairment may result in:

- significant reduction in ability to hear speech in background noise;
- diminished ability to use two ears for sound localization and for separation of signals from noise; and
- reduced **temporal processing** of auditory information.

The ability of the auditory system to deal with timing aspects of speech perception is called **temporal processing**.

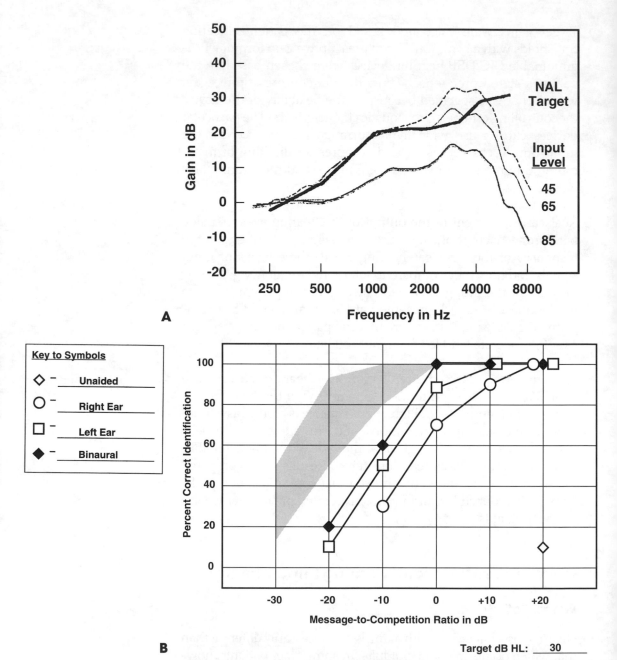

Figure 13-1. Aided results in a 54-year-old man with bilateral sensorineural hearing loss. Hearing aid response measurements (A) from the right ear are compared to a frequency gain target. Speech-recognition results (B) show good aided performance.

Hearing aid amplification, then, must be targeted either to overcome these problems or to reduce the impact of their influence. When fitting hearing aids on older individuals, the audiologist must remember that sound emanating from the hearing devices needs to be processed by the auditory nervous system. When the nervous system is intact, the hearing devices need to overcome the peripheral cochlear deficit. However, as people age, so too do their auditory nervous systems, and this aging process is not without consequences. Audiologists are often confronted in the clinic with the impact of the aging auditory nervous system on hearing ability in general and on conventional hearing device use in particular. It appears that patients with demonstrable deficits from **senescent** changes in the auditory nervous system do not benefit as much from conventional hearing devices as their younger counterparts.

Senescent changes are changes that occur due to the aging process.

Rehabilitative Strategies

Clinical experience with older individuals suggests that the more that can be done to ease the burden of listening in background noise, whether by sophisticated signal processing in an ear-level hearing device or by use of a remote microphone, the more likely the patient will benefit from hearing-device amplification. Another important challenge in fitting hearing aids in older individuals is the difficulty involved in the physical manipulation of the device.

Hearing Aid Selection. The technical advances designed to enhance signal-to-noise ratio are, of course, no different for the elderly than for younger patients, but their application is probably more important. The use of binaural hearing aids, **directional microphones**, and advanced signal processing appear to be key elements in successful fitting.

A **directional microphone** focuses on sounds in front of the listener.

Gain and output characteristics should be similar to those prescribed for younger adults. Dynamic range compression is indicated, particularly for those with mild to moderate degrees of sensorineural hearing loss. Programmable hearing aids should be considered because of their flexibility in matching responses to target gain.

ITE hearing aids are better for older individuals than BTE devices. Although perhaps counterintuitive because of relative size, custom hearing aids are easier for older patients to insert and remove than BTE hearing aids with earmolds. Most ITE devices can be ordered with an extraction handle, which can be quite helpful to a patient with limited fine-motor control.

Remote controls can be quite useful to some older patients with poor dexterity but a burden to others who are not technologically oriented or who have difficulty remembering where they place things.

Although binaural hearing aids are indicated in most cases, some older individuals have significant ear asymmetries in speech perception and cannot successfully wear two hearing aids. In fact, in some rare cases, fitting a hearing aid on the poorly functioning ear can make binaural ability with hearing aids poorer than the best monaural performance.

Hearing Aid Fitting and Verification. As in younger adults, gain targets should be matched and verified with probe-microphone measurements. Loudness judgments can be obtained reliably in most older patients and should be used to verify that soft sounds are audible and loud sounds not uncomfortable. Finally, verification can be confirmed in many older adult patients with sensorineural hearing loss with speech quality or speech intelligibility judgments. However, this can be a difficult perceptual task for some older listeners who have difficulty assigning a quality or intelligibility ranking.

Hearing Aid Validation. Aided speech recognition testing is very important in older patients to help determine if both ears can be aided effectively. Here a comparison should be made of right monaural, left monaural, and binaural speech recognition ability. If binaural ability is poorer than the best monaural ability, then consideration should be given to fitting only one hearing aid. This, however, will only occur in the exceptional patient. A self-assessment scale should prove useful in pre- and postfitting assessment of communication abilities and need. Assessment by a spouse or significant other can also be quite useful in this age range.

Rehabilitation Treatment Plan. Despite all of the technical advances in conventional hearing aids, some older individuals cannot make use of conventional hearing aids. In such cases, the use of remote-microphone technology for the enhancement of the signal-to-noise ratio has been a successful approach. Many audiologists believe that it is good practice to familiarize older patients with personal FM systems and other ALDs during the orientation process so that if hearing aid benefit declines, they will be aware of an alternative solution to their hearing problems.

Illustrative Case

Illustrative Case 13–2 is an elderly patient with a long-standing sensorineural hearing loss. The patient is a 78-year-old woman with bilateral sensorineural hearing impairment that has progressed slowly over the past 15 years. She has worn a hearing aid for the past 10 years, and has an annual audiologic re-evaluation each year.

An audiological assessment revealed normal middle ear function; a bilateral, symmetric, moderate, sloping, sensorineural hearing loss; and speech-recognition ability that is substantially reduced, consistent with the patient's age. She also shows evidence of a dichotic deficit, with reduced performance in the left ear. Results are shown in Figure 13–2A.

A rehabilitation assessment showed that the patient has difficulty in communicating with her grandchildren and in trying to hear in noisy cafeterias and restaurants. Results of the hearing handicap assessment show that she has communication problems a significant proportion of the time in most listening environments, especially those involving background noise. She has slightly reduced motoric function, but no other disabilities. Her current hearing aid is 3 years old. She reports that, although a hearing aid worked well for her at the beginning, she is not receiving the benefit from it that she did when she was first fitted with amplification 10 years ago.

Electroacoustic analysis of the patient's hearing aid showed it to be functioning as expected. It is a programmable ITE hearing aid that was adjusted adequately to her degree of hearing sensitivity loss, which had changed little over the ensuing years. This patient may benefit from assistive listening devices, and a consultation to discuss these alternatives was recommended.

The first decision was to try to complete the binaural fitting. For whatever reason, this was not done initially. The first step in the process of trying to meet her needs is to give her back both of her ears to try to help her hear more effectively in noisy environments. A device for the left ear was chosen that matched the frequency gain, input-output, and output limiting characteristics of her other hearing aid.

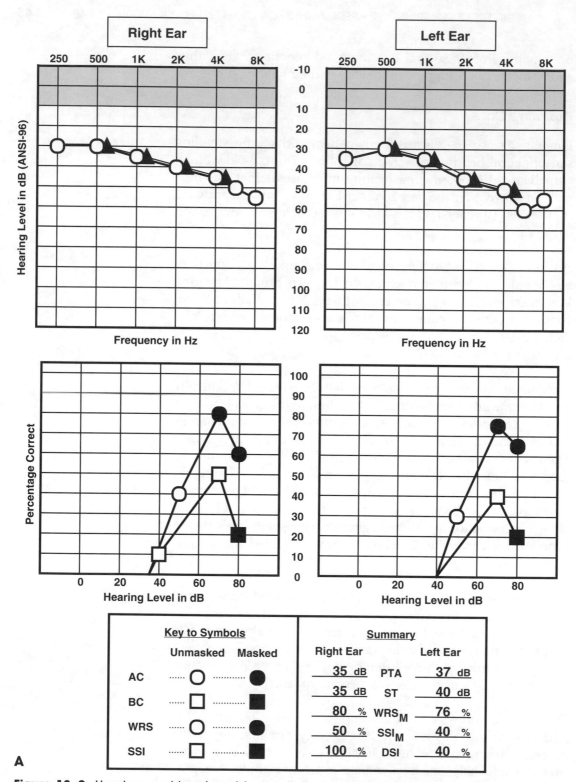

Figure 13-2. Hearing- and hearing-aid consultation results in a 78-year-old woman with long-standing, progressive hearing loss. Pure-tone and speech audiometric results (A) show bilateral, symmetric, moderate, sensorineural hearing loss and reduced speech recognition ability. Aided speech-recognition results (B) show adequate aided performance.

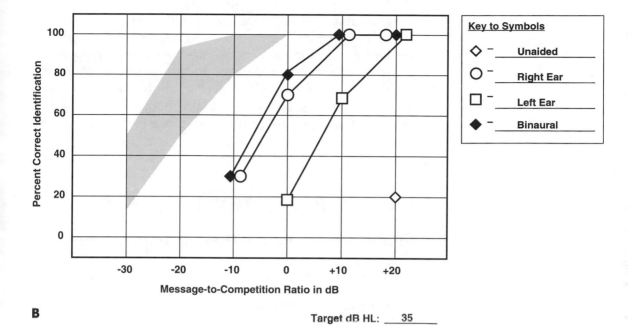

B

Target dB HL: ___35___

Frequency gain was adjusted by adjusting real-ear responses measured by a probe microphone to targets for soft, moderate, and loud sounds. The hearing aids were then readjusted according to her loudness estimates to speech presented at levels of 45, 65, and 85 dB SPL. The gain of her older hearing aid had to be reduced because of the increased apparent gain achieved from having binaural input.

At the time of completion of the binaural fitting, the patient was familiarized with the use of a personal FM system. The device was used during all informational counseling prior to the completion of hearing aid fitting.

Validation was assessed after 1 month of hearing aid use. The patient's speech-recognition performance with the hearing aids is shown in Figure 13–2B. Results showed that the patient performed fairly well with both hearing aids. In addition, the self-assessment scale that was given when she was using only one hearing aid was re-administered. Results were compared to the earlier evaluation and showed that communication problems were reduced for her in most listening environments with two hearing aids.

Despite the relative advantages shown with the self-assessment scale and her adequate performance with hearing aids, this patient was not demonstrating the benefit from hearing aid use to an extent that might be expected of a younger person with the same degree of hearing loss. At the time of the follow-up evaluation, the patient was encouraged to try to use an FM system coupled to her hearing aids, especially during luncheons and other social activities. Following a trial period, she purchased an FM system. She now uses hearing aids alone in quiet situations, the FM system alone to watch television, and both hearing aids and the FM system in noisy situations.

PEDIATRIC POPULATIONS

Pediatric Sensorineural Hearing Impairment

Rehabilitative Goals

The rehabilitative goal for young children is to maximize the use of residual auditory ability to ensure the best possible hearing for the development of oral language and speech. The specific aims are to provide the best hearing aids possible, supplemented with assistive listening devices when indicated, and to provide maximum exposure to language stimulation opportunities.

Hearing impairment in children results in the following problems:

- loss of hearing sensitivity, so that soft sounds need to be amplified to become audible;
- degree of sensitivity loss that varies with frequency and is generally greater in the higher frequencies;
- reduced dynamic range from the threshold of sensitivity to the threshold of discomfort;
- nonlinearity of loudness growth.

You will notice immediately that these are the same problems faced by adults. Thus, in meeting the specific aim related to hearing aids, the actual hearing loss challenges are not different than those of adults. That is, sensorineural hearing loss in young children is essentially the same as sensorineural hearing loss in adults. The difference in the challenge is that we are seldom able to quantify it with the same precision or to verify our amplification solutions to the same extent.

Rehabilitative Strategies

Hearing aid selection and fitting in children with sensorineural hearing impairment is a challenging business for various reasons.

One is that audiometric levels may be known only generally at the beginning of the fitting process. Another is that children are less likely or able to participate in the selection and fitting process. Still another is that hearing may be more variable in young children due to progression or to fluctuation secondary to otitis media. Following are general guidelines for fitting children.

Hearing Aid Selection. Children should always be fitted with binaural hearing aids unless contraindicated by medical factors or extreme hearing asymmetries. The goal is to maximize residual hearing, and two ears will accomplish that better than one.

Because the auricle and ear canal grow in size, the custom part of the hearing aid will need to be changed frequently while the child is young. As a result, most audiologists choose to fit BTE hearing aids and change the earmolds as indicated rather than having an ITE case changed.

Programmable hearing aids are indicated for young children for at least three reasons. First, the degree and configuration of hearing loss may be known only generally at the beginning of the fitting process. The final frequency gain characteristics may only resemble those tried initially. Programmable hearing aids provide a larger range for making such changes. Second, hearing is likely to fluctuate if the child has bouts of **otitis media** with effusion, and flexibility again will be required. Third, hearing loss can be progressive in children, and a programmable hearing aid can be adjusted to some extent to keep up with the changes.

Otitis media with effusion is middle ear inflammation with the presence of fluid.

Gain and output characteristics should be similar to those in adults, but targets will be more difficult to determine because of limited audiometric data. Fortunately, algorithms have been developed to predict targets for frequency-specific gain to low-level and high-level input from audiometric data of children.

Hearing Aid Fitting and Verification. Fitting challenges start with the making of earmold impressions. The audiologist who is thinking ahead will make ear impressions while the child is undergoing ABR verification of hearing loss and is sedated. Otherwise, the making of ear impressions in young children can be as much a matter of will as of technical ability.

Although target gains can be estimated from audiometric data, they are not often easy to verify with probe-microphone measurements in children due to their lack of cooperation with probe-microphone insertion. Verification often depends on measurement of functional gain. Functional gain targets for children have been estimated from threshold data and can be used to serve as a guideline for fitting verification. Discomfort levels can be estimated similarly.

Hearing Aid Validation. Depending on the child's age and language ability, validation can be made with speech audiometric measures. The procedure is not unlike that used in adults, wherein speech targets are presented in the presence of background competition and the child attempts to identify the speech, usually through a picture pointing task. Aided results can be compared to unaided results and to expectations for normal hearing ability under similar circumstances. Otherwise, validation depends on directed observation of hearing ability by the parents, teachers, therapists, and audiologist.

Rehabilitation Treatment Plan. Once the hearing aid has been fitted, treatment begins. Depending on the degree of hearing loss, intensive auditory training, language stimulation, and speech therapy are introduced in an effort to maximize language development.

Children are likely to use remote-microphone systems in classrooms at school, and proper fitting and orientation are imperative. Many parents find that supplemental use of an FM system at home can greatly enhance the language stimulation opportunities as well.

Illustrative Case

Illustrative Case 13–3 is a young child with a fluctuating, mild-to-severe sensorineural hearing impairment bilaterally. The patient is a 4-year-old girl. The hearing impairment appears to be caused by CMV or cytomegalic inclusion disease, a viral infection usually transmitted in utero. There is no family history of hearing loss and no other significant medical history.

An audiological evaluation showed normal middle ear function; a bilateral, mild-to-severe, sensorineural hearing loss; and speech-recognition ability that was congruous with the degree and configuration of hearing loss. Results are shown in Figure 13–3A.

The child's age and the fluctuating nature of the hearing loss were two major factors in the decision about type of amplification device to use. The first decision was that the child will wear two hearing aids. Nothing about her ears or hearing loss contraindi-

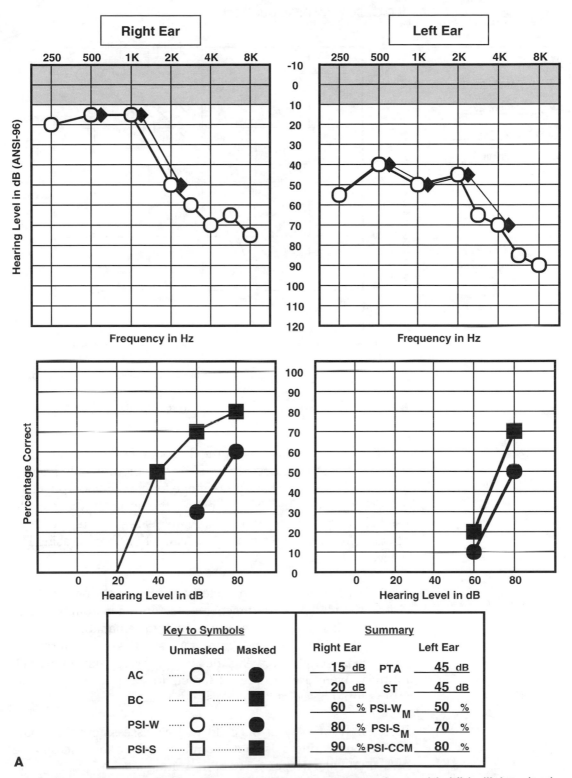

Figure 13-3. Hearing- and hearing-aid consultation results in a 4-year-old child with hearing loss secondary to CMV infection. Pure-tone and speech audiometric results (A) show bilateral mild-to-severe sensorineural hearing loss and speech-recognition ability consistent with the loss. Aided speech-recognition results (B) show appropriate aided performance.

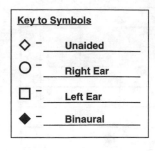

Key to Symbols

◇ – Unaided

○ – Right Ear

□ – Left Ear

◆ – Binaural

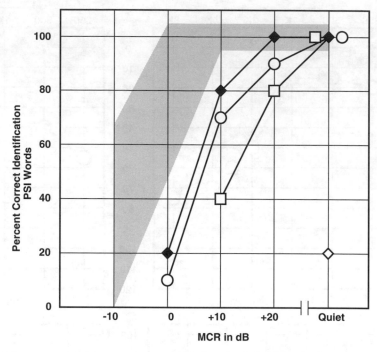

B

Target dB HL: ___30___

cates this decision. Because of the fluctuating nature of her hearing loss, the second decision was to try programmable hearing aids, which generally have more range for changing output characteristics. Finally, because of her age, the decision was made to use behind-the-ear hearing aids. As her ears grow, replacement of earmolds is usually a more practical option than recasing ITE devices.

With regard to the other characteristics of the hearing aid, a decision was made to use directional microphones in an effort to enhance the signal-to-noise ratio of sounds emanating from the front of the child. Frequency gain characteristics were determined based on prescriptive targets. The DSL, or desired sensation level, formulae were used to predict targets for both gain and maximum output based on the child's audiogram.

Fortunately for a 4-year-old child, real-ear assessment of the output of the hearing aids could be made with probe-microphone measurements. Responses of both hearing aids to moderate and high input signals were compared to the targeted frequency gains and adjusted to approximate them. Adjustments were made to ensure that the patient was not provided with too much output for her comfort.

Validation was assessed at the time of initial fitting. The patient's speech-recognition performance with the hearing aids is shown in Figure 13–3B. Here, materials were used that were age-appropriate for the child. Results show very good speech-recognition performance in the aided conditions.

Validation was also assessed as part of an ongoing follow-up process to ensure that the child was receiving adequate aided gain and to assess the impact of any hearing fluctuation on performance with the hearing aids. When this child enters school, the use of classroom amplification will become important. Her hearing aids have t-coils built in to be used with a neck loop on an FM system for classroom use.

This patient had access to speech and oral language development prior to the initial reduction in her hearing. However, she is now at risk for developing speech and academic-achievement problems and needs to be monitored carefully.

Central Auditory Processing Disorder

Rehabilitative Goals

CAPD is an auditory disorder that has as one of its main components difficulty in understanding speech in background noise. Rehabilitative goals that focus on this component are often effective in forestalling or changing the expected outcome related to the presence of CAPD.

Intervention strategies directed toward enhancement of signal-to-noise ratio have proven successful in the treatment of children with CAPD. There are at least two approaches to this type of intervention. The first approach is to alter the acoustic environment to enhance the listening situation. Environmental alterations include practical approaches such as preferential seating in the classroom and manipulation of the home environment so that the child is placed in more favorable listening situations. Alterations may also include equipping the classroom with sound-field speakers to provide amplification of the teacher's speech.

It is not uncommon in children with CAPD for the diagnosis itself to serve as the treatment. That is, once parents and teachers become aware of the nature of the child's problem and that the solution is one of enhancement of the signal-to-noise ratio, they manipulate the environment so that the problem situations are eliminated, and the child's auditory processing difficulties become inconsequential.

In other cases, however, when severity of the auditory processing disorder is greater, the use of remote microphone technology may be indicated.

Rehabilitative Strategies

The main challenge in treating children with CAPD is to assist them in overcoming their difficulties in understanding speech in background noise. The main focus of their problems is the classroom setting. In some areas, classrooms have amplification systems that can be used to overcome these problems. If not, the child may benefit from amplification designed to enhance the signal-to-noise ratio.

Hearing Aid Selection. Conventional hearing aids do not appear to be indicated for children with CAPD. Even mild gain amplification with sophisticated signal processing and noise reduction circuitry may be insufficient to reduce background noise to the extent necessary for children with CAPD. Here the selection process is focused on finding the right remote microphone configuration for the child. Generally that means the use of a personal FM system. These systems can be designed to provide a flat frequency response with minimal gain delivered to the ear and low maximum output levels to protect the normal hearing ear from damaging noise levels.

The amplified signal is usually delivered to the ear through small headphones to both ears or an ear coupler to one ear.

Hearing Aid Fitting and Verification. Probe microphone measurements can be made of the output of the remote-microphone device to ensure minimal gain and low maximum output.

Speech recognition testing should be used to verify that the child can take advantage of enhanced signal-to-noise ratios. A common approach is to present speech signals at a fixed intensity level from a loudspeaker placed in front of a patient, with background competition of some kind delivered from a speaker above or behind. Performance in recognizing the speech targets is then measured, and the competition intensity level is varied to assess ability at various signal-to-noise ratios. Testing is carried out without a device and with the remote microphone in close proximity to the loudspeaker from which the targets are being presented. Performance should increase substantially with the remote-microphone device.

Hearing Aid Validation. Validation of success with this fitting strategy is made with teacher and parental questionnaires designed to assess the benefit of device use in the classroom and at home. Successful questionnaires include assessment of listening skills, general behavior, apparent hearing ability, and general academic achievement before and after implementation of device usage. The questionnaire also addresses the emotional impact of device use in the classroom.

Rehabilitation Treatment Plan. Children with CAPD may also benefit from auditory-training therapy directed toward enhancement of the ability to process auditory information and toward development of compensatory skills.

Because children with CAPD often have **concomitant deficits** in speech, language, attention, learning, and cognition, comprehensive approaches to treatment are recommended. Treatment for memory, vocabulary, comprehension, listening, reading, and spelling are often necessary in children with multiple involvement.

Concomitant deficits are those that occur together.

Illustrative Case

Illustrative Case 13–4 is a young child with central auditory processing disorder. The patient is a 6-year-old girl with a history of chronic otitis media. Although her parents have always suspected that she had a hearing problem, pure-tone screenings in the past revealed hearing sensitivity within normal limits. Tympanometric screenings revealed type B tympanograms during periods of otitis media and normal tympanograms during times of remission from otitis media.

An audiological evaluation showed normal middle ear function, normal hearing sensitivity, abnormal speech-recognition ability, and abnormal auditory evoked potentials. Results are summarized in Figure 13–4A.

A rehabilitation assessment showed that this child has substantial difficulty hearing in noisy and distracting environments. She is likely to be at risk for academic achievement problems if her learning environment is not structured to be a quiet one.

Initially, the parents were provided with information about the nature of the disorder and the strategies that can be used to alter listening environments in ways that might be useful to this child.

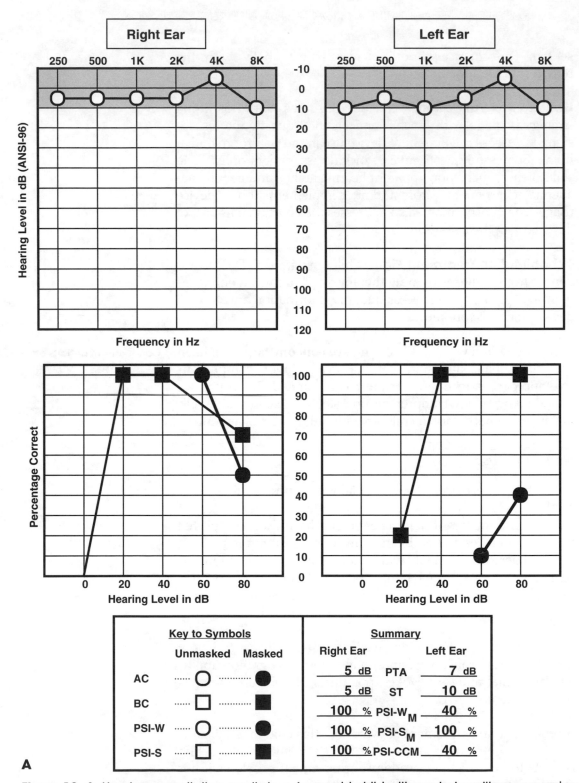

Figure 13-4. Hearing-consultation results in a 6-year-old child with central auditory processing disorder. Pure-tone and speech audiometric results (A) show normal hearing sensitivity and abnormal speech-recognition ability. Aided results (B) show good speech-recognition performance with an FM system in a sound field.

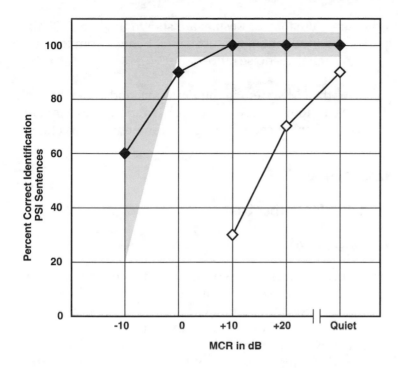

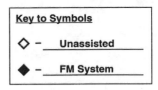

Target dB HL: 20

B

The parents found this information to be quite useful and to go a long way in solving the patient's communication needs in the home environment. However, once the child entered school, the hearing problem resurfaced.

A re-evaluation showed little change in the patient's processing ability. Consultation with the parents and teacher led to a decision to try the use of a personal FM system in the classroom.

Personal FM systems for use with those who have normal hearing sensitivity generally provide a flat frequency response with very little gain across the frequency range. The input-output is generally linear. Output limiting is of little concern because of the minimal gain characteristics. A set of contemporary headphones were used, a solution that tends to be acceptable if not enviable in today's classroom.

Performance with the FM system was assessed by measuring speech-recognition in the sound field with the microphone located at the child's ear and in proximity to the loudspeaker from which the target emanated. Results are shown in Figure 13–4B. As expected, the patient enjoys substantial benefit from the enhancement of signal-to-noise ratio.

The child uses the FM system in the classroom and under certain circumstances at home. Parent and teacher reports substantiate the benefits of an enhanced listening environment for this child.

OTHER POPULATIONS

Conductive Hearing Loss

Rehabilitative Goals

Conductive hearing loss results from disorders of the outer or middle ears. In most cases, these disorders can be treated medically or surgically, and little residual hearing impairment remains. In a small percentage of patients, however, the disorder cannot be treated. For example, a patient who has experienced multiple surgical procedures for protracted otitis media and **mastoiditis** might end up with middle ear disorder that is beyond surgical repair. In such cases, a hearing aid might be the only realistic form of rehabilitation. As another example, patients with **congenital atresia** have hearing loss due to lack of an external auditory meatus. Although this condition is surgically treatable, it is usually not carried out in children until they are older. In such cases, hearing aid use will be necessary during the presurgical years.

Inflammation of the bony process behind the auricle is called **mastoiditis**.

Congenital atresia is the absence at birth of the opening of the external auditory meatus.

The rehabilitative goal in the treatment of intractable conductive hearing loss is to maximize the use of residual hearing with hearing aid amplification. A conductive hearing loss acts as a sound attenuator, with little reduction in suprathreshold hearing once sound is made audible. Hearing aid amplification, then, is targeted at this primary manifestation of conductive hearing impairment.

Rehabilitative Strategies

Overcoming the attenuating effects of conductive hearing loss is relatively simple from a signal processing strategy. The challenge in this population is more often related to providing a satisfactory physical fit for the amplification device.

Hearing Aid Selection. Patients with permanent conductive hearing loss in both ears should be fitted with binaural hearing aids as a means of enhancing gain.

A permanent conductive loss is usually flat in configuration, requiring a broad, flat frequency gain response. Target gain should be increased by approximately 25% of the air-bone gap at a given frequency. Loudness growth in a conductive hearing loss is equivalent to that of a normal ear, making linear amplification the input-output characteristic of choice. There is little need for output limitation, because the attenuation effect of the conductive hearing loss serves as a protective measure.

The style of hearing aid depends on the nature of the disorder causing the conductive hearing loss. For example, permanent conductive hearing loss secondary to chronically draining ears requires a BTE hearing aid with sufficient venting due to the drainage. Because a conductive hearing loss requires more gain than a sensorineural hearing loss, this venting must be done carefully to avoid feedback problems.

As another example, bilateral atresia requires the use of a bone-conduction hearing aid. In a bone-conduction hearing aid, the normal receiver is replaced with a bone vibrator that is designed to stimulate the cochlea directly, bypassing the closed ear canal.

Hearing Aid Fitting and Verification. Fitting of a conventional hearing aid can often be done with probe-microphone measures, depending on the physical status of the ear canal. The frequency gain and maximum output characteristics can then be adjusted to meet target gain estimates. Because the loss is conductive, the only other important measure is to ensure that soft sounds are audible. Assessing discomfort levels and speech perception is largely unnecessary.

Fitting of bone conduction hearing aids requires functional gain measurement for output verification. The output of the hearing aid can be adjusted until targeted functional gain levels are met.

Hearing Aid Validation. Aided speech recognition testing can be used to ensure that speech recognition meets expectations for the loss. A self-assessment scale will prove useful in pre- and postfitting assessment of communication abilities and needs.

Rehabilitation Treatment Plan. Other rehabilitation needs are often unnecessary for those with permanent conductive hearing loss. The exception is the child with congenital, bilateral atresia, who, until proven otherwise, will need all of the intensive hearing and language stimulation training of children with sensorineural hearing impairment. The efficiency with which such training can be accomplished is likely to be better in the child with atresia because of normal cochlear function.

Illustrative Case

Illustrative Case 13–5 is a young patient with bilateral conductive hearing loss due to long-standing untreated middle ear disorder. The patient is a 19-year-old woman. As a child, she experienced chronic otitis media with effusion that was not treated because of restricted access to appropriate health care. As a result of the chronic nature of the disease process, her middle ear structures eroded to a point that surgical attempts to reconstruct the middle ears failed. Although there was no longer any active disease process, the conductive hearing loss remained. She used a telephone amplifier to communicate on the phone and a personal amplifier on certain occasions to communicate with friends. She was interested in going to college and felt that she might stand a better chance of succeeding if she used hearing aids.

An audiological assessment revealed a bilateral, symmetric, flat conductive hearing loss and good suprathreshold speech-recognition ability. Results are shown in Figure 13–5A.

A rehabilitation assessment showed that the patient has significant communication needs, especially in terms of her desire to pursue a college education. Results of a hearing handicap assessment showed that she has communication problems a significant proportion of the time that she spends in certain listening environments, especially those in which the speaker has a soft voice or is at a distance. She has no motoric or other physical disabilities.

The hearing aid fitting in this patient was relatively straightforward. She needed linear gain and lots of it, and output limiting was not important. Her need for gain dictated that she use either a tightly fitted ITE or a BTE with a tightly fitted earmold. Because of the gain requirements and the need to provide some degree of venting, a BTE configuration was chosen. Target gains were calculated based on the patient's hearing thresholds with a commonly used prescriptive gain formula and a correction factor of 25% of the air-bone gap. Nonprogrammable, linear hearing aids within the targeted gain range were chosen.

Real-ear assessment of the output of the hearing aid was made with functional gain measurements. Figure 13–5B shows the aided responses.

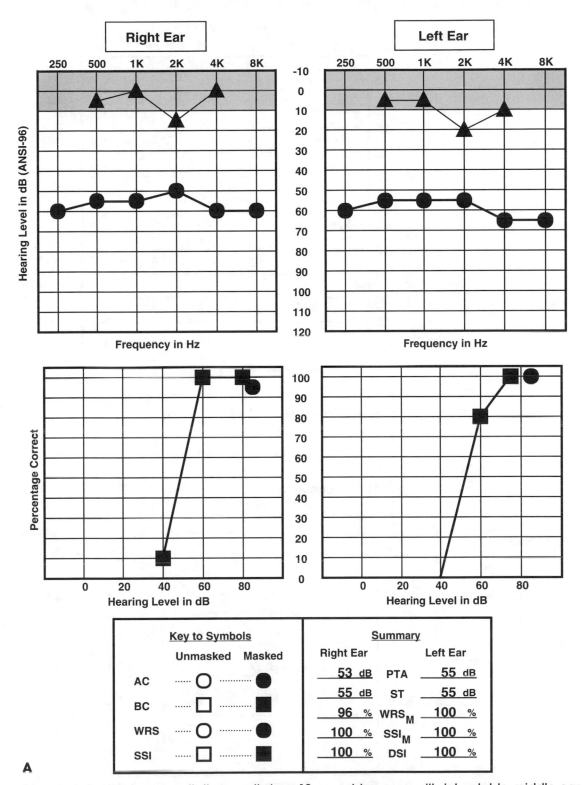

Figure 13-5. Hearing-consultation results in a 19-year-old woman with intractable middle ear disorder. Pure-tone and speech audiometric results (A) show flat conductive hearing loss and good suprathreshold speech-recognition ability bilaterally. Functional gain measurements (B) show appropriate real-ear gain. Speech-recognition results (C) show good aided performance.

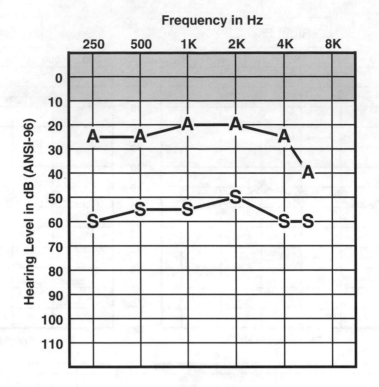

Frequency in Hz

Functional Gain Assessment

Unaided soundfield thresholds .... **S**

Aided soundfield thresholds .... **A**

B

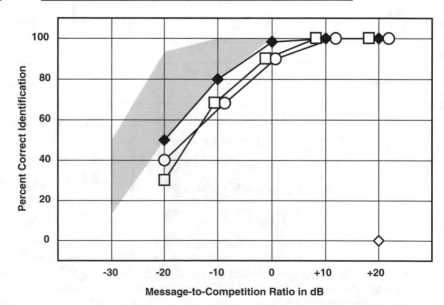

Key to Symbols

◇ — Unaided

○ — Right Ear

□ — Left Ear

◆ — Binaural

C

Target dB HL: ___30___

Validation was assessed after 1 month of hearing aid use. The patient's speech-recognition performance with the hearing aids is shown in Figure 13–5C. Here, performance is plotted as a function of message-to-competition ratio. In addition, the self-assessment scale that was given at the time of the initial rehabilitation assessment was readministered. Results were compared to the earlier evaluation and showed that the patient's communication problems were reduced in most listening environments with the hearing aids.

Profound Sensorineural Deafness

Rehabilitative Goals

Profound hearing impairment in children or adults substantially limits the use of the auditory channel for communication purposes. Even with very powerful hearing aids, auditory function may be limited to awareness of environmental sounds or, at best, serve as an aid to lipreading.

In young children, the prognosis for learning speech and oral language is quite low. Most children born with profound hearing loss communicate in sign language and have little or no verbal communication ability.

In adults with adventitious profound hearing impairment, reception of verbal communication can be limited, and speech skills can erode due to an inability to monitor vocal output.

The most common first step in hearing rehabilitation in this population is trial use of conventional amplification, followed by cochlear implantation. The rehabilitative goal is the same: maximize hearing in an effort to ameliorate the communication disorder caused by the hearing loss.

Rehabilitative Strategies

Cochlear implantation is the primary hearing rehabilitation strategy for patients with profound deafness. In young children, candidacy for cochlear implantation includes the following criteria:

■ profound bilateral sensorineural hearing loss
■ little or no benefit from hearing aids or vibrotactile devices
■ no medical contraindications

■ educational placement in a program that emphasizes audition
■ family support
■ appropriate expectations

In adults, candidacy for cochlear implantation includes the following criteria:

■ severe to profound bilateral sensorineural hearing loss
■ limited benefit from appropriate hearing aids
■ hearing loss acquired after learning oral speech and language
■ no medical contraindication
■ motivation to be part of the hearing culture

Patients with profound deafness who are not candidates for cochlear implantation may benefit to a limited extent from powerful conventional hearing aids. The selection and fitting strategies for power hearing aids are challenging but straightforward. Binaural hearing aids are used to provide the most gain possible. Hearing aids are BTE devices with tight-fitting earmolds. Gain targets are generated and met as usual. Dynamic range is usually quite limited, and maximum output must be carefully adjusted. Hearing aids use analog processing and have linear input-output characteristics.

One other strategy that may be tried is the use of a vibrotactile device. A vibrotactile device is a lot like a bone-conduction hearing aid in that the receiver of a conventional hearing aid is replaced by a vibrating device, in this case a sophisticated array of electrodes that translate acoustic information into vibratory patterns that are delivered to the skin. Perception of sound is vibrotactile and can serve as an alerting device and as a valuable adjunct to lipreading.

The remainder of this section will address cochlear implantation as the strategy for hearing rehabilitation of this population.

Cochlear Implant Selection. Once candidacy has been determined, decisions related to strategy are limited mostly to which ear to implant and which brand of device to implant. The former decision is an important one. In general, there is a tendency to implant the better ear if there is a difference in function between ears, assuming that prognosis will be best for successful neural stimulation in that ear.

Most of the selection process is completed once this decision is made. Different manufacturers use different processing strategies, most of which have been implemented with equivalent success. Often this issue is resolved by choosing the manufacturer with the latest technological advance.

Device Fitting and Verification. Programming of the cochlear implant processor varies by manufacturer and by processing strategy, but some generalizations can be made. One of the first steps is to determine if activation of a given electrode in the implanted array results in the perception of hearing. If so, then the threshold and dynamic range of that electrode are determined. Once this is done for the entire array, a "map" of these values is created across electrodes. From these basic data, determination is made of which electrodes are to receive frequency and intensity information, depending on the processing strategy that is chosen.

This process of "mapping" the electrodes is an ongoing one that can take several sessions to complete in adults and can take months to complete in young children.

Verification of the map is usually accomplished with the use of speech perception testing. Large batteries of tests have been developed for both children and adults to assess performance with the implant devices.

Device Validation. Validation of successful cochlear implantation use is similar to that described for conventional hearing devices. In adults, it is not uncommon to use speech recognition measures and benefit questionnaires to assess outcomes. In young children, outcomes can also be assessed with speech recognition measures, depending on language ability, or by directed observation of hearing ability by the parents, teachers, therapists, and the audiologist.

Rehabilitation Treatment Plan. Similarly, rehabilitation treatment planning is the same as that described for conventional hearing devices. Adults may benefit from supplemental use of remote microphone input and other assistive devices. They might also benefit from courses in speechreading. For young children, implantation simply marks the beginning of the process of speech and language stimulation.

Illustrative Cases

Illustrative Case 13–6. Case 6 is an adult patient with profound bilateral sensorineural hearing impairment that has progressed over the last 10 years. The patient is a 44-year-old woman. Based on familial history, her hearing impairment is thought to be caused by dominant progressive hereditary hearing loss. She is an accountant in a large insurance firm and, although much of her work is computer based, she feels that she is being left behind professionally and socially because of her substantial hearing impairment.

An audiological assessment shows a profound, primarily sensorineural hearing loss. Speech-recognition ability is poor, consistent with the degree of hearing loss. Performance with binaural hearing aids shows some achievable aided gain, but little benefit in speech-recognition ability. Results are shown in Figure 13–6A.

A rehabilitation assessment showed the patient to be an excellent candidate for hearing rehabilitation. She was in good health and has strong support from her family, friends, and employer. She judges her communication needs and her communication disorder to be substantial.

After evaluation of her unaided and aided performance, a decision was made to pursue the use of a cochlear implant. A multichannel device was selected and implanted in her right ear.

Approximately 6 weeks following implantation, the device was activated through the speech processor, and the processor was programmed to stimulate the electrodes that were considered distinctly usable. Programming was accomplished by setting thresholds of detectability of electrical currents delivered to each electrode. Comfort levels were also set for each electrode or group of electrodes. The exact processing strategy was determined from the proprietary strategies available for the specific implant that was chosen.

Performance with the device was assessed by comparing pre- and postimplant performance on a range of speech-recognition measures. Results on several selected tests are shown in Figure 13–6B. Results indicated that the cochlear implant was providing substantial improvement over aided performance.

A self-assessment scale showed that the patient is receiving substantial benefit from the cochlear implant and that, with the implant, her communication problems are reduced in most listening environments.

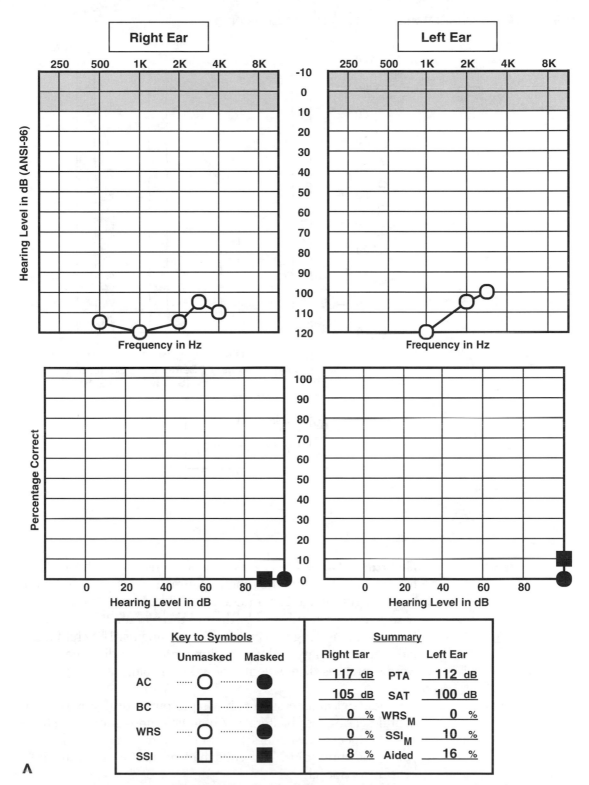

Figure 13-6. Hearing-consultation results in a 44-year-old woman with profound hearing loss. Pure-tone and speech audiometric results (A) show bilateral hearing loss, poor speech-recognition ability, and little benefit from binaural hearing aids. Pre- and postimplant results (B) show significant improvement in performance on selected speech-recognition measures.

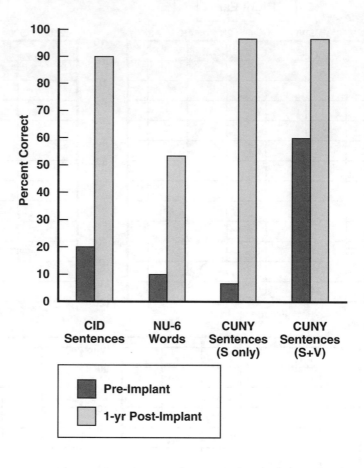

B

Illustrative Case 13-7. Case 7 is a young boy with profound bilateral sensorineural hearing impairment, secondary to a bout of meningitis at age 18 months. The child passed a routine newborn hearing screening at birth, and the parents had no reason to suspect a hearing loss prior to the meningitis. The child had a growing vocabulary and was beginning to use rudimentary two-word sentences. The patient is now 3 years old.

An audiological assessment shows profound, primarily sensorineural hearing loss bilaterally. An audiogram is shown in Figure 13–7A. Speech awareness thresholds were in agreement with pure-tone thresholds. The child had no useful suprathreshold hearing for speech.

At age 20 months, the child was fitted binaurally with power BTE hearing aids and enrolled in an aural habilitation program that stressed use of audition for the learning of language. The child

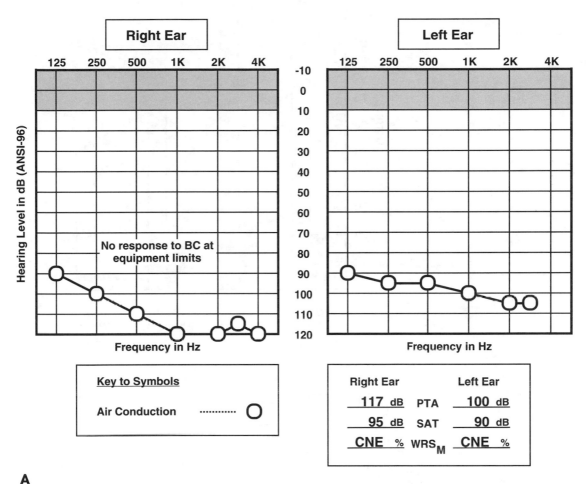

Figure 13-7. Hearing-consultation results in a 3-year-old child with profound hearing loss. Pure-tone audiometric results (A) show bilateral hearing loss and no measurable suprathreshold speech-recognition ability. Pre- and postimplant results (B) show significant improvement in performance on selected speech- and sound-recognition measures.

received some usable gain from the hearing aids, but was not progressing in speech and language development at a rate that was acceptable to the parents or educators.

After a great deal of consideration, the parents decided that the child should receive a cochlear implant. The device was implanted at age 28 months. Following recovery, the speech processor was programmed and reprogrammed in an effort to achieve the best speech and sound recognition ability available from the device. The programming efforts took approximately 3 months to complete.

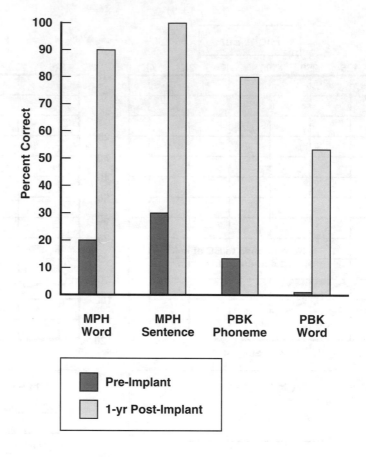

B

During the programming period, the child showed substantial improvement in his ability to function through the auditory channel. Anecdotal reports from the parents and teachers suggested that his speech improved and the ease with which he was learning language was dramatically enhanced.

Selected speech- and sound-recognition results at age 36 months are shown in Figure 13–7B. Substantial improvements were noted between the child's ability to perceive sound with the cochlear implant over conventional hearing aid amplification.

The child remains enrolled in the aural habilitation program, although the parents plan to enroll him on a part-time basis in a "mainstreamed" capacity at a local preschool when he reaches age 4 years.

SUMMARY

☐ Although the overall goal of any hearing rehabilitation strategy is to reduce hearing handicap by maximizing the use of residual hearing, the approach used to reach that goal can vary across patients.

☐ The approach chosen to evaluate and fit hearing aids is sometimes related to patient factors such as age, type of hearing disorder, and patient need.

☐ Adult patients with sensorineural hearing impairment tend to be both easy and challenging in terms of hearing aid selection and fitting—easy because they are cooperative and can provide insightful feedback throughout the fitting process and challenging because there is not much to limit the audiologist's options.

☐ The most important variables in this population are the degree and configuration of hearing loss.

☐ With older individuals, the more that can be done to ease the burden of listening in background noise, whether by sophisticated signal processing in an ear-level hearing device or by use of a remote microphone, the more likely the patient will benefit from hearing-device amplification.

■ Another important challenge in fitting hearing aids in older individuals is the difficulty involved in the physical manipulation of the device.

☐ Hearing aid selection and fitting in children with sensorineural hearing impairment is a challenging business for various reasons. One is that audiometric levels may be known only generally at the beginning of the fitting process.

■ Another is that children are less likely or able to participate in the selection and fitting process.

☐ Still another is that hearing may be more variable in young children due to progression or to fluctuation secondary to otitis media.

■ The main challenge in treating children with CAPD is to assist them in overcoming their difficulties in understanding speech in background noise.

■ A child with CAPD may benefit from amplification designed to enhance the signal-to-noise ratio.

☐ Overcoming the attenuating effects of conductive hearing loss is relatively simple from a signal processing strategy. The challenge in this population is more often related to providing a satisfactory physical fit for the amplification device.

■ Cochlear implantation is the primary hearing rehabilitation strategy for patients with profound deafness.

SUGGESTED READINGS

Alpiner, J. G., & McCarthy, P. A. (1993). *Rehabilitative audiology: Children and adults* (2nd ed.). Baltimore: Williams & Wilkins.

Clark, G., Cowan, R., & Dowell, R. (1997). *Advances in cochlear implants for infants and children.* San Diego: Singular Publishing Group.

Crandell, C. C., Smaldino, J. J., & Flexer, C. (1995). *Sound-field FM amplification.* San Diego: Singular Publishing Group.

Sandlin, R. E. (Ed.). (1992). *Handbook of hearing aid amplification. Volume II: Clinical considerations and fitting practices.* San Diego: Singular Publishing Group.

Valente, M. (Ed.). (1994). *Strategies for selecting and verifying hearing aid fittings.* New York: Thieme Medical Publishing.

Index